T0251861

POCKET GUIDE ALSO AVAILABLE:

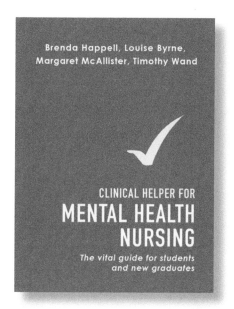

Brenda Happell, Louise Byrne,
Margaret McAllister, Timothy Wand

CLINICAL HELPER FOR
**MENTAL HEALTH
NURSING**
*The vital guide for students
and new graduates*

Are you anxious about your mental health placement?
Do you need help remembering the terms, therapies and guidelines?

The *Clinical Helper for Mental Health Nursing* is a quick and reliable
reference for students and new graduates to reduce stress and
boost confidence in the clinical setting.

Covering the key information you must have at your fingertips, this pocket
guide is essential for all nurses entering mental health practice and an aid or
ideal companion to *Introducing Mental Health Nursing*, 2nd edition.

ISBN: 9781743316993

Brenda Happell • Leanne Cowin
Cath Roper • Richard Lakeman • Leonie Cox

Introducing Mental Health Nursing

A service user-oriented approach

2ND EDITION

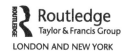

Routledge
Taylor & Francis Group

LONDON AND NEW YORK

First published 2008 by Allen & Unwin

Published 2020 by Routledge
2 Park Square, Milton Park, Abingdon, Oxon OX14 4RN
605 Third Avenue, New York, NY 10017

Routledge is an imprint of the Taylor & Francis Group, an informa business

Cataloguing-in-Publication details are available
from the National Library of Australia
www.trove.nla.gov.au

Index by Puddingburn Publishing Services
Set in 11/13 pt Berkeley by Midland Typesetters, Australia

ISBN-13: 9781743312681 (pbk)

About the authors

Professor Brenda Happell is Professor (Engaged Research Chair) of Mental Health Nursing, Director of the Institute for Health and Social Science Research and Director of the recently established Centre for Mental Health Nursing Innovation at CQUniversity, Australia. She has considerable expertise in mental health nursing education, including teaching, curriculum development and evaluation, at the undergraduate, postgraduate and higher degree levels. Brenda pioneered the introduction of the consumer academic position in her former position as Director of the Centre for Psychiatric Nursing Research and Practice at the University of Melbourne, and more recently at CQUniversity. She is nationally and internationally recognised for her expertise in mental health nursing and has published widely in nursing and related health journals. She is widely published in a number of areas, including service user participation and mental health nursing education. Brenda is currently Editor of the *International Journal of Mental Health Nursing* and Associate Editor of *Issues in Mental Health Nursing*.

Dr Leanne Cowin is currently Head of Program for the Master of Nursing course at the University of Western Sydney. She continues to teach in the undergraduate and postgraduate nursing and medical program. Leanne is a keen researcher whose growing body of work reflects a commitment to generating new professional directions in nursing as well as investigating current workforce and workplace issues within the health-care professions. Leanne has recently completed a Masters degree in statistics, and leads a joint academic and clinical nursing research team committed to examining and enhancing the new graduate nurse experience. She publishes regularly in national and international journals.

Cath Roper is a consumer academic with the Centre for Psychiatric Nursing and a lecturer in the Department of Nursing, University of Melbourne. She held one of four pioneering staff consumer consultant positions established in 1995 in Victorian mental health services. Following this, she became the first person to occupy a consumer academic role in Australia. Cath experienced annual involuntary admissions to mental health services over a thirteen year period and uses this perspective in her work. She has a strong interest in working alongside clinicians towards practices that support the self-determination of people subject to mental health legislation. Cath has a BA, DipEd and an MA in Social Health.

Dr Richard Lakeman has worked as mental health nurse, teacher and researcher in Australia, New Zealand and Ireland. He is presently a Senior Lecturer at Southern Cross University. He has extensive practice experience working with people with complex needs, and has worked in the homeless sector and in assertive community mental health teams. He currently works part time providing psychotherapy in the Mental Health Nurse Incentive Program. He has researched, published and presented extensively on a range of mental health issues, including suicide, recovery, the impact of trauma on caregivers, clinical supervision, stigma, migration, nursing identity and ethics. He has been a vocal critic of pharmaco-centric approaches to mental health care and works to promote alternatives through advocacy, teaching and participation in organisations such as The International Society for Psychological and Social Approaches to Psychosis.

Dr Leonie Cox is a Senior Lecturer in the School of Nursing, Queensland University of Technology, Brisbane. Leonie is a medical and social anthropologist whose ethnographic work with Aboriginal people and Torres Strait Islanders focuses on the intersection of colonial history, contemporary policy and practice, knowledge, power, class, race relations and well-being. Leonie also has extensive clinical nursing experience in the mental health field, and she teaches and publishes on the relationship between history, society, culture and health. Her take on this relationship embraces the philosophy of cultural safety, promoting a social justice approach to how nurses work with marginalised people in society. Leonie is the lead author for chapters 8 and 14 which embrace these issues.

About the chapter contributors

Ali Drummond is a Dauareb man from the Torres Straits who has ancestral connections to the Wuthathi and Yadaigana people of Cape York Peninsula. He is a Registered Nurse with a Bachelor of Nursing Science and is currently working in public policy. Ali is an Adjunct Senior Lecturer with the James Cook University and guest lectures on Torres Strait Island knowledge in the Bachelor of Nursing Program at Queensland University of Technology. Ali also serves on the Board of Directors of the Lowitja Institute for Aboriginal and Torres Strait Islander Health Research.

Melissa Walker is a Palawa Aboriginal woman, lecturer at the Queensland University of Technology and has over 21 year's Indigenous nursing experience. She is a recognised international ambassador, credentialed mental health nurse, Indigenous researcher and well-respected Aboriginal and Torres Strait Islander women's leader. Melissa has presented her work on national, international and community-based levels, and she has recently been an invited keynote speaker at both the 2012 International Network of Indigenous Health Knowledge and Development (INIHKD) Conference and the 23rd International Nurses Research Conference. Her research outputs to date focus on Aboriginal and Torres Strait Islanders' mental health, including addressing social and emotional well-being and wellness risk factors, preventative population education, chronic disease prevention and health program development. Recently Melissa has been acknowledged for her outstanding community-based mental health program development and implementation, receiving the prestigious Stan Alchin Award at the 2012 International Mental Health Nursing Conference. She has previously been a member of the Indigenous Participatory Advisory Group that reports to the Minister of Indigenous Affairs.

Contents

Figures and tables

Acknowledgements

We owe a particular debt of gratitude to our colleagues Kim Foster, Associate Professor in Mental Health Nursing at the University of Sydney, and Ms Rose McMaster, Senior Lecturer in Nursing at the Australian Catholic University. Professor Foster and Ms McMaster were contributing authors to the first edition, and made a vital contribution to the development of the thinking on which this book is based.

Preface

This is a mental health nursing textbook unlike any others you may have seen. We hope our somewhat different approach to discussing mental health nursing provides a fresh and exciting perspective from which to embark on your study of this specialised field. Throughout the text, we have sought to address comprehensively the attitudes, knowledge and skills required by nurses to provide care for service users experiencing mental health problems across all health-care settings, with a particular emphasis on mental health services.

The text does not follow a traditional biomedical format where nursing care is discussed in terms of psychiatric diagnosis. Many texts state that mental health nursing involves an appreciation of, and response to, the uniqueness of each individual experiencing a mental health problem, yet they reflect a biomedical approach. These texts generally devote chapters (or parts of them) to psychiatric diagnoses and present nursing interventions as dependent on diagnoses rather than the specific and individual needs of the service user. While a biomedical perspective reflects a prevailing approach to mental health care, it is not the only—or indeed the most appropriate—approach to take in a text that is about the science and art of mental health nursing. In particular, this book recognises the lived experience of being diagnosed with a mental illness and of mental health service use as knowledge that is at least equally valuable to scientific and medical knowledge. Therefore, while we have included the biomedical approach, we have also included a social model of health and emphasised service users' individual experience of mental health challenges. In addition, we have focused particularly on the nurse as a vital member of the mental health team, with an active role in facilitating the recovery of individuals who have been diagnosed with a mental illness.

The five authors of this Australian-based text are four mental health nurses—Brenda Happell, Leanne Cowin, Richard Lakeman and Leonie Cox—with considerable experience in both practice and academia, and a user of mental health services—Cath Roper. A number of other nursing and mental health texts include the service user voice; however, most have service users writing specific sections or chapters only. In this text,

Cath has had input into all chapters of the book. This reflects the desire to present a service user perspective throughout the text, to enable you to more fully appreciate the potential impact (both positive and negative) of nursing care on the users of services, and a desire to demonstrate and recognise that a service user perspective is an essential part of health education and practice. Cath Roper, the service user author, holds the position of consumer academic at the Centre for Psychiatric Nursing. She has substantial experience in mental health nursing education, and is one of only two known mental health service users to hold an academic position of this type in Australia.

A primary aim of this book is to encourage you to think critically about mental health nursing, and the care and treatment provided in mental health settings. We have included a number of critical thinking exercises designed to assist you to reflect on various aspects of mental health care, and the impact of our practices on service users. There is also a specific chapter on addressing mental health issues within the broader health-care system. You may find in your reading of the text that there will be times where it seems the service user and clinical/health professional views or perspectives presented have clashed. It may be helpful to remember that one 'truth' or perspective does not cancel out the other. Instead, we invite you to engage with such dilemmas, and understand there is space for many—and even competing—perspectives. We take the view that an awareness of contradictory 'truths' provides room for more honest, less fearful responses from both health professionals and service users alike.

Another important difference is our use of language. Instead of the commonly used terms 'patient' or 'client', we use the term 'service user' to describe a person who is using a health service. This is the 'language of the day' in health care, and we provide a specific definition for our use of the term in the introductory chapter. We also use the term 'person diagnosed with a mental illness' in preference to pejorative language such as 'the mentally ill' or 'person suffering from a mental illness'. 'Person first' language is particularly important to mental health service users in differentiating the person from any health condition they may have. The pronoun 'we' is sometimes used to refer to service users and to express the vantage point of service user perspective.

In most cases, we use the terminology 'mental health problems' in preference to 'mental illness'. This decision acknowledges the fact that the understanding of one's mental health is highly subjective, and therefore a person can experience a mental health problem without necessarily being diagnosed with a mental illness. Furthermore, nurses will find themselves caring for people who experience mental health-related symptoms that do not meet the criteria for a specific diagnosis, but nevertheless trouble the person. When we use the term 'mental illness', it is generally in relation to mental health legislation or psychiatric diagnosis, where it is important to make a distinction between mental illness and mental health problems.

We have intended that when you use this text as part of your formal mental health nursing studies (theory and clinical), it will assist you to: appreciate the importance of mental health nursing skills for any clinical setting; understand that there are many approaches to and perspectives on mental health and illness; appreciate the importance of service user perspective in nursing in general and in mental health nursing in particular; overcome any fears you might have about working with people experiencing a mental illness; regard mental health nursing as a valuable and realistic area of nursing practice—even if it isn't where you want to work in the future; and most importantly, learn a lot and enjoy yourself.

Brenda Happell

Leanne Cowin

Cath Roper

Richard Lakeman

Leonie Cox

PART I

BACKGROUND AND CONTEXT TO MENTAL HEALTH NURSING

1

Introduction

Main points
- Mental health nursing is an important, exciting and rewarding nursing specialty.
- Mental illness is a common health problem; therefore, mental health nursing knowledge and skills are necessary for all areas of nursing practice.
- Language is important in shaping our attitudes to people experiencing a mental illness.
- Consumers of mental health services should be actively involved in all aspects of mental health service delivery.

Definitions
Mental health nursing: A specialised field of nursing providing care and treatment specifically for people experiencing mental illness or significant mental health problems.
Mental health service user: A person who uses, has used, or attempted to use mental health services.
Mental health services: Specialist services designed to provide care and treatment for people with mental illness.

WHY STUDY MENTAL HEALTH NURSING?
The purpose of this book is to introduce you to the field of mental health nursing, and to the skills and knowledge you will require in providing care for people experiencing a mental health problem.

Many of you may be asking 'Why do I have to study this subject?' There is now a substantial body of literature indicating that most nursing students do not start their course with an interest in working in the mental health area (Happell & Cutcliffe 2011; Hoekstra, van Meijel & van der Hooft-Leemans 2010). The literature also tells us that one of the main reasons for this disinterest is a fear of people experiencing mental health problems. Commonly cited issues include fears that the nurse will become physically hurt by violent and aggressive acts, and fear of becoming emotionally damaged because of exposure to people's pain and distress. If you currently share such feelings, it is important to know that you are not alone. It is also important to keep in mind that by the time you have completed the theoretical and clinical components of this subject, your fears about being with people experiencing mental health problems are likely to be significantly reduced or even to disappear altogether (Happell 2008).

Mental health nursing is a fantastic profession: it provides the opportunity to make a difference in the lives of people from diverse backgrounds, with differing needs and experiences. You have the opportunity to learn more about the interactions between people, their environment and their experiences, and through this you will learn a lot about your own thoughts, feelings and behaviours as well. As you will discover, mental health nursing offers many opportunities to practise in a variety of settings and to use a broad range of skills.

To answer the question 'Why study mental health nursing?'—particularly for those who want to work in another field such as medical/surgical, paediatrics, midwifery, critical care or operating theatre—it is important to look at mental health nursing more broadly. There is no doubt that this field requires highly specialised skills and knowledge, but the principles of mental health nursing are not limited to mental health settings. In whatever areas of nursing you choose to practise during your career, as well as in your own life, you will encounter people experiencing mental illness or mental health problems, and it is crucial that you feel comfortable and confident with these issues. There are a number of factors involved in the delivery of mental health care in Australia, including changes to care settings, awareness of holistic health-care needs and provision of holistic nursing care. You will be introduced to these concepts in this chapter, and many will be dealt with in greater detail in other parts of this book.

MENTAL HEALTH-CARE SETTINGS

Changes in the delivery of public mental health services in Australia have occurred over the past 30–40 years (see Chapter 4). Most large psychiatric hospitals have now closed as the result of processes known as deinstitutionalisation and mainstreaming (Ash et al. 2012). People experiencing a mental health problem are now more likely to receive care and treatment from a community-based program or within in-patient units located in general hospitals. These changes to the model of mental health service delivery mean that more people experiencing mental health problems are accessing general hospital and community-based services.

HOLISM

It is likely that during your nursing course you have already been introduced to the concept of holistic nursing care. The underlying principle of holism is that the nurse provides care for the person as a total person, encompassing all aspects of physical, social and psychological well-being (Cowling 2011; Povlsen & Borup 2011). What this means for you as a nurse is that, although you may specialise in a particular area of practice (for example, midwifery), you must constantly remember that the needs of the people for whom you care very rarely fit into neat categories. For example, a pregnant woman requires the expertise and knowledge of a qualified and experienced midwife during the antenatal, labour and post-natal periods of childbirth. Parenthood is not always a planned event, and even when it is, the expectations of childbirth and parenthood often involve anxieties about the future—questions such as 'Will my child be healthy?' or 'Will I be a good mother?' Attending to these needs is just as important as meeting the physical needs of the pregnant mother. The expectant mother may also experience a mental health problem prior to, during or related to pregnancy or childbirth, such as post-natal depression. The midwife must be able to assess the woman for signs and symptoms of mental health challenges, and provide appropriate care to ensure optimal physical and emotional health for the woman and her family at all stages of contact.

Approximately one in five Australians will experience a mental health challenge at some stage in their lives (Wynaden 2010). The percentage has been found to be higher in people accessing the health-care system. Mental health problems within the general health-care system are covered in detail in Chapter 16. As you progress through the theory and practice of mental health nursing, remember that what you learn during this time will be invaluable to your further career as a nurse, irrespective of where you choose to work in the future. For some of you, the experience of mental health nursing will be considerably more positive than you expected. Despite the reservations you may have at present, some of you will choose this as the area in which you wish to work in the future. Whatever the outcome, keep your mind open, view this as a useful learning experience and, above all, enjoy the challenges you will encounter as you study mental health nursing.

As well as preparing you to better meet the mental health needs of the people for whom you care across a broad range of health-care settings, the study and practice of mental health nursing is likely to bring personal rewards. You will learn more about yourself as a person, and how you relate to the people with whom you live, work and socialise. A student nurse made the following statement after completing a mental health/psychiatric nursing subject: 'I thoroughly enjoyed the semester of psych nursing. I felt it was not only beneficial for nursing, but for life.'

LANGUAGE IN MENTAL HEALTH CARE

The language used in Australia to refer to people experiencing a mental health problem varies between different mental health settings and service providers, and across policy documents. There is no single term that has currency over any other; however, many Australian health policy documents continue to use the term 'consumer' to refer to people who use health services, and this is also true of mental health.

What is a consumer?

'Consumerism' is the health and human services language of the day, and it is reflected in current health policies and guidelines. The terminology comes from a business model, and the focus is not on the 'condition' of the customer, but on the quality of the transaction between the consumer and service.

A business framework is useful when it comes to describing the sorts of things all customers or consumers should reasonably expect in any business transaction, including the right to complain if a service is less than satisfactory, and the right to choose within a competitive market. The term 'consumer' is now used widely by people who have become more knowledgeable about health rights and activism, and who see themselves as citizens with a right to expect a partnership from health-care professionals—including being properly informed throughout all contact with health services. The relatively recent shift from provider as 'expert' to provider as 'partner' in a person's health concerns means that people expect to be fully informed and empowered to make decisions and choices. Knowing how to communicate respectfully, negotiate and impart knowledge in ways that people can grasp are now key skills for all health providers.

One limitation of the business model when it is applied to mental health service use is that it cannot adequately describe circumstances surrounding an involuntary admission to hospital or treatment patterns that do not involve free choice, as occurs when a person is governed by mental health legislation—that is, when they are hospitalised on an involuntary basis.

Self-identification

While 'consumer' is currently used in mental health policy, the merits or otherwise of this term continue to be hotly debated. Another way to think about language use is the way people choose to individually identify themselves. Paralleling black pride/gay pride movements is 'mad pride' where people adopt terms that were historically experienced as discriminatory or oppressive, in new empowering ways. Reclamation of language in this sense includes such self chosen terms as 'batty', 'nutter' or 'mad'. In mental health, the term 'survivor' is self-chosen, meaning someone who is *a survivor of the mental health system*—rather than someone surviving or recovering from a mental health problem. People who identify themselves as survivors have usually experienced mental health services involuntarily. While some people do not like the term 'patient' because of the connotations of passivity, and medical 'paternalism', others prefer this term as it is the terminology most often used in general health. Some prefer the term 'client' because it seems to accurately describe a professional relationship with a practitioner, while others do not have a strong opinion about it either way. More recently, the term 'lived experience' has been used to describe first-hand experience of using mental health services and/or experiencing mental health problems.

In this book, we primarily adopt the term 'service user', defined as a person who uses, has used or has attempted to use mental health services. This term is commonly used internationally, and we adopt it here in preference to the term 'consumer' because it maintains the focus on service provision while also allowing reference to involuntary service use.

SERVICE USER LEADERSHIP IN MENTAL HEALTH SERVICES

There is a growing trend across the health industry towards recognising that people who use health services are well placed to give advice and direction about how services should be developed and provided. This approach is intended to ensure that what is delivered is more closely aligned with what communities want, need and expect. Historically, such activities have been known as 'consumer participation'. Gordon (2005) uses the term 'consumer leadership' to describe activities undertaken by service users working within mental health services across such areas as service planning, delivery, monitoring and evaluation. Most of these activities emphasise a 'systems approach', looking at the way organisations work, and using a 'quality improvement' approach to achieve positive change. These circumstances mean that most health providers will be working alongside service users at some time in their careers.

In mental health, there is a long tradition of service user leadership in service reform, largely because of sustained activism resulting in policy influence. This tradition has impacted in a number of ways—for example, Commonwealth mental health policies from the 1990s onwards have specified the right of service users to be involved in care and treatment decisions, and the right of service users and carers to be involved meaningfully in service reforms. There are service user and carer consultants, advisers and advocates in most mental health services across the country. More recently, there has been a growth in the number of peer support roles across the specialist mental health and non-government sectors.

CONSUMER/SURVIVOR MOVEMENT

The consumer/survivor movement is an international social movement sharing histor-ical ties with the American Civil Rights Movement and other social movements emerging in the 1960s and 1970s. For many service users, the experience of being detained and/or treated against their will is life-defining, leading to an interest in social and political activism. The movement is characterised by loose networks of people, from local groups to international networks (as with most social/political movements). The consumer/ survivor movement typically is concerned with ending discrimination and oppression, and promoting citizenship, equality, self-determination, social justice and pride in being who we are. The consumer/survivor movement, its origins and concerns are discussed in more detail in Chapter 3.

SERVICE USER PERSPECTIVE

Perhaps the easiest way to understand the service user perspective is to view it as based on experience of service use, leading to a conscious way of viewing the world. When we talk about our own experiences of services, our legitimacy comes from our subjective or 'lived experience', so cannot be judged as right or wrong.

Anyone can develop an appreciation of service user perspective by listening to and attempting to understand the experience and views a person has about using services. The service user perspective is captured in Epstein and Shaw's classic account as:

> Something which has developed out of a collective consciousness and political solidarity that grew from the consumer/survivor movement. That is to say that it is an identity shaped through an awareness of 'belonging' to a group of people who are marginalized and discriminated against, who have an experience of oppression from more powerful elements in society that is part of the pattern of the way they (we) live. (Epstein & Shaw 1997, p. 13)

In this text, the term 'service user perspective' will be used to reflect the above definition while 'lived experience' is a broader, more inclusive term that highlights the value of personal, subjective experience in contrast to professional knowledge and expertise.

The service user perspective grew from a political/social movement, but it can now also be understood as a discipline in its own right that, although yet to be fully articulated, nevertheless has its own theoretical approaches and underpinning philosophies. Many service user perspective activities are well developed—for example, the service user perspective is recognised as essential to developing and delivering mental health education (Cowling et al. 2006), and in the development and conduct of research (Sweeney et al. 2009).

The service user perspective recognises that although we should be the agents of our own lives, once we have been diagnosed with a psychiatric or mental health condition, we are often left out of decision-making. Hence the principle 'nothing about us without us'—long championed by disability activists—is also a basic tenet of the service user perspective, indicating there is no aspect of mental health—from individual treatment decision-making to policy development—that would not benefit from first-person knowledge and expertise based on lived experience.

In the service user perspective, 'person first' language is very important. A person has a diagnosis of something—the person is not the diagnosis itself. So we would say, 'She has been diagnosed with schizophrenia', rather than, 'She is a schizophrenic'. The reason behind this is that, historically, service users have been discussed and written about as though they were not actual people, living real lives, but rather collections of symptoms. Respectful language is all the more important to us because there can be prejudice towards people who have been diagnosed with mental health problems.

The concept of service user perspective is open to debate, and probably always will be. However, it is possible to describe certain characteristics of service user perspective as a discipline in that it tends to:

- acknowledge that social, personal and legal authority is real and has impact
- understand oppression, social exclusion, poverty, minority status, injustice, discrimination and disadvantage
- emphasise the importance of subjective experience and self-determination, and acknowledge a multiplicity of views and beliefs
- be linked with action (speaking out, training, service reform)
- be reflective/critical
- value lived experience as a knowledge base
- recognise that our social/economic context plays a vital role in our recovery prospects
- posit that recovery is possible for all people, whether or not symptoms are present.

CRITICAL THINKING

The following is a list of terms that have been used to refer to people with mental health problems:

consumer	unwell	mentally retarded
lunatic	mentally ill	crazy
survivor	client	patient.
mad	psycho eccentric	

- What does our choice of language reveal about: how we understand things; what we want to communicate to others?
- What difference does it make if the term is self-chosen rather than being used to describe others?
- *Listen* for how/whether the people you meet self-identify.

RECOVERY

Mental health problems traditionally have been regarded as degenerative 'life sentences' from which people were unlikely to recover. Mental health services operated from the idea that mental illness was lifelong, permanent and disabling. The idea that a diagnosis of mental illness is not a life sentence is a significant positive development in the mental health field, and contemporary mental health care is based on the expectation that people do recover. Australia's National Mental Health Policy defines recovery as:

> A personal process of changing one's attitudes, values, feelings, goals, skills and /or roles. It involves the development of new meaning and purpose and a satisfying, hopeful and contributing life as the person grows beyond the effects of psychiatric disability. The process of recovery must be supported by individually identified essential services and resources. (Commonwealth of Australia 2009b, p. 31)

There is considerable hope for people who have experienced mental illness and, consequently, the people and services that support them must reorient their focus towards recovery. Recovery is the subject of Chapter 3.

MENTAL HEALTH NURSING IN AUSTRALIA

In order to give you some idea of how mental health care and mental health nursing have developed, this section outlines some of the major advancements in nursing and mental health care service provision in Australia.

Historical overview

Understanding the history of mental health nursing promotes increased awareness of the social and intellectual origins of the discipline (McAllister, Happell & Bradshaw 2010). This knowledge provides a better basis from which both students and practising mental health nurses can meet the mental health needs of the community—not just in the present, but in anticipation of the changes that are likely to occur in the short and longer term future.

Nursing generally is acknowledged as a highly complex and diverse profession, providing care to people across the lifespan who are experiencing a variety of health-care problems. However, interestingly, mental health nursing is not often reflected by historical accounts, as histories of the nursing profession tend to focus on the care of people experiencing physical illness or injury. Mental health nursing is either totally absent from or receives only superficial mention within these historical texts.

This situation may be explained partly by the fact that madness historically was viewed as the result of factors such as possession, 'bad blood' or inherent character flaws rather than as an illness (Singh et al. 2007). Furthermore, there was a greater emphasis on the custodial rather than the caring role in the treatment of people experiencing a mental illness—an approach that is not often considered to be characteristic of nursing. However, if we are to provide education for nurses that is genuinely comprehensive, greater attention must be devoted to the history of all branches of nursing. To exclude mental health nursing may be interpreted as reflecting the view that this specialty is not as important or not of equal status to other areas of nursing practice, which runs the risk of further stigmatising people who experience mental health-related problems.

The history of mental health nursing in Australia differs significantly from the history of other branches of nursing. The history reflects a primarily custodial approach to the treatment of people experiencing a mental illness. This kind of approach to care includes the control and supervision of people with mental illness and attention to their basic needs, but little or no use of therapeutic approaches to their illness. The first Australian lunatic asylum was opened at Castle Hill (New South Wales) in 1811, staffed by untrained mental attendants. Large numbers of 'disturbed' people were usually restrained as a means to maintain control. There was virtually no attention to treatment (Keane 1987).

In response to overcrowding of the Castle Hill Asylum, a new asylum was erected at Tarban Creek (New South Wales) in 1837. It continued to be the only place where people experiencing a mental illness were housed until the opening of Yarra Bend Asylum in 1848. The Yarra Bend Asylum was opened at Kew in the Port Phillip district (Melbourne, Victoria). Immediately, ten 'mental patients' were transferred there from prison. A lay superintendent administered Yarra Bend; his wife occupied the position of matron, for which she received approximately half of his salary (McCoppin & Gardiner 1995). Asylums subsequently were opened in other colonies of Australia.

The early approach in Australia to the treatment of people experiencing a mental illness followed the British model, and tended to reflect the views of medical superintendents who migrated to the colonies to oversee the asylums. The philosophy was one of humane care; however, the considerable overcrowding of the asylums frequently led to a more custodial approach, which involved the restriction of freedom in preference to active care and treatment. A number of Royal Commissions during the nineteenth century failed to substantially address the problems identified (Singh et al. 2007).

In 1867, an Act of Parliament was passed that made it mandatory for persons showing signs of mental impairment to be sent to a lunatic asylum rather than a prison (Keane 1987). By 1900, people experiencing a mental illness were separated from the 'mentally retarded'. The 'nursing' in the mental asylums continued to be delivered predominantly by male attendants, and the care continued to be custodial, delivered by untrained staff until the medical staff of the institutions started providing lectures to the attendants. The idea of employing female attendants then began to receive serious consideration (Keane 1987).

The period from the 1950s to the 1980s saw rapid changes within the healthcare industry that dramatically altered the practice of nursing. The knowledge base required for nursing expanded enormously, and could no longer be included in general nursing curricula—hence the commencement of specialisation and the development of nursing specialties (Bessant 1999).

Advances in medical science similarly affected the practice of mental health nursing. Mental impairment increasingly became considered an illness, and considerable attention was devoted to finding a cure for specific illnesses (Cade 1979). The 1950s were particularly famous for the first use of major tranquillisers, which meant that the former heavy reliance on the straitjacket and other forms of physical restraint was no longer necessary. Psychiatric nurses were able to establish therapeutic relationships with service users, involving both group and individual therapy (Cade 1979).

Further changes to psychiatric/mental health nursing occurred during the 1970s and 1980s, when large psychiatric institutions (previously known as asylums) were scaled down, then later closed and replaced by smaller units within general hospitals and an increase in community-based care. This movement, known as 'deinstitutionalisation', has seen enormous reductions in the length of stay in psychiatric hospitals, and a significant number of people experiencing a mental illness are now never admitted to hospital.

Criticisms of deinstitutionalisation tend to reflect the view that not enough funding has been provided to ensure that adequate supports are available for people experiencing mental health problems and their families in the community. Community services are therefore not sufficiently well resourced to ensure an optimum level of care. The strongest critics suggest that deinstitutionalisation has meant relocating the institutions from hospitals to boarding houses or special accommodation facilities (Hamden et al. 2011). There is no doubt this is true in some cases, and community services require further development and additional funding in order to realise their full potential. Despite the different views regarding the extent to which the deinstitutionalisation movement has been successful, there is wide support for the idea behind caring for people with mental health problems with the least possible restriction to their freedom.

The current perspective

Changing views about mental illness have gradually led to the understanding that the isolation of people experiencing mental health problems within institutions was not a satisfactory arrangement. Major changes to the structure of mental health services represent the outcome of this movement. While there is variation between the states and territories of Australia, deinstitutionalisation has resulted in the scaling down and in most cases the closure, of large institutions, and an increase in community-based services. This reflected the belief that people experiencing a mental illness should, where possible, receive care within their own family and community settings.

The development of community-based services was celebrated as a significant advance. However, the separation of mental health services from the broader health-care system continued to be an issue of concern. The release of the National Mental Health Plan (Australian Health Ministers, 1992) signalled one of the major reforms to mental health services in Australian history. The focus of official policy moved towards promoting the maintenance of mental health as opposed to a primary focus on the treatment of what was frequently termed 'serious mental illness'. The process of deinstitutionalisation was a central focus of the report of the National Inquiry into Human Rights and Mental Illness (HREOC 1993). Commonly known as the Burdekin Report, it highlighted problems that affected service users, their carers and members of the public as it detailed the incidence and effects of mental illness and the available treatments. The policy focus of care and treatment in the least restrictive environment has been maintained in the subsequent policy documents, including the most current Mental Health Plan (Commonwealth of Australia 2009).

One of the most significant outcomes of this new policy direction was the introduction of a process known as 'mainstreaming'. This refers to the integration of mental health services within the general health-care system, and is discussed further in Chapter 4. In most instances, mainstreaming has meant that units providing in-patient care for people experiencing a mental illness are now located within a general hospital. The desire to produce a responsive health-care system capable of responding to a broad range of health-care issues, and to reduce the stigma frequently associated with accessing mental health services, were the primary reasons for the introduction of mainstreamed services.

These reforms to mental health services have not developed uniformly throughout Australia. In Victoria, for example, all the large institutions have now been closed and all in-patient facilities are located within general hospitals (with the exception of Thomas Embling Hospital, which provides in-patient beds as part of the Victorian Institute for Forensic Mental Health). A number of other states, such as New South Wales, Queensland and Western Australia, currently have units located within general hospitals as well as separate institutions specifically for the provision of mental health care, although these are now considerably smaller in terms of bed numbers than they were historically. A more detailed coverage of mental health services in Australia is presented in Chapter 4.

MENTAL HEALTH NURSING EDUCATION IN AUSTRALIA
An historical perspective
Historically, mental health nursing was viewed as a separate branch of nursing. In order to become registered as a mental health (or psychiatric) nurse, a student undertook a three-year hospital-based course. General nurses could complete specific post-registration training to register as a psychiatric nurse. The student was employed by the hospital and undertook clinical experience as a paid staff member of the organisation. At the conclusion of the course, the student sat state-based examinations. Students were

required to pass the examinations and complete the specified clinical experience, and to demonstrate competence through the satisfactory completion of clinical objectives and practical examinations. People registered as mental health or psychiatric nurses were only able to practise within their specialty area.

The course you are currently undertaking is based on a model of comprehensive education that represents a significant change to the structure of nursing education. Rather than specialising in a specific area of nursing, this course is designed to prepare a generic nurse with sufficient skills to practise at a beginning level in a variety of health-care settings, including the mental health area. For you, this means that after completing your course you are legally able to seek employment as a mental health nurse. It is also expected that you are competent to meet the basic mental health needs of the person across a variety of health-care settings.

The extent to which existing courses are truly comprehensive has been the subject of much debate. Australian research suggests that the vision has not been fully realised. Most undergraduate nursing curricula remains highly focused on hospital-based medical–surgical care, with significantly less attention devoted to areas such as mental health and care of older people (Wynaden 2010).

To further develop the skills and expertise required for specialisation in the mental health field, postgraduate courses in mental health nursing have been developed throughout Australia. While postgraduate mental health nursing courses have grown in numbers in recent years, the current system of nursing registration does not require a nurse to complete such a course if they wish to work in the mental health field

WHAT DO MENTAL HEALTH NURSES DO?

The precise role of the mental health nurse is often difficult to appreciate for students and registered nurses who are not familiar with the mental health environment. Many aspects of mental health nursing care differ from the roles performed in other areas of the health-care sector. These differences are often emphasised at the expense of the many similarities in nursing practice across all settings. The aim of this section is to provide an overview of the role of mental health nurses, and the specific contribution that nursing makes to the care of people experiencing mental health problems. Having said that, it is by no means as easy a task as it may appear to be. The nursing profession as a whole has struggled to define what it brings to health care, particularly when attempting to emphasise the unique contribution of nursing. Mental health nursing is no exception. One definition of mental health nursing is offered by the Australian and New Zealand College of Mental Health Nurses (now called the Australian College of Mental Health Nurses), the professional organisation for mental health nurses in Australia:

A Mental Health Nurse is a registered nurse who holds a recognised specialist qualification in mental health. Taking a holistic approach, guided by evidence, the mental health nurse works in collaboration with people who have mental health issues, their family and community, towards recovery as defined by the individual. (Australian College of Mental Health Nurses Inc. 2010, p. 5)

The relationship between mental health nurses and service users is pivotal. This is not to suggest that the relationships between nurses and the people they care for is not important in all practice settings—if nursing is truly to be a caring profession, the nurse–service user relationship must always form the basis for the provision of that care. However, the very nature of nursing practice in the mental health field places greater emphasis on this relationship than in any other field of nursing.

You may well be struck by the different environment within which mental health nursing operates, compared with the other areas where you have gained your clinical experience to date. The environment is much less technical than areas where physical illness and injury are treated. Consequently, mental health nurses tend to focus much less on tasks. Although there has been a conscious intention to reduce the task-oriented nature of nursing within the general health system, there remains many tasks that need to be done, such as attending to hygiene and nutritional needs, dressing wounds and monitoring intravenous therapy. While people experiencing mental health problems share many of these needs, the ways in which these needs are met vary considerably in the mental health environment. For example, people experiencing mental health problems generally have fewer physical limitations than people receiving care within the general health-care environment.

The relationship between nursing and the broader multidisciplinary team also differs substantially from other areas of nursing. Again, nurses in all settings work within a team environment. However, within the general health-care environment, each discipline—such as medicine, physiotherapy or social work—tends to have defined roles and functions, which are clearly distinguishable from one another and from the role of the nurse. Where nurses take on the roles of other disciplines, it is generally outside of usual working hours. For example, the nurse in the medical–surgical setting may perform physiotherapy interventions during the evenings, nights and over the weekend.

MENTAL HEALTH SETTINGS AND THE NURSE'S ROLE

Within the mental health setting, the five main disciplines are identified as nursing, psychiatry, psychology, occupational therapy and social work—although contributions of other professional groups, such as physiotherapy and speech therapy, are more apparent in specific specialist areas such as aged care, and child and adolescent psychiatry respectively. The roles of the various disciplines are, however, not so easy to define. This is particularly apparent within community settings. If you were to observe a community team, you may have trouble distinguishing the nurse from the social worker. Although each professional group brings its specific area of expertise to the team, the boundaries between roles are often not clear. This is largely due to the importance attached to the role of the case manager, case coordinator or service coordinator within the mental health field. The case manager works collaboratively with service users and carers to ensure that the optimal standard of individually based care and treatment is provided for people experiencing a mental health problem. Nurses and allied health staff frequently adopt the role of case manager, and in so doing share many tasks that traditionally may be performed by other health professionals, although they may consult with other members of the team when their specific area of expertise is required.

Mental health nursing care will be described in greater detail in Chapter 12, where these differences in approaches will be explored further. However, it is important to bear in mind the similarities that mental health nursing shares with other aspects of the nursing profession. Like all fields of nursing, mental health nursing is underpinned by the desire to provide the highest possible standard of care for people. It involves working with people from a broad variety of backgrounds, who are experiencing a variety of health problems. The differences in the health problems experienced, the reaction to these problems and the individual personalities of the people concerned require the nurse to be involved in the provision of individually based care, which reflects the specific needs of each individual. Furthermore, all areas of nursing should not focus purely on the illness itself, but should encompass a philosophy of health promotion, education and illness prevention.

ESSENTIAL QUALITIES OF A MENTAL HEALTH NURSE

One reason nursing students give for not wanting to pursue a career in mental health nursing is their belief that they do not have what it takes (Happell 2001). This view gives the impression that there is only one certain kind of person who can be a mental health nurse. While there are definitely some characteristics that are considered essential, this field of work also thrives on variety. Just as the people we care for are not the same in their personalities, interests and needs, it is important that nurses reflect this diversity and bring their individual personalities to the nursing relationship.

On the other hand, one may argue that the attributes required of a mental health nurse are essentially similar to the attributes required of any nurse. Nurses need to be motivated by a desire to help, to care for or to tend to others in a time of great need. A compassionate, caring nature and a non-judgemental attitude are crucial. Traditionally, these characteristics were seen as the most important—and perhaps even the only— ones required of a good nurse. As a result of the development of nursing practice, more than ever nursing requires a high level of intelligence and the ability to reflect and think critically.

CRITICAL THINKING

- What images come to mind when you think of a mental health nurse? Where do you think you may have gained these impressions—for instance, media representations of mental health nurses, knowing someone who is a mental health nurse?
- What do you consider are the specific characteristics and qualities that a mental health nurse should have? What are the implications if not all mental health nurses have these?
- 'Mental health nurses are born, not made.' Do you agree with this statement? Give reasons to support your answer.

We hope that the thousands of students who, every year, commence their undergraduate nursing program will possess these attributes, irrespective of the field of nursing in which they wish to practise in the future. However, every student—like every nurse currently registered—will have particular personality traits. Mental health nursing is no exception. Some characteristics that may be particularly beneficial include a good sense of humour and a well-developed sense of fun. This is not to suggest that mental health nursing is not a serious discipline, nor that it is not taken seriously, but the ability to laugh and have fun is important within any therapeutic environment.

It is difficult to say briefly what makes a good mental health nurse, but whether or not you consider this area of practice in the future should not be limited by your preconceived ideas about what it takes. As a starting point, make the most of your clinical placement, and let decisions about the type of nursing to which you are best suited come later.

MAKING THE MOST OF YOUR CLINICAL PLACEMENT

It is not unusual to feel apprehensive about your clinical placement. Set aside your fears and look at your forthcoming clinical experience as a positive learning opportunity. Australian research shows that the clinical placement is the most important factor in influencing students' attitudes towards mental health nursing (O'Brien, Buxton & Gillies 2008).

To get the most out of this experience:

- Remember that whatever area of nursing you choose to practise in, you will be providing care for people experiencing mental health challenges, and that the skills and knowledge you develop in this setting will better equip you for this aspect of your role.

- View this experience as a challenge. You will have the opportunity to learn about, and provide care for, people experiencing mental health problems. You will discover that they are people much like you and your family and friends, with particular interests, needs and issues that are not exclusively related to their mental health.

Remember that you will work with experienced mental health nurses, with a broad range of skills, knowledge and experience.

The mental health setting offers the opportunity to be exposed to a very different aspect of nursing. Although nursing relationships are based on principles that apply across all health-care settings, many aspects are different within the mental health environment. It is likely that you will have more opportunity to be with the people for whom you are caring. There is less emphasis on doing things for your clients in mental health, as it is more about being with and doing things with them. Therefore, forming relationships with your clients on a mental health placement is an important part of the experience—always remembering that it is the client's needs that are at the centre of such relationships, not your own. For many nursing students, the differences in environment are striking. Some students mistakenly assume that mental health nurses do not do anything; they talk to the clients, or engage in other 'casual' activities such as playing pool or going for a walk. While it is very different from the role of the nurse in a busy surgical unit, talking and listening do not mean doing nothing. Through spending time and engaging with people experiencing a mental illness, the nurse builds trust, which will enable them to work together towards recovery for the person experiencing mental health problems. It is equally as important as the more technologically driven interventions more commonly observed within the general health-care environment.

Above all, you are encouraged to view your mental health placement as an exciting and challenging opportunity. In order to make the most of this experience, it is important that you are as prepared as you possibly can be. It is equally important not to place too much pressure on yourself. You are a student undertaking a course that requires you to learn about a broad range of nursing practices and health-care settings. You cannot reasonably be expected to know everything about them all.

It is likely that your clinical placement will be supervised either by a clinical teacher employed by the hospital or a clinical facilitator employed by the university. This person has a key role to play in supporting and guiding you during your clinical experience. The relationship you establish with this person is crucial. The following tips may assist you in ensuring that this relationship is a positive one:

- Continually demonstrate interest.
- Be clear about the learning objectives you are expected to achieve. Seek assistance and clarification from your preceptor/clinical teacher when you are unsure or require assistance.
- Familiarise yourself with practical expectations, such as punctuality and appropriate dress requirements.
- Attend handovers, intake meetings, team meetings and clinical reviews, which will enable you to achieve a greater understanding of the professional practices and the specific issues facing the recipients of services.
- Where possible, plan your placement in advance. It is likely that within each setting there will be a diary or activity board that outlines specific activities. Once you have decided what you are most interested in attending, negotiate with the person responsible for coordinating the activity for the opportunity to become involved.
- Be aware of your limitations. If you feel uncertain at any time, do not hesitate to ask for help. Do not be tempted to bluff your way through due to the fear that you will appear foolish if you ask.
- Be aware of your own feelings. If you feel uncomfortable at any time, it is import-ant to understand why this may be so. Does it reflect your own lack of knowledge of experience? Or does it indicate fear about caring for people experiencing mental health challenges? Is it something to do with your health or that of someone you know? Either way, do remember that it is nothing to be ashamed of. By being aware of and reflecting upon these feelings, you will have the opportunity to work through your fears and concerns. Merely ignoring these feelings will not make them go away, and will reduce your ability to learn from them and grow, both professionally and personally. You might find it useful to keep a journal through-out the clinical experience.
- Become familiar with the setting, including policies and procedures, and safety issues. The importance of asking questions when you are not sure about something cannot be over-emphasised.
- Although the relationship with your clinical facilitator/clinical teacher is crucial, do not restrict your interactions to just this person. By working with others, you will have the opportunity to observe a number of different styles and approaches. This will increase your ability to identify and develop your own style that complements your individual personality and your own specific attributes. This does not need to be restricted to nurses. It is likely that members of other professional disciplines will be pleased to involve you in aspects of their activities.
- Seek regular feedback. Do not be afraid to ask your clinical facilitator/clinical teacher for their impressions of how you are progressing throughout your placement.

If they identify areas where you need further development, seek their expertise and guidance as to how this can be achieved.

- Regular debriefing should be provided by your clinical facilitator/clinical teacher. However, if you encounter situations you find disturbing or disconcerting, seek the opportunity to debrief. It is crucial that you have the opportunity to work through these issues, and do not continue to carry them with you. If you are not satisfied with the opportunities provided to you, contact your university lecturer in order to achieve a more satisfactory outcome.

- Take as many opportunities as you can to become involved in the many and varied activities offered by the setting. Be guided by your clinical learning objectives, but do not be restricted by them. If there is something else happening, seek advice from your preceptor/clinical teacher as to how you might become involved.

- Remember that the most important aspect of this clinical experience is the opportunity to spend time with and increase your understanding of people experiencing mental health challenges.

PURPOSE OF THIS TEXT

As stated at the beginning of the chapter, the aim of this book is to introduce you to the field of mental health nursing. The authors hope to interest you in this specialised field as you undertake both the theoretical and practical components of mental health nursing. It is, however, important to remember that both this book and your course will provide an introduction to mental health nursing. They have not been designed to make you an expert or specialist in this field. What we do hope is that at the end of your course you have gained an appreciation of the role and the valuable contributions that mental health nurses make through working closely with people experiencing mental health problems. A few of you may already want to become mental health nurses. We hope that, as a result of the education you are receiving, many more of you will plan to do so. Above all, it is hoped that you will gain a much broader understanding of mental health issues, and feel more comfortable and confident about providing care for people experiencing a mental health problem in whatever area of health care you choose to work in the future.

Good luck, learn a lot, and above all enjoy yourself!

REFERENCES

Ash, D., Bland, R., Brown, P., Oakley Browne, M., Burvill, P., Davies, J. et al. (2012). Mental health services in the Australian states and territories. In G. Meadows, J. Farhall, E. Fossey, M. Grigg, F. McDermott & B. Singh (eds), *Mental Health in Australia: collaborative community practice* (3rd ed.). Melbourne: Oxford University Press, pp. 118–54.

Australian College of Mental Health Nurses Inc. (2010). *Standards of Practice for Australian Mental Health Nurses 2010*. Canberra: ACMHN.

Australian Health Ministers (1992). *National Mental Health Policy*. Canberra: Australian Government Publishing Service.

Bessant B. (1999). *Milestones in Australian nursing*. Collegian, 6(4), insert.

Cade J.F.J. (1979). *Mending the Mind: a short history of twentieth century psychiatry*. Melbourne: Sun Books.

Commonwealth of Australia. (2009). *National Mental Health Policy 2008*. Viewed 20 February 2013, <www.health.gov.au/internet/main/publishing.nsf/content/532CBE92A8323E03CA25756E001203BF/$File/finpol08.pdf>.

Cowling W.R. III (2011). The global presence of holistic nursing. *Journal of Holistic Nursing*, 29(2), 89–90.

Cowling, V., Edan, V., Cuff, R., Armitage, P. & Herszberg, D. (2006). Mental health consumer and carer participation in professional education: 'getting there together' for children of parents with mental illness and their families. *Australian Social Work*, 59(4), 406–21.

Epstein, M. & Shaw, J. (1997). *Developing Effective Consumer Participation in Mental Health Services*. Melbourne: Victorian Mental Illness Awareness Council (VMIAC).

Gordon, S. (2005). The role of the consumer in the leadership and management of mental health services. *Australasian Psychiatry*, 13(4), 362–5.

Hamden, A., Newton, R., McCauley-Elsom, K. & Cross, W. (2011). Is deinstitutionalization working in our community? *International Journal of Mental Health Nursing*, 20, 274–83.

Happell, B. (2001). Comprehensive nursing education in Victoria: rhetoric or reality? *Journal of Psychiatric and Mental Health Nursing*, 8(6), 507–16.

—— (2008). The importance of clinical experience for mental health nursing—part 1: undergraduate nursing students' attitudes, preparedness and satisfaction. *International Journal of Mental Health Nursing*, 17(5), 326–32.

Happell, B. & Cutcliffe, J.R. (2011). A broken promise? Exploring the lack of evidence for the benefits of comprehensive nursing education. *International Journal of Mental Health Nursing*, 20(5), 328–36.

Hoekstra, H.J., van Meijel, B.B. & van der Hooft-Leemans, T.G. (2010). A nursing career in mental health care: choices and motives of nursing students. *Nurse Education Today*, 30(1), 4–8.

Human Rights and Equal Opportunity Commission (HREOC) (1993). *Human Rights and Mental Illness: report of the National Inquiry into the Human Rights of People with Mental Illness*. Canberra: Australian Government Publishing Service.

Keane, B. (1987). Study of Mental Health Nursing in Australia: report to the Nursing and Health Services Workforce Branch. Canberra: Australian Government Publishing Service.

McAllister, M., Happell, B. & Bradshaw, J. (2010). Making us what we are: noteworthy people and achievements in Queensland mental health nursing. *International Journal of Mental Health Nursing*, 19(4), 250–6.

McCoppin, B. & Gardiner, H. (1995). *Tradition and reality: Nursing and politics in Australia*. Melbourne: Churchill Livingston.

O'Brien, L., Buxton, M. & Gillies, D. (2008). Improving the undergraduate clinical placement experience in mental health nursing. *Issues in Mental Health Nursing*, 29(5), 505–22.

Povlsen, L. & Borup, I.K. (2011). Holism in nursing and health promotion: distinct or related perspectives? A literature review. *Scandinavian Journal of Caring Sciences*, 25(4), 798–805.

Singh, B., Benson, A., Weir, W., Rosen, A. & Ash, D. (2007). The history of mental health services in Australia. In G. Meadows, B. Singh & M. Grigg (eds), *Mental Health in Australia: collaborative community practice* (2nd edn). Melbourne: Oxford University Press, pp. 65–75.

Sweeney, A., Beresford, P., Faulkner, A., Nettle, M. & Rose, D. (2009). *This is survivor research*. Hereford-shire: PCCC Books

Wynaden, D. (2010). There is no health without mental health: are we educating Australian nurses to care for the health consumer of the 21st century? *International Journal of Mental Health Nursing*, 19(3), 203–9.

2

Conceptual frameworks guiding mental health nursing

Main points
- Theories of mental illness can provide perspectives on how and why mental illness may occur.
- Nursing theories incorporate multiple sources of knowledge to create a structure for mental health nursing practice.
- Ways of knowing and understanding nursing are linked together, forming conceptual frameworks.
- Conceptual models help to reveal the substance of a theory in a symbolic format.
- Nursing and contemporary theories of mental health care continue to evolve and expand.
- Models of practice help to organise, identify and clarify caring nursing practices.
- Theory in practice is how knowledge and research cross over into everyday practices.

Definitions
Theory: A self-contained network of definitions, concepts and ideas that link together, thereby forming an understanding and specific knowledge of a phenomenon.

Concept: An abstract notion or idea that is a symbolic representation.

Conceptual models: A series of concepts that link together to form a symbolic representation of a phenomenon.

Construct: A complex psychological view or impression—may be the underlying subject or theme.

INTRODUCTION
In this chapter, we explore theories, conceptual frameworks and conceptual models, models of nursing practice, new and emerging theories and models, and evidence-based

practice to the extent that these topics fit with your growing understanding of the unique and special practice skills that make up mental health nursing care. As with any new topic to which you are introduced in the book, we recommend further reading if you are particularly interested in the topic or are likely to be developing an essay or presentation.

Before embarking on providing mental health nursing care, it is important to have some understanding of 'why and how we do what we do'—or, in theory terms, concepts and models of practice. In any area of nursing, there is an over-arching need to formulate or construct a framework for your caregiving—for example, what is within your scope of caregiving, what are the general aspects of this caregiving, how might it be altered to best serve those receiving your care?

In order to organise nursing care so that it is consistent, focused and evidence based, it is common to utilise theories of nursing. More than many other specialties, mental health nursing has explicit theories that relate specifically to communication, and to interpersonal and therapeutic relationships. This is because mental health nurses are often most reliant on their communication and interaction skills to provide care. To assist you in thinking about nursing theories, the following section explores what a nursing theory is; explores specific nursing theories relating to mental health nursing; and finally, examines how nursing theory informs and shapes our nursing care.

There are a number of theories that relate to why people do what they do (psychology), to mental illness (biological, genetic and sociological) and to mental health (health maintenance and promotion). These theories can assist you to better understand why people think and act in certain ways. Some theories can challenge your understandings of genetics and society, while others can help you to understand the ways in which people interact in families and in the broader community. Most of these theories are developed and will continue to evolve through the research and writings of nurse researchers, sociologists, psychologists, psychiatrists, even geneticists. Further reading for theories on behaviour, interpersonal relationships, cognitive, behavioural and biogenic theories can assist you in providing mental health nursing care.

As stated above, nursing care is embedded in or constructed out of a theory for providing health care. Many nursing theories that relate to nursing in general (that is, medical–surgical nursing) will contain generic or non-specific features that can also apply to mental health nursing. This includes nursing theories on physical and disease processes.

The unique feature of mental health nursing, as opposed to general nursing, is the significance of the interpersonal relationship between the nurse and the service user. It is important to remember that the interpersonal relationship is fundamental to all nursing; however, it is the central feature of mental health nursing. Therefore, mental health nursing theory primarily relates to the development and maintenance of interpersonal relationships.

CASE STUDY

Joanne was nervous, so she arrived at the Mental Health Acute Care Unit early on her first day. On her way to the unit, Joanne had been fretting over her perceived lack of knowledge of mental health care, particularly on how her nursing skills might benefit clients, or be utilised or even challenged. Joanne reflected back to her student nurse practicum where she had spent just one clinical week in a mental health-care facility. The week had flown by so quickly, and Joanne struggled to recall the highlights of her student experience. Joanne's biggest concern as she entered the front doors of the unit was whether she had the skills and knowledge required to provide good nursing care. She wondered what models of nursing care she should call upon for mental health nursing, and what life skills might be most helpful to the clientele.

WHAT IS A THEORY?

Whenever you ask why something is so, how it works, what the history is and what the connection to other knowledge is, what you are really thinking about is *theorising*. Theories can provide that in-depth knowledge of how, when, where and why that can assist a person to make an informed start on any project. Theories can act as a 'user's manual', a 'help file' or a comprehensive 'think' about a particular phenomenon. Theories contain concepts or a series of ideas that link together to form an understanding. An example can be taken from understanding ourselves. Theory about the 'self' contains concepts such as self-concept, self-knowledge and self-worth. Another example of a theory and the concepts that may lie within is personality theory and the concepts of personal integration, maturity and ego development.

A theory is an abstract or 'intellectual thinking' method of summarising and organising knowledge of a particular event or phenomenon (Meleis 2012). As such, theory is a very handy tool for describing and exploring or even adding knowledge to that event or phenomenon. While a theory may represent what knowledge existed at a particular point in time, it can evolve and can also become defunct or disproved as our evolving knowledge is tested and reshaped by our search for new understandings.

Nursing theory is a title for a body of knowledge that informs and structures the practices of nursing. Nursing theories are developed from a wide variety of sources, including nursing research, nursing experiences and theories from related professions such as medicine, psychology, sociology and biology. Nursing theory then relates specifically to the person, the environment and health.

Theories in general aim to demonstrate and even organise relations between information so that they assist us by informing our actions. Nursing theories fulfil a similar function in that, according to Meleis (2012), they contain specific elements such as concepts that help to describe, predict and explore nursing phenomena. Examples of nursing phenomena that you may already have examined are caring, wellness, illness and recovery. Nursing theories continue to increase in number and complexity as the profession of nursing embraces the idea of examining what nursing is.

WHAT IS A NURSING THEORY?

Nursing theory assists nurses to make informed choices about their nursing practice (Chinn & Kramer 2008) by incorporating an evidence basis, a rationale for nursing tasks and a basis for professional development. Therefore, if a nursing theory significantly contributes to the professional evolution of nursing, it is also of great importance for mental health nursing as a sub-branch of nursing. Knowing about nursing practices is only the first step towards providing safe and competent mental health nursing care (Varcarolis 2010). Understanding the process and being aware of patterns in knowledge and in practice are also important features of a theory-driven mental health nursing practice. Figure 2.1 shows the structure of the theories in mental health nursing.

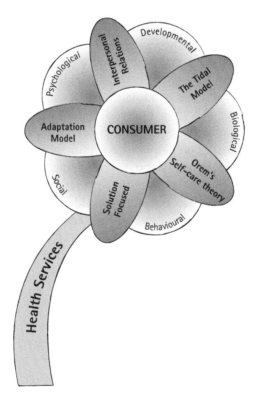

Figure 2.1 Theories used in mental health nursing

Table 2.1 Theories relating to the human condition that continue to influence contemporary nursing theory

Theory	Name attributed	Relevance to nursing
Psychological 1 Psychoanalytic 2 Psychodynamic	Sigmund Freud Anna Freud Melanie Klein	Unconscious processes direct human behaviour and deviance. Mental illness occurs from conflict (anxiety) through predominantly unconscious processes. Symptoms are symbolic of conflict and lack of developmental resolution.
Developmental	Jean Piaget Erik Erickson John Bowlby Lawrence Kohlberg Aaron Beck Carol Gilligan Mary Ainsworth	Defines and relates stages of human cognitive, moral, physical, spiritual and social development to connectedness. Development follows predictable pathways so that deviation or distortions are recognisable. Assists in locating sources of anxiety and impact on interpersonal skills, self-esteem and trust.
Biological	Rene Descartes Emil Kraeplin	Mental health problems result from a biological source such as disease, genetics or environmental processes. Symptoms are related to abnormality in neuroanatomy and/or neurophysiology. Diagnosis requires classification, which describes clinical features. Neurobiology and psychopharmacology are central tenets.
Behavioural	Abraham Maslow B.F. Skinner Ivan Pavlov Albert Bandura	Includes basic need, existential and behavioural theories. Classic conditioning initiates behaviour and modifying or reinforcing aspects of behaviour results in desired responses. Behaviourist principles can reduce maladaptive and undesired behaviours.
Social	Margaret Mead Madeleine Leininger Murray Bowen Carl Jung Thomas Szasz Herbert Blumer	Includes numerous theories such as family dynamics and theory, role theory and symbolic interaction, thereby placing individual behaviour into the larger societal perspective. Family and cultural norms are significant. The social realm is central to understanding appropriate care, as are rituals, symbols and spirituality derived from social effects. Cultural knowledge, awareness and skill lead to culturally sound/safe practices. Symbolic interaction means that people's actions are defined by the meaning that events, things and impressions have for the individual.
Interpersonal	Harry Stack Sullivan Adolf Meyer Eric Fromm Hildegard Peplau Alfred Adler Karen Horney	Human processes/interactions occur through the interrelational network and not in isolation from people or environments. Attachment relates to personal and social development. Relationship health results from hope, self-esteem and self-worth, dignity and interpersonal skills.

Mental health nurses may take a pluralistic approach to nursing theories. For example, mental health nursing does not simply base practices on one particular nursing theory; rather, the nurse bases their nursing practice on a variety of nursing theories while predominantly using the nursing theory that pertains to the nurse–client relationship. Although nursing theory has been informed by broader social theories, a mental health nursing theory also is informed by, and in part evolves from, broader psychological, social and human development theories. Therefore, a mental health nursing theory will contain concepts that have a genesis (or beginning) in other non-nursing professions. For example, the bio-psycho-social model of care (LeVine 2012), the unity model (Song & Shih 2009) and the mediational model (Barrett et al. 2010) begin with the generic basis of recovery theory.

Consequently, if mental health nursing theory is influenced by many different nursing and non-nursing theories, can there be one theory that guides and informs mental health nursing? The answer to this question is yes in the historic sense, and no in the contemporary sense. First, no discussion on mental health nursing theory should bypass the contributions of Hildegard Peplau, and the section on nursing theorists later in the chapter will focus on the legacy of Peplau for mental health nursing. Second, exciting new mental health nursing theories are evolving and will be discussed as contemporary theories.

CONCEPTUAL FRAMEWORKS

Another term to consider in this chapter is 'conceptual frameworks'. These represent a way of viewing, knowing and understanding a particular perspective on the world. You may be used to the idea of a framework being something that you construct in order to house or hold the content you wish to put in it. Take the building of a house as an example. In order to separate your house from the space surrounding it, you build a structure—or, in this scenario, a frame. This has now provided you with an area in which to continue building your house. The framework provides you with structural supports and specific areas to become rooms.

In a metaphorical sense, the conceptual framework houses your theoretical terms, meanings and even the set of assumptions and phenomena about the nature of the theory that is being housed. All these elements are networked together within your conceptual framework.

There are a number of conceptual frameworks that may be relevant to our work as mental health nurses. You might picture your house framework as not the only house frame on the street block—in fact, your house framework might constitute just one segment of a street full of house frameworks, or a cluster of mental health nursing conceptual frameworks in a suburb called 'nursing conceptual frameworks'.

CONCEPTUAL MODELS

Theories contain definitions, purposes, abstraction and concepts (LoBiondo-Wood & Haber 2010). Many cognitive and behavioural theories, such as in psychology and sociology, are complex. Consequently, it can be difficult to gain a sense of meaning and relevance to clinical practice. Using the most simplistic of explanations, conceptual models are one method of portraying or revealing the substance of a theory, and contain concepts and realities in a symbolic format to represent the abstract ideas within the theory. Fawcett and Karban define conceptual models as:

> A set of relatively abstract and general concepts that address the phenomena of central interest to a discipline, the propositions that broadly describe those concepts, and the propositions that state relatively abstract and general relations between two or more of the concepts. (Fawcett & Karban 2005, p.16)

A detailed account of conceptual models is beyond the scope of this text, and you are directed to Meleis (2012) as one example of a good account of concept models. From a conceptual model, we can perhaps gain a better grasp of the components of a concept or the concepts within a theory. Figure 2.2 presents a well-known example of a conceptual model.

Conceptual models are abstract, as they represent theory rather than stating it. They are constructed or patterned to best represent reasoning in a logical chain; by doing so, the relationships between constructs are made clear. Modelling refers to a process of developing or generating a chain of reasoning to represent a phenomenon.

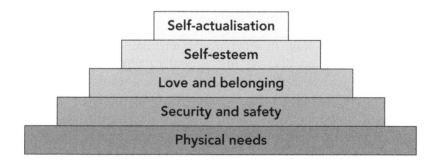

Figure 2.2 Maslow's hierarchy of needs
Source: Adapted from Maslow (1970).

CRITICAL THINKING

Maslow's theory of a hierarchy of human needs lends itself to being quickly grasped or comprehended when in the shape of a model as in Figure 2.2. There are many conceptual models created from theories of nursing. Before reading further, take the time to consult a nursing theory text and make a list of the theories that you think may be relevant to mental health nursing. As you create this list, you could think about some of the potential problems that may arise from the generation of these conceptual models.

For example, Jacobson and Greenley (2001) have developed a conceptual model of recovery from mental illness. The model contains internal conditions such as experiences, attitudes and processes of change, as well as external conditions such as events, policies and practices that promote and guide recovery. The internal and external conditions begin, maintain and create recovery in the Jacobson and Greenley model.

CRITICAL THINKING

The image created by the Jacobson and Greenley recovery model can be drawn. Create your vision of this model on a sheet of paper. Where in this model will you put essential features such as hope, human rights, empowerment, control, responsibility and connection?

THE MEDICAL MODEL

Diseases have a biological core. In other words, anything that goes wrong with the human condition has a biological cause. In philosophical terms, the mind and body are separate entities, and modern medicine 'treats' the body in a manner similar to a car that has broken down. The medical model, according to Turner (1987, p. 213), 'underlies the basis of institutionalised, scientific, technologically directed medicine'.

The medical model operates on the basis of the scientific or empirical knowledge of 'cause and effect', and this fact alone may provide the main focus of limitations for this model. The addition of the prefix 'bio' to 'medical' further limits the model to that which is organically derived. You may find that the terms 'medical model' and 'biomedical model' are often used interchangeably in literature.

Features of the medical (biomedical) model include the following:

- Diseases have a physical cause.
- The focus is on classifying (diagnosing) and treating disease and illness.
- Organic aspects of disease take precedence.
- Pathways of cure are for physically based illness (mind–body split).
- The treatment focus is on physical invasion from disease (bypassing the human situation).
- Detection and destruction of disease are best achieved by hospitalisation.
- Individualised health care parallels the rise of capitalism.
- Health-care resources, provision and research are dominated by a prestigious medical profession. (Adapted from Kermode 2004, p. 13)

Medical model of disability

People influenced by the medical model may regard people with disabilities as 'suffering' and in need of medical treatment. This has led to beliefs that society ought to care for people with disabilities in residential institutions and hospitals, and experts being seen as in the best position to determine treatment—and even how and where people spend their lives. This ideology is still evident in the way we think about people with disabilities, how we behave towards them and how we often fail to allow access to education, leisure, work and relationships. This way of thinking has been challenged by people with disabilities as disempowering. Traditionally, psychiatric disability has described the social aspects of living with a 'mental illness'—if the 'illness' describes the presence of a biological disease, then 'disability' describes what it is like to live with the disease.

INFLUENCE OF THE MEDICAL MODEL ON NURSING

The core principles of the medical model are the diagnosis, treatment and cure of disease; hence the values and attitudes engendered by the medical model may be different from the values and attitudes of nurses. The 'diagnose, treat and cure' process may be at odds with contemporary nursing practice in that it tends to neglect the individual within the model, or to limit the role of the individual within their own health care. This is perhaps more obvious in mental health care than in the more generic nursing situations such as medical–surgical nursing. As Pearson, Vaughan & Fitzgerald (2005) point out, the invisible and not clearly curing aspects of nursing, such as psycho-social and spiritual care, may not rate as important nursing interventions under the medical model. Instead, providing medication and an aseptic technique may be understood as the most important tasks for nurses because they are more consistent with the values and attitudes of the medical model.

The influence of the medical model on nursing is substantial—and even, in some cases, insidious. The effects of the model filter through the various levels of nursing

(Carlyle, Crowe & Deering 2012) from an over-valuation of the more technical and physical tasks to reducing time and skills available for more psycho-social care. The notion of a nursing-led and managed health service periodically arises in the Australian health-care setting, but its demise is often due to the broader health-care organisation's dependence on the medical model where cure is valued and resourced, whereas care—being often invisible—lacks the power to maintain its independence (Bennetts, Cross & Bloomer 2011)

LIMITATIONS OF THE MEDICAL (BIOMEDICAL) MODEL

While advances in some aspects of health care throughout the past century have indelibly been linked to the rise of the medical model, the argument claiming that the medical model is becoming less relevant to current health care in the twenty-first century is becoming louder and stronger. Nursing theory has been influenced by this model, particularly in relation to the disease and cure aspects; however, it is here that we gain a sense of the 'living component' of nursing theories as they continue to evolve and move away from the confines of the medical model, and adopt a more humanistic and holistic model for health-care provision.

Potential limitations are summarised as:

- decreases in new microbes, meaning increasing irrelevance to the current human condition
- an increase in iatrogenesis (Vincent 2010)
- the inability to incorporate spirituality, emotions and psychological distress
- a linear approach to health, which can misconstrue complex multi-causal illnesses
- a lack of relevance for 'incurable' conditions
- culturally bound views (predominantly Western civilisations) (Small 2006)
- a preoccupation with quantity of life as opposed to quality of life
- an hierarchically structured system—that is, one determined by the 'patient role' as opposed to 'client', 'consumer' or 'service user' (Kermode 2004).

If the central focus of the current medical model in mental health care is the use of pharmacological agents (new and old), we may need to re-examine the use of this model. In fact, Ramon and Williams (2005, p. 14) refer to the model as the 'biochemical model of mental illness'. Table 2.2 compares the conditions of diabetes and depression. Our understanding and health care of these conditions is different, and this is reflected in the table.

Table 2.2 Why comparisons between diabetes and depression (or schizophrenia or manic depression) are untenable

Diabetes	Depression
Precision potential of medication	
Very refined; down to precision of single-unit dose calculation	Continuing investigations, currently blunt; single-strength dose for all
Mode of action of medication	
Thoroughly known and understood	Postulated: not at all clear: So far, the neurochemical underpinnings of mood disorders are not known. Although serotonin has long been thought to be central to their aetiology, some of the newer treatments have no effect on serotonin.
	For more than 30 years, the dominant hypotheses of the biological basis for depression have been related to noradrenaline and serotonin. Note the word 'hypotheses', not 'established facts'.
	Acceptance of the biological basis of depression (as fact) on the basis of unproven hypothesis? Why are no other hypotheses pursued with equal vigour?
Specificity of treatment	
Highly specific to diabetes	Not at all specific. Used widely for anxiety, panic, phobias, shyness, social anxiety, obsessive-compulsion, anorexia, post-traumatic conditions
Monitoring: early stages	
Intensive; blood sugar tests several times an hour is not unusual	No tests carried out because no tests exist
Response to treatment	
Swift: effect of insulin treatment measurable within minutes	Best estimates claim to take two to three weeks to respond to treatment. No test or laboratory method to monitor or oversee individual response to treatment
Adverse effects of treatment	
Very few, due to precision of replacing like with like (i.e. insulin with insulin)	Many: not replacing what is missing
Monitoring: ongoing	
Regular blood and urine tests. So refined that recipients can carry out the tests themselves daily with sophisticated blood glucose-monitoring equipment at home	No tests exist, so no monitoring of levels of supposed biochemical abnormality

continued

Diabetes	Depression
Response to no treatment	
Swift: rapidly rising or falling blood glucose (measurable) leading to diabetic coma	Effects of cessation of treatment on supposed biochemical abnormality unknown, not measurable
Effectiveness of treatment	
100 per cent	50–60 per cent (claims by the Royal College of Psychiatrists)
Response to placebo	
None	45–50 per cent success rate
Response to counselling	
None	40–60 per cent success rate
Duration of treatment	
For life: as well as regular monitoring of blood sugar levels	Three to nine months: levels of supposed biochemical abnormality are never measured
Life off treatment	
Impossible: insulin is for life	Frequent: But where did the biochemical abnormality go? How can we be sure it was ever there? If the medication was correcting a biochemical abnormality all along, has the abnormality spontaneously disappeared? How can the medication be stopped without any assessment of levels of the supposed biochemical abnormality, if the condition is fundamentally biochemical?

Source: Adapted from Gray (2005, p. 36).

PSYCHO-SOCIAL THEORY

Good health is more than physical well-being, and you are asked to consider the notion that good health is a combination of psychological, social, physical and spiritual well-being. Therefore, consideration in nursing theory is given to how a person's psycho-social health relates to their overall health. The term 'psycho-social', when broken down, means a combination of psychological and social factors. A person's psychological state interacts with their social development and position within society to influence the person's overall well-being.

Have you ever wondered why some health and life crises are easy to manage, whereas others seem like the very last straw? In psycho-social theory, the interactions of the mind and body are continuous and complex. Illness, for example, is influenced by psycho-social development and needs, as well as by the physical pathology. One of the strengths of nursing is that we can go beyond a biomedical (disease-oriented) focus. For example, nursing care is not (and should not be) limited just to care of the body or care of the mind.

It is difficult to define a theory as broad as psycho-social theory. This may be because it is not so much a theory as a method or approach to understanding people. Psycho-social theory asks us to think about people as a melting pot of psychological and social events. Our biogenetic endowment (inheritance), along with the effects of our significant relationships, combines with the impact of societal and cultural experiences to form our unique view of life. Clearly, this method of understanding people is not the contribution of any one theorist, and has developed over many years. A range of social science authors have used terms such as 'psycho-situational', 'psycho-social', 'psycho-cultural' and 'psycho-political'. People are the product of interactions between inherent dispositions and their environment. Psycho-social theory provides a dynamic or evolving view of how an individual integrates with their society as seen in the following summaries:

- Psycho-social theory provides a lifespan view of human development. Desires and goals of both the individual and society are important for conceptualising human development.
- Each life stage involves crises and triumphs. These are caused by differences between individual desires and resources and what society expects of the individual at each life stage. People develop and change as each new challenge is met and their successes are carried forward into the next life stage.
- The style, resources and circle of important relationships carried forward by a person through the psycho-social stages of life are a measure of their individual and social development. Progression is usually consistent.
- Social behaviour, new ideas and actions that occur as a person progresses through life are triggered by contact and interaction with society. New and evolving relationships help to open new directions in life.

THE PSYCHO-SOCIAL AND BIO-PSYCHO-SOCIAL MODELS

The term 'psycho-social model' has been in use now for over 50 years (attributed to Pearlman 1957, cited in Ramon & Williams 2005). As the term implies, it is the combination of psychological and social concepts within the model. Other conceptual frameworks, such as the 'bio-psycho-social model' simply refer to the aspects of biological functioning added to psychological and social functioning. It is important to understand that one theory, conceptual framework or model is not exclusive of all others. One of the main criticisms of the medical model is its lack of 'the human element', and it is here that the psycho-social model of mental health care can contribute vital concepts.

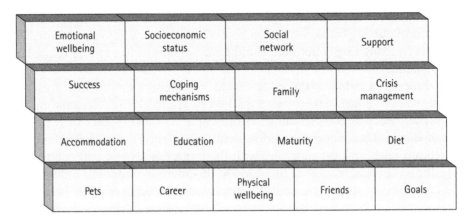

Figure 2.3 Interlocking psycho-social influences

Source: Cowin, in Wilkinson & Van Leuven (2007, p. 188).

Features of the bio-psycho-social model of mental health care include:

- Influences on illness include biological, psychological and social aspects of a person.
- The course and clinical pathways of illness, health and recovery include biological, psychological and social phenomena.
- Biological, psychological and social aspects are not equal; rather, significant effects of each will depend on the individual's circumstances.

New theories evolve into models, with some gaining traction in our health-care systems and others gradually fading away due to a lack of relevance in the current socio-political environment. The embodied-socio-psychological model (Delefosse 2011) is an example of adjustments to the bio-psycho-social model. The author states that it is based 'on the patients' accounts of the emergence of the illness and its daily evolution, in which they mention a deep modification of their being in the world' (2011, p. 221).

SOCIAL MODEL OF DISABILITY

The social model of disability has been articulated by disabled people themselves. The model asserts that it is not the individual's impairment that causes or equates with disability; rather, disability occurs as a result of social barriers that restrict the activities of people with impairments (Oliver 1997). These barriers may be encountered daily, such as discriminatory attitudes where people's skills and attributes may be overlooked, and their potential may be limited by prejudice and social exclusion:

In the main, it is not the impairment that is the problem, or the disabled person, rather it is society's failure to take into account our diverse needs. The Social Model shifts policy away from a medical, charity, care agenda into a rights led, equalities agenda . . . The Social Model in its simplest changes the focus away from people's impairments and towards removing the barriers that disabled people face in everyday life. (Birmingham City Council 2012)

Any social factor—whether attitudinal or environmental—can either contribute to the experience of disability (obstacles to well-being) or reduce the experience of disability (facilitating well-being).

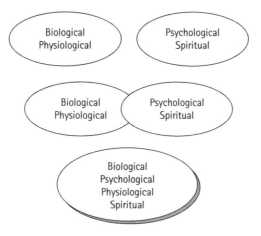

Figure 2.4 Bio-psycho-social: from separate to fully integrated models

---

CRITICAL THINKING
Think of a recent news story that you have seen regarding a person/people with a psychiatric diagnosis. Do you think the story would have contributed to or hampered a better understanding and appreciation of the lives and experiences of service users? How?

EVIDENCE-BASED MODELS OF CARE
Evidence-based practice (EBP) is now central to the deliberation, construction and delivery of good nursing care. There are a number of terms here, such as 'evidence-based medicine (EBM), evidence-based nursing (EBN) and, more recently, evidence-based

health care (EBHC)' (Hudson et al. 2008, p. 409). Evidence-based health care means the deliberate and sensible use of evidence (the best available at that time) to support all decision-making processes used to care for health-care service users. As you can imagine, evidence-based medicine means that the focus of evidence and decision-making is on the strength of medical treatments and their outcomes. Evidence-based nursing also refers to a culture within the workplace that supports the incorporation of EBP into all aspects of nursing care.

Decisions on care must be based on good and solid evidence, and not on tradition or questionable practices. Models of care that encourage a culture of supporting the incorporation of EBP into all aspects of nursing care form the basis of a definition of evidence-based models of care. However, an important—if not the most important—form of evidence should be based upon the individual's own lived experience, and their goals and aspirations for their individual recovery. This important principle of nursing practice can be lost if there is too much focus on scientific evidence (Fisher & Happell 2009).

CRITICAL THINKING

- How is EBP different from other models of care?
- What are the important features covered in EBM models that will have a direct effect on your nursing practice?

HOLISM

The philosophy and theory of holism are discussed in this chapter, as they provide an excellent example of how we may build upon various aspects of philosophy, theory and conceptual models to encompass the needs of the service user rather than simply the dictates of a theory. Holism is defined by Pearson et al. (2005, p. 66) as a philosophical view in which a person will 'respond as a unified whole' and where a person is 'different from and more than the sum of their parts'. As such, holistic health care is a non-medical philosophy incorporating a physical, mental and spiritual focus, where the emphasis is on the interconnectedness of the person and spirituality binds these aspects together (Townsend 2011; Barker & Buchanan-Barker 2010).

A holistic model of mental health care includes:

- differences in healing and curing—where curing may still end in death but healing brings about a transition from illness to wellness
- a self-reflective practice in order to assist self-reflection in others
- circumstances and situation viewed as learning events instead of 'victimology'
- an investment and focus on hope and clear goals

- comprehension of the whole person, not just a collection of problems or symptoms
- equal recognition given to various approaches to health care.

A THEORY OF MENTAL HEALTH NURSING: HILDEGARD PEPLAU

There are a number of relevant and even competing theories of nursing, and at any time in any nursing situation we may find ourselves drawing aspects of these more general nursing theories into our nursing care. However, mental health nursing has relatively few specific nursing theorists. The most famous of the mental health nursing theorists is Hildegard Peplau. Indeed, it is impossible to discuss nursing theory without first being aware of the contributions of Peplau. Her legacy includes a specific theory for mental health nurses that centres on the nurse–patient relationship.

Table 2.3 A comparison of common health-care models

Medical model		Holistic model
Patients	versus	Persons
Disease	versus	Illness
Understanding the biological situation	versus	Understanding the personal situation
Diagnosis	versus	Clinical judgement
Curing	versus	Healing
Treatment	versus	Collaboration
Eradicating sickness	versus	Achieving health

Source: Adapted from Barbour (1995, p. 32).

Hildegard Peplau (1908–99) was born in the north-eastern United States and had a long and illustrious career that included being president of the American Nurses Association (the largest nurse organisation in the world) and a member of the International Council of Nurses (ICN). Labelled by some nursing authors as the 'mother of psychiatric nursing', Peplau's contribution to an integrated theory of mental health nursing began with the publication of her book, *Interpersonal Relations in Nursing*, in 1952. Having started her nursing career as a staff nurse, Peplau gained a Bachelor's degree in interpersonal psychology, and was heavily influenced by eminent psychologists such as Erich Fromm and Harry Stack Sullivan (Pearson et al. 2005). While much of Peplau's later career was spent in nursing education, research and academia, the focus of publications and ongoing writings help to clarify the interpersonal model first explored in her 1952 publication.

Table 2.4 Health promotion: shifting the focus

Biomedical focus	Holistic focus
Risk factors for disease	Supportive factors for health
Supportive factors for health	Purpose in life
Total cholesterol	Spiritual connections
HDL cholesterol	Social support
LDL cholesterol	Meaning in work (paid/unpaid)
Total cholesterol/HDL ratio	Ability to experience emotions
Triglycerides	Ability to express emotions
Smoking	Optimism and hopefulness
Drinking	Perceived happiness
Cardiovascular fitness	Perceived health
Abdominal strength	Intellectual stimulation
Upper body strength	Restful sleep
Flexibility	Time alone
Back care	Pleasure and play
Weight	Financial resources
Fat intake	Laughter and humour
Sodium intake	Movement/physical resilience
Sugar intake	Abundant/varied food supply
Fibre intake	Contact with nature

Source: Adapted from Robison (2004, p. 5).

Peplau's theory of mental health nursing relates to the core of the mental health nurse's practice: the nurse–patient relationship. This is achieved by framing the stages of the relationship and by visualising the relationship as a two-way dynamic circumstance. Perhaps for the first time in a nursing theory, it was proposed by Peplau that the nurse gives and receives from the relationship at the same time that the service user receives and gives. This notion was innovative, controversial and even daring in the 1950s.

Peplau utilised several theories in building her unique and specific theory for mental health nursing. Interpersonal relations incorporates aspects of human needs theory as well as developmental and interactionist theories (Pearson et al. 2005). Because of the thoroughness of nursing theorists such as Peplau, a well-investigated road map for the development of therapeutic relationships in nursing now exists. The stages of a therapeutic relationship as developed by Peplau can be summed up as an introductory phase, a middle working phase and a termination phase (Mohr & Tasman 2011). Further details on nurse therapeutic relationships first developed by Peplau (1952, 1954, 1960, 1962, 1964, 1991, 1992, 1993) include the following:

- Therapeutic relationships are planned to meet the needs of the service user.
- The basic tool of the therapeutic relationship is communication.
- The mental health nurse uses personality as an integral tool.
- The mental health nurse uses involvement such as 'being there' as a tool to develop the relationship.

CONTEMPORARY THEORIES
The tidal model
The tidal model of Barker and Buchanan-Barker (2004) represents a new theory of and current model for mental health care provision. The central and critical feature of this theory is 'person-centred care'. At the heart of the tidal model is the idea that the journey of mental illness through to recovery is assisted by health care professionals caring 'with' the person through an ocean of experiences. The tidal model reflects a metaphor of ebbs and flows, as seen by the ocean tide as it rises and falls. As a part of the ocean, the tide is an analogy for the flow of experiences through our lives. Barker (2001, p. 235) explains this as 'life is a journey undertaken on an ocean of experiences'. The tidal model emerged in response to a perceived increase in custodial type care, inadequately trained staff, crisis management, increasing violence and restraint, and the decreasing resource allocation that plagues mental health services throughout the world.

Major points within the tidal model theory are the following:

- It relocates the service user to the centre of the caring process.
- Service user experiences define and clarify their own understanding of their journey.
- Professional caring relationships are shaped by collaboration and shared decision-making.
- It involves holistic assessment, as opposed to pre-existing 'one size fits all' theory.
- There is facilitation of the reconstruction or 're-authoring' of life to 'get going again'.
- It features centre-staging of interpersonal interactions.
- It challenges paternalistic medically driven models of mental health care.
- It involves practical demonstrations of positive regard that focus on the person, not the illness.
- It gives voice to personal stories and guides relationship development. (Barker & Buchanan-Barker 2004, 2010)

An idea that was first put into print by Carl Rogers, the creator of client-centred therapy, and was nurtured and further developed by Peplau in her development of interpersonal relations and therapeutic nursing care, forms the focus or centre of the Tidal Model. Rogers called it 'unconditional positive regard' (Rogers 1990). In Rogers' definition, unconditional positive regard is the carer's belief that the service user is a worthy, valuable and capable person, even if the service user does not act or feel that way:

> The therapist [nurse] experiences a warm acceptance of the client's [patient's] experience as being a part of the client as a person, and places no conditions on his [sic] acceptance and warmth. He [sic] prizes the client in a total rather than a conditional way. He does not accept certain feelings in the client and disapprove others. He feels an unconditional positive regard or warmth for this person. This is an outgoing, positive feeling without reservations and without evaluations. It means not making judgements. It involves as much feeling of acceptance for the client's expression of good, positive, mature feelings . . . It is a non-possessive caring for the client as a separate person. (Rogers 1967, in Rogers 1990, p. 103)

Peplau also asks nurses to consider ways of being with clients. The Tidal Model asks that we refocus on the primary goal of helping, being respectful and being human. By gaining insight into the experiences of psychosis and how it is a unique and individual experience, we come to a place of knowing and sharing in our nursing care, enabling us to support rather than impose.

Mainstream mental health theories can become entrenched and inflexible, particularly those framed in the dominant medical model. Mental health care, which was initially viewed as exciting, liberating and humanistic in its conception, can become lost or buried as theories become entrenched and stretched to suit every circumstance and every person experiencing an episode of mental illness. The very enlightening features that drew us to a theory can become a barrier that may prevent a nurse from seeing the person behind or through the illness. Ebbs and eddies in the flow of nursing theories mean that we embrace philosophical shifts and continually re-examine what is important in the provision of nursing care.

MODELS OF PRACTICE

By this point in the chapter, you will likely have reached the conclusion that many theories may influence our approach to providing mental health nursing care. The model of practice that we may use is likely to vary from one nurse to another, and will be influenced by their education and experience (Wimpenny 2002), as well as the influence of the type of health service from which the nursing care is provided.

A good method you might consider here is thinking about whether your choice for model of practice will be influenced by the type of problems and issues of concern presented by the service user and carer. For example, if we were working in an Early Intervention and Prevention team we may want to utilise a model of practice that is based on developing therapeutic communication and relevance with younger persons, adolescents and their families, and facilitating mental health promotion programs. In short, models of practice vary according to the current dominant theory and according to the service user's needs.

Models of nursing practice continue to evolve, with some becoming redundant while new directions are developed (Wimpenny 2002). The key to nursing models is their relevance to the care we provide. Models of practice can provide organisation of nursing theory-based actions; create shared understanding; put a spotlight on service user needs and issues; clarify purpose; and identify care directions.

There are numerous models we could choose to influence and direct our mental health nursing practices, such as Peplau's nurse–client relationship, Roy's Adaptation Model or Orem's Self-Care Model and further reading of these can be found in texts such as Meleis (2012). You may wish to investigate a new model of practice that can challenge many of our previous broader-based models such as the Medical Model by reading about McAllister's Solution Focused Nursing Practice (McAllister 2007).

The Solution Focused approach offers an alternative to the frequently used problem-based approach to nursing practice. In problem-based approaches, the first emphasis is on locating and diagnosing the potential problem. The nursing process uses a problem-based approach to reach potential solutions. This model highlights deficits, uses a deductive process, and categorises and focuses on processes and procedures (McAllister 2007).

Six principles of Solution Focused Nursing

1. The person, not the problem, is at the centre of inquiry.
2. Problems and strengths may be present at all times. Looking for and then developing inner strengths and resources will be affirming, and assist in coping and adapting. Working with what is going right can enhance the service user's hope, optimism and self-belief.
3. Resilience is as important as vulnerability.
4. The nurse's role moves beyond an illness-care role to one of adaptations and recovery.
5. Goals have three parts: service user, nursing and society. Nurses are required to move beyond individual-focused care towards valuing the role of society and culture. Practices that might be unhelpful or unjust are altered so they empower and enable. Such strategies are achieved by being active, involved and committed.

6. Being with service users means being proactive rather than reactive. Care involves three phases of joining: getting to know the person rather than the diagnosis; building and developing skills and resources that the service user can use to recover and adapt; and extending the opportunity for the service user to practise these new skills and to connect with further social supports. (Adapted from McAllister 2007, p. 2)

Trauma-informed models

Trauma-informed approaches to practice are relatively recent, having evolved as a hybrid through work with World War II veterans and victims of domestic violence. There is increasing interest in the effect that trauma has on both children and adults and its relationship with mental health. Consideration of trauma and serious life events adds a new dimension to psycho-social understandings of a presenting problem. This is especially so for people who come to the attention of mental health services, because studies consistently report the incidence of childhood trauma/abuse at between 50 and 80 per cent for this group (Read et al. 2004; see also Chapter 12).

Despite this, it is not routine in mental health services to assess or screen for histories including trauma, or to assess for post-traumatic stress. Many researchers and practitioners are arguing for the need to assess for trauma in every person who presents for help, and to provide specific interventions that are responsive to trauma.

Trauma-informed models of care begin by using trauma assessments that establish whether the trauma is current or historical, what the nature of the trauma was and what the immediate safety needs are. Then all care planning stems from this. Approaches include:

- having one person conduct the assessment/ interviews with the service user
- advance directives (for end-of-life issues), safety plans and de-escalation
- communicating and using preferences
- mapping individual concerns such as possible re-triggers (reactivation)
- being aware that hospitalisation can be re-traumatising
- attending to unit culture (beliefs, values and understandings held by the unit health-care staff)
- organisational commitment to all staff being trained in trauma approaches
- availability of additional expertise as needed
- access to supervision for health-care staff. (Adapted from NETI 2005)

CRITICAL THINKING

- Compare your understanding of the problem-based approach to nursing practice with the six principles of Solution Focused Nursing, keeping your developing understanding of what is important in mental health nursing foremost in your mind.
- Mental health nursing is usually provided from within a multidisciplinary team (a team including other carers such as doctors, psychologists, occupational therapists, etc.). What model of care will suit the whole team?

MENTAL HEALTH NURSING MODEL OF PRACTICE

Nursing theories of any type can be meaningless unless they relate to, or are used to guide and direct, nursing practice. You may have found that the question often arising in your classroom is 'Of what relevance is this information to me when I will be faced with the daily realities of service provision that appear to have little connection to theorising about nursing?' While nursing theory can make no sense without the realities of the clinical setting, it is also true that nursing practice lacks evidence and credibility if it is not analysed and theorised.

The quality of and best practices in nursing care are built first on reflection and theorising about nursing. However, mental health nurses may not always recognise the theory that underlies their practice (Munnukka et al. 2002). Our goal in using theory in practice is to transform the theories discussed briefly in this chapter into nursing actions. For example, if we understand the theories associated with Barker's concepts of 'oceans of experiences ebbing and flowing', and are aware that the service user is the centre of the caring process, then we should be able to understand how a therapeutic relationship using Barker's Tidal Model should develop. We will be able to describe and explore these concepts with our colleagues and service users, and share in understanding the effects of specific actions that are generated from utilising these theories.

Use of theories (nursing and others) will depend on what issues arise in the clinical area (Boyd 2008; Fawcett et al. 2012). For example, Peplau's therapeutic relationship theory will be useful in setting about developing a therapeutic relationship with a new service user, and Barker's Tidal Model theory will be useful when developing a collaborative care plan with your new service user. Other more generic nursing theories, such as Orem's self-care theory and Neuman's systems theory (Meleis 2012), may help the service user to meet their needs and understand their response to stressors by gaining resilience. You may even find Benner's theory of nursing skills and knowledge development (Meleis 2012) useful in helping you to understand your professional growth and development in clinical areas.

A few considerations that might assist you in using theory in practice include the following:

- *Reflection*: Spend time thinking about the goals of the mental health nurse that are unique to each clinical setting and how to link your knowledge of theories to practice.
- *Acknowledgement*: Realise early that mental health nursing is evolving, and that it is sensitive to societal and political changes alongside our increasing understanding of mental illness.
- *Flexibility*: Be open and adaptable, because mental health nursing theories cover a broad range of care perspectives and the clinical area is often full of competing as well as complementary practices.

CONCLUSION

There is a potential for a chapter on theories to leave out much of what might interest you or more fully explain details of particular theories. This chapter has introduced theories of mental illness, nursing theory, conceptual frameworks and models that relate to mental health nursing. Further reading and investigation can provide you with more detail.

CASE STUDY: ORGANISING, IDENTIFYING AND CLARIFYING CARING PRACTICES

A new graduate nurse was about to start in the mental health care team, and Alison was to be a mentor for the first time. What sorts of things might the new graduate nurse need in order to start fitting into the care team?

Much of what the team currently did in terms of mental health care depended on the approach to care it had worked hard on developing. After the close of longer term services in the area, it had taken many months of consultation with service users, carers and clinicians to find a particular flexible model of care that seemed to provide the sort of assistance needed by people in this neighbourhood and health catchment area. The starting point for the development of a model of care was on the person's understanding of what was happening to them, and the very next step taken by this team was on how to use this information to develop a personalised plan of care. Such a plan can take into account the person's unique understandings, and helps to work out where to go and what to do next instead of taking a 'one-size fits all' or a disease-oriented approach. Where possible, the service user is encouraged to participate in the construction and development of their own nursing care plan, and to even take home a copy to assist with recovery.

Critical thinking

- What sort of model of care would you describe here?
- How can Alison sum up this approach of care to the new graduate nurse?

CASE STUDY: LINKING KNOWING AND UNDERSTANDING
Uncle Sam has been admitted to your unit overnight, and you will need to start developing a care plan and strategies including discharge. Uncle Sam has gained this nickname through his many admissions over the past five years during his manic and depressive phases of a bipolar mood disorder. Several stressful events have already occurred as Uncle Sam settles into the unit. It seems that every time Uncle Sam is admitted, he presents with different circumstances and unique issues.

Critical thinking

- How can you best link previous care with current and future strategies?
- What differences between theory and practice are likely to occur with Uncle Sam?

REFERENCES

Barbour, A.B. (1995). *Caring for Patients: a critique of the medical model*. Stanford, CA: Stanford University Press.

Barker, P. (2001). The tidal model: Developing a person centred approach to psychiatric and mental health nursing. *Perspectives in Psychiatric Care*, 37, 79–87.

Barker, P.J. & Buchanan-Barker, P. (2004). *The Tidal Model: a guide for mental health professionals*. Abingdon: Routledge.

—— (2010). The tidal model of mental health recovery and reclamation: application in acute care settings. *Issues in Mental Health Nursing*, 31, 171–80.

Barrett, B., Young, M. S., Teague, G. B., Winarski, J. T., Moore, K. A., & Ochshorn, E. (2010). Recovery orientation of treatment, consumer empowerment, and satisfaction with services: A mediational model. *Psychiatric Rehabilitation Journal*, 34(2), 153–6.

Bennetts, W., Cross, W. & Bloomer, M. (2011). Understanding consumer participation in mental health: issues of power and change. *International Journal of Mental Health Nursing*, 20(3), 155–64.

Birmingham City Council (2012). Website. Viewed 20 February 2013, <www.birmingham.gov.uk>.

Boyd, M.A. (2008). *Psychiatric Nursing: contemporary practice* (4th edn). Philadelphia, PA: Lippincott Williams & Wilkins.

Carlyle, D., Crowe, M. & Deering, D. (2012). Models of care delivery in mental health nursing practice: a mixed method study. *Journal of Psychiatric and Mental Health Nursing*, 19(3), 221–30.

Chinn, P.L. & Kramer, M.K. (2008). *Integrated Theory and Knowledge Development in Nursing* (7th edn). St Louis, MO: Mosby.

Delefosse, M.S. (2011). An embodied-socio-psychological perspective in health psychology? *Social and Personality Psychology Compass* 5(5), 220–30.

Fawcett, B. & Karban, K. (2005). *Contemporary Mental Health: theory, policy and practice*. London: Routledge.

Fawcett, B., Nicholson, S. & Weber, Z. (2012). *International Perspectives on Mental Health: critical issues across the lifespan*. Basingstoke: Palgrave Macmillan.

Fisher, J.E. & Happell, B. (2009). Implications of evidence-based practice for mental health nursing. *International Journal of Mental Health Nursing*, 18, 179–85.

Gray, P. (2005). Beyond the medical model . . . Terry Lynch. *Therapy Today*, 16(10), 33–6.

Hudson, K., Duke, G., Haas, B., & Varnell, G. (2008). Navigating the evidence-based practice maze. Journal of Nursing Management, 16(4), 409–16.

Jacobson, N., & Greenley, D. (2001). What is recovery? A conceptual model and explication. *Psychiatric Services*. 52(4), 482–5.

Kermode, S. (2004). *Foundation Concepts for Holistic Health* (2nd edn). Sydney: Pearson.

LeVine, E. S. (2012). Facilitating recovery for people with serious mental illness employing a psycho-biosocial model of care. *Professional Psychology: Research and Practice*, 43(1), 58–64.

LoBiondo-Wood, G. & Haber, J. (2010). *Nursing Research: methods and critical appraisal for evidence-based practice* (7th edn). St Louis, MO: Mosby.

McAllister, M. (2007). *Solution Focused Nursing: rethinking practice*. Basingstoke: Palgrave Macmillan.

Maslow, A.H. (1970). *Motivation and Personality*. Englewood Cliffs, NJ: Prentice Hall.

Meleis, A.I. (2012). *Theoretical Nursing: development and progress* (5th edn). Philadelphia, PA: Wolters Kluwer Health/Lippincott Williams & Wilkins.

Mohr, W.K. & Tasman, A. (2011). *Fundamentals of Psychiatry*. Oxford: Wiley-Blackwell.

Munnukka, T., Pukuri, T., Linnainmaa, P. & Kilkku, N. (2002). Integration of theory and practice in learning mental health nursing. *Journal of Psychiatric and Mental Health Nursing*, 9, 5–14.

National Executive Training Institute (NETI) (2005). *Training Curriculum for Reduction of Seclusion and Restraint*. Draft curriculum manual. Alexandria, VA: National Association of State Mental Health Program Directors (NASMHPD), National Technical Assistance Center for State Mental Health Planning (NTAC).

Oliver, M. (1997). *The politics of disablement*. London: Palgrave Macmillan.

Pearson, A., Vaughan, B., Fitzgerald, M. (2005). *Nursing Models for Practice* (3rd edn). Edinburgh: Butterworth Heinemann.

Peplau, H.E. (1952). *Interpersonal Relations in Nursing*. New York: G.P. Putnam's Sons.

—— (1954). Utilizing themes in nursing situations. *American Journal of Nursing*, 54(3), 325–8.

—— (1960). Talking with patients. *American Journal of Nursing*, 60(7), 964–6.

—— (1962). Interpersonal techniques: the crux of psychiatric nursing. *American Journal of Nursing*, 62, 50–4.

—— (1964). Basic Principles of Patient Counseling: a conceptual framework of reference for psycho-dynamic nursing. New York: Springer.

—— (1991). *Interpersonal Relations in Nursing*. New York: G.P. Putnam's Sons.

—— (1992). Interpersonal relations: A theoretical framework for application in nursing practice. *Nursing Science Quarterly*, 5, 13–18.

—— (1993). Nursing pioneers: the Peplau legacy (Interview by Phil Barker). *Nursing Times*, 89(11), 48–51.

Ramon, S. & Williams, J.E. (eds) (2005). *Mental Health at the Crossroads: the promise of the psycho-social approach*. Aldershot: Ashgate.

Read, J., Mosher, L. & Bentall, R. (2004). *Models of Madness*. New York: Brunner-Routledge.

Robison, J. (2004). Toward a New Science. *WELCOA's Absolute Advantage Magazine*, 3(7), 2–5.

Rogers, C.R. (1990). *The Carl Rogers Reader* (edited by Howard Kirschenbaum and Valerie Land). London: Constable.

Small, M. F. (2006). *The Culture of our Discontent: beyond the medical model of mental illness*. Washington, DC: Joseph Henry Press.

Song, L. Y., & Shih, C. I. (2009). Factors, process and outcomes of recovery from psychiatric disability: The unity model. *International Journal of Social Psychiatry*, 55(4): 348–60.

Townsend, M.C. (2011), *Psychiatric Mental Health Nursing: concepts of care in evidence-based practice*. Philadelphia, PA: F.A. Davis.

Turner, B.S. (1987). *Medical Power and Social Knowledge*. London: Sage.

Varcarolis, E.M. (2010). *Foundations of Psychiatric Mental Health Nursing*: a clinical approach (6th edn). St Louis, MO: Saunders.

Vincent, C. (2010). *Patient Safety* (2nd edn). Hoboken, NJ: Wiley-Blackwell.

Wilkinson, J.M. & Van Leuven, K. (2007). *Fundamentals of Nursing*. Philadelphia, PA: F.A. Davis

Wimpenny, P. (2002). The meaning of models of nursing to practising nurses. *Journal of Advanced Nursing*, 40(3), 346–54.

3

Recovery

Main points
- Recovery is a process that is defined, owned, and directed by an individual, acknowledging the person's right to be self-determining.
- Learning how the person understands what is happening to them is a fundamental feature of recovery approaches.
- In a recovery approach, 'helpers' support the person as they find their own meaning and purpose, and regain control over their life.
- Recovery approaches incorporate attending to the social conditions necessary for well-being, personal growth and citizenship.
- In Australia, mental health services are in a process of transformation to a recovery orientation.
- Peer-led approaches have a vital role in the range of alternatives available to mental health service users.

Definitions
Self-determination: The right to be in control of one's own life, to act in accordance with one's own aspirations—the concept can be applied both to individuals and groups.

Emancipatory conditions: The external elements or environmental features that are conducive to people being able to exercise self-determination and empowerment such as social, economic and personal supports.

Lived experience: First-hand experience (used here to mean using mental health services and/or experiencing mental health problems at first hand).

Paradigm: A commonly accepted framework containing its own basic assumptions, values and ways of thinking.

Paradigm shift: A dramatic transformation from one way of thinking to another.

INTRODUCTION

Contemporary mental health policy, practice and service orientation are based on the idea that people diagnosed with mental illness can expect to recover. Although the term 'recovery' is now pervasive in mental health, it has a variety of very different meanings and is used in a number of different ways. For now, let's imagine that there are two distinctive branches of knowledge about recovery. Down one path is a medical view of recovery, where it is usual to think of it as equating with anticipated and measurable improvements in an individual's health or functioning following illness—similar to what we would expect with physical illness. In mental health, this way of understanding recovery has been called 'clinical recovery' (Slade 2009) or 'recovery from' (Davidson & Roe 2007). Criteria for 'clinical' recovery generally include symptom remission and social functioning—such as having employment, independent living, activities and friends (Slade 2009). Down the other path is knowledge about recovery generated by people who have themselves experienced mental distress and who have used mental health services (lived experience knowledge). The axiomatic principle differentiating 'lived experience' notions of recovery from the clinical criteria is the idea that recovery is not dependent on or defined by whether or not 'symptoms' are present—symptoms cease to be the defining factor.

In this chapter, we privilege the collective lived experience body of knowledge about recovery. We assume that this emergent body of knowledge provides important concepts and a framework for understanding processes of recovery and the conditions likely to facilitate it. Much of the lived experience knowledge has been articulated through the consumer/survivor movement, so this chapter traces the movement's origins and concerns. Lived experience knowledge has also been generated from diverse narratives about what it is like to experience 'mental illness' at first hand. A selection of 'first-person' narratives and other resources is listed at the end of this chapter.

Underpinning the lived experience framework of recovery is the concept of self-determination: to be in control of one's life and destiny. The framework provides a way of analysing the extent to which social/cultural attitudes, mental health service systems, social and health policies and laws, mental health services systems and mental health practice either enhance or limit self-determination. Adopting this view of recovery necessitates thinking beyond individual well-being to considering the social conditions necessary for healing and personal growth. Once you are familiar with this framework, you will be able to tell whether a work practice, attitude or aspect of a service is really recovery focused by analysing the extent to which it promotes or limits people's dignity and self-determination. You will be able to analyse social attitudes and arrangements by the degree to which they limit or promote citizenship and equality for people experiencing mental health problems. Finally, you will be able to think critically about the extent to which our everyday communities are able to tolerate and celebrate the fullest expression of psychological diversity.

A PARADIGM SHIFT

In his book, *Personal Recovery and Mental Illness* (2009, p. 3), Slade argues that 'the primary goal of mental health services needs to change, from its current focus on treating illness in order to produce clinical recovery, to a new focus on supporting personal recovery by promoting well being'. Adopting a recovery framework presents a radical challenge to traditional ways of understanding and helping with people's experiences of mental distress. For a recovery agenda to be genuine, embedded and enduring, some traditional attitudes, practices and ideologies need to be jettisoned, while past practices and current power structures need to be critiqued (Masterson & Owen 2006). Examples are psychiatry's tradition of holding low expectations about what service users are capable of, assuming they will make unwise decisions and taking over decision-making. Indeed, if professional concerns are oriented primarily to accurate diagnosis, adherence to medication and risk-management, they will be incompatible with a recovery framework (Pilgrim 2008). No service can be called recovery oriented unless it embodies and promotes the attitude that hope, healing, empowerment and connection are possible (Jacobson & Greenley 2001, p. 485). If the development of policy and service delivery is not predicated on lived experience, wisdom and the leadership of service users, recovery orientation cannot be realised.

The transformation to recovery-oriented practices means working with service users in a new way: from being the holder of knowledge and expertise to being a facilitator, helping people discover and achieve their own aspirations:

> recovery is *lived* and *experienced* by individuals, what recovery-orientated services do is provide supports and interventions to facilitate people in recovering. In other words, recovery cannot be done *to* or *for* someone. (Meadows et al. 2012, p. 502)

As a facilitator of recovery, your practice aims to promote people's autonomy and self-management (Turton et al. 2011). This requires privileging the person's self-knowledge—their experiences, needs and choices—over standardised models and forms of clinical care, and broadening ideas about well-being beyond medicalised views (Smith-Merry, Freeman & Sturdy 2011). Rather than only viewing experience of mental distress as an individual medical problem that needs medical intervention, a recovery framework stresses the inherent value and meaning within subjective experience (Glover 2005). If you can maintain an appreciation of and openness to the diversity of language and ideas people use to describe their feelings, thoughts and experiences, this will be an important clinical asset. Because self-determination is at the heart of a recovery framework, your clinical practice ultimately will be directed towards assisting people to regain control of their own lives, arriving at their own choices and decisions in ways that make sense to them.

Table 3.1 Recovery approaches contrasted with traditional medical approaches

Practitioner using recovery orientation	Practitioner using traditional approaches
We see your strengths.	We need to find out what's wrong with you.
You are the holder of expertise.	We are the experts.
We ask you what does and doesn't work.	We know what's wrong with you (diagnosis) and how to help (treatment).
We support you to achieve what you want.	We will encourage realistic goals.
We ask: Is this where you want to be in your life?	We will help maintain/improve your functioning.
We know you are unique.	You have diagnosis x and this is the evidence-based treatment.
We expect that you will take charge of your choices and your life.	We need to protect you from yourself.
We value what your experience of distress means for you.	Mental illness is something you suffer from.
We would like to understand how you regard what's happening to you.	You lack insight into your illness and need psych-education.

CLINICAL RECOVERY: CHALLENGING THE 'PROGNOSIS OF DOOM'

Before exploring lived experience knowledge about recovery, we will take a short detour down the 'clinical recovery road' to bust any remaining myths that to have a diagnosis of a mental illness such as schizophrenia is to have a lifelong disabling and degenerative condition. From a medical perspective, optimism about the prospect of whether or not madness can be 'cured' or whether the 'insane' can recover has waxed and waned. Taking schizophrenia as an example, after psychiatry first became a medical specialty, the expected prognosis was 'incurability' and lifelong degeneration. This belief remained influential in psychiatry until well into the latter decades of the twentieth century, and arguably still has influence. However, empirical research has long since demonstrated that *improvement* is more likely than deterioration in people who are diagnosed with schizophrenia, that it is not a permanent disabling condition, is not all pervasive in a person's life and it is not uniform in course or outcome (Calabrese & Corrigan 2005; Davidson & Roe 2007).

Interestingly, in the late 1960s the World Health Organization (WHO) commissioned a research study on schizophrenia in culturally diverse cohorts of people across nine countries. This study found that the course and outcome of schizophrenia was better for people in developing societies than for those in North America and Europe. The results were so surprising that a second WHO study was conducted using more rigorous criteria; it produced similar findings (Hopper et al. 2007). How could it be that rich countries with sophisticated health-care systems and treatments were doing worse (Calabrese & Corrigan 2005)?

CRITICAL THINKING

What do you think might be reasons for the WHO study results?

So, even if we limit our understanding of recovery in mental health to 'clinical' recovery, longitudinal and cross cultural studies have shown that recovery is the most likely outcome for people diagnosed, for example, with schizophrenia.

EMERGENCE OF THE CONSUMER SURVIVOR MOVEMENT

At roughly the same time that clinical evidence about recovery was emerging which would challenge the 'prognosis of doom' attached to diagnoses of mental illness, people who had been hospitalised as 'mental patients' had begun to speak out about their experiences, often seeing themselves as 'living proof' of recovery—frequently despite, not because of, the treatment they had received (Chamberlin 1990). The consumer/ survivor movement is a global social movement characterised by networks of formal and informal groups at local, national and international levels. There were several influences shaping the movement during the 1960s and 1970s, from which the recovery movement later flowed. The emancipation movements of black civil rights campaigns in the United States were a fundamental influence, spawning many other social movements worldwide as marginalised groups began to fight for their own freedoms, equality and citizenship.

CRITICAL THINKING

Talk to someone who was an adult during the 1960s and early 1970s, or investigate online:

- What major social/political events were occurring in the 1960s and early 1970s? Where?
- What rights movements/protest movements/social movements emerged at this time?
- What ideas lay behind the protest movements of this historical period?

During this period, institutional power was being questioned, and the field of psychiatry was no exception. Interest in alternatives to, and critiques of, psychiatry's role as a form of social control, the integrity of the profession and coercive treatment all came from within psychiatry's own ranks thanks to such figures as David Cooper, R.D. Laing, Thomas Szasz and Roland Littlewood (Crossley 2006). Scholars Michel Foucault and Erving Goffman also turned a critical gaze on institutional psychiatry (Lakeman, McGowan & Walsh 2007). Later, the media would open the door on human rights abuses in mental health services—for example, in the film *One Flew Over the Cuckoo's Nest*.

Mutual self-help

A formative aspect of the consumer/survivor movement was the growth of mutual self-help groups inspired by programs such as Alcoholics Anonymous (Davidson & Roe 2007). The tradition of mutual self-help is underpinned by the idea that working for the recovery of others facilitates personal recovery, and in helping oneself, one helps others (Finn, Bishop & Sparrow 2009). In mutual self-help groups, peer support is given and found among people who have walked a similar path by coming together to share their experiences with one another; knowing that they will be understood, that they are not alone and that it is a safe place to be. Peer support is unique because it draws on tried and true helpful knowledge and techniques that derive from the experiences people have had. It is characterised by reciprocity, and mutual acceptance and respect (Davidson et al, 1999; Clay, 2005; Deegan, 2006).

CRITICAL THINKING

Go to the website of GROW at <www.grow.net.au> for an example of an Australian mutual self-help group grassroots organisation

---

Consciousness-raising

The consumer/survivor movement drew strength and political techniques from other social movements such as 'consciousness-raising' taken up by the women's movement. This political technique began with small groups of women sharing stories about their lives with each other. As they did so, they began to realise that the social order itself subjugated women 'as a group' through assumptions and attitudes about what women should be like and expectations about what they could and couldn't do. Rather than centring on individual stories about how awful it was to be a woman, the focus of consciousness-raising was to begin to realise how legal, economic and social arrangements were often constructed so that they benefited men 'as a group'—often at the expense of women 'as a group'. Freire (1970) calls this type of social arrangement an 'unjust order' or a situation of oppression. Under such conditions, people's 'vocation to be more fully human' is interfered with (1970, p. 56), inevitably resulting in a struggle on the part of the oppressed to pursue the right to be human. Consciousness-raising historically has been instrumental for marginalised social groups because it is a political process that occurs when people's stories of oppression are shared, and it becomes evident that many struggles that seemed personal are in fact structural, and are thus more likely to need political solutions rather than individual solutions.

People who had been individually labelled 'mental patients' started to share experiences of having their freedoms and dignity taken away, being forced to accept treatment, and feeling as though their pain and distress were being ignored. Groups emerged spontaneously and simultaneously in different countries and cities as people began to grow angry about their treatment in hospitals—what they saw as the human rights abuses and treatments that did not help, but rather harmed them. Such groups began to identify needs that had not been met by traditional mental health services, and they began to value the unique knowledge and expertise they shared. In the consumer/survivor movement, people began to understand their experiences collectively through the lens of oppression, and also began to appreciate the social and political significance of those experiences:

> My feelings began to change when I discovered the existence of the Mental Patients' Liberation Project in New York, one of the earliest mental patients' liberation groups. We talked about our experiences and discovered how similar they were. (Chamberlin 1977, p. 67)

People did not want to be discriminated against on the basis of being diagnosed with mental illness. Once shared, what had been an individual experience could be transformed into socio/political analysis: Why were people so afraid of madness? Why did they insist that a hopeful future was not possible? Why did people get locked up when they were mad? Why were they the only people who could be forced to accept medical treatments without consent? Why did nobody seem to want to hear about or understand people's pain and distress? How could social conditions that produced inequality and prejudice be changed? It was the exploration of questions like these that would later form both the basis of a political agenda for the movement and the articulation of a recovery approach in mental health. These groups developed different purposes, from drafting human rights charters, starting up newsletters and organising protests outside mental health hospitals and providing mutual support through 'phone trees', crisis centres and other alternatives to traditional mental health services, to operating small businesses (Chamberlin 1977).

Self-determination

For groups who have experienced oppression, the quest for self-determination is a search for social justice and equality of opportunity. In individual terms, it is the right to be in control of one's own life, to act in accordance with one's own aspirations (Onken et al. 2007). The concept of self-determination is used not only at the level of the individual, but also at the level of the collective—for example, indigenous groups have also used this concept to describe liberation from ruling groups, following histories of colonisation. Groups who identify with this concept tend to have had direct experience of inequality, powerlessness and marginalisation. Not surprisingly, then, a vital aspect of self-determination is speaking up rather than being spoken on behalf of.

CRITICAL THINKING
When and how does your course of study involve a service user perspective?

Many in the consumer/survivor movement had experienced discrimination, and had been treated and hospitalised against their will, so choice, self-determination, human rights and citizenship were central concerns, later becoming foundational principles of recovery. For example, the principle that the individual must be the one who decides what constitutes their own recovery has its roots in self-determination.

INFLUENCE OF THE DISABILITY MOVEMENT

The consumer/survivor movement was highly influenced by the disability movement, and benefited greatly from the political gains and later the intellectual work arising from it. Self-determination is a concept that is fundamental to the disability movement. Activists sought to reframe social views away from a paternalistic, medical, charitable view of people with disabilities towards a rights- and equality-based social agenda (Thomas 1999). The slogan 'nothing about us without us' that was adopted by the consumer/survivor movement reflected the strong desire for political participation and participation in all decisions involving the person. The concept of self-determination gave voice to the idea that all people with disabilities should be in control of their own lives, and have rights and freedoms on an equal basis with others—including the right to live lives free from discrimination. A focus on self-determination places importance on what has to be provided to the individual or group in order to obtain equality of opportunity.

Social analysis

Champions within the consumer/survivor movement, such as Pat Deegan and Judi Chamberlin, saw similarities between the aims of the disability movement and the consumer/survivor movement; the task was to ensure the equality of human, citizenship and social/economic rights of all persons.

CRITICAL THINKING

For further background, take a look at these websites:

- for Deegan's critique of rehabilitation services and her vision of freedom: <www.patdeegan.com/sites/default/files/files/rethinking_rehabilitation.pdf>
- for Chamberlin's speech on citizenship rights and psychiatric disability: <www.power2u.org/articles/empower/citizenship.html>.

Disability activists had already been successful in ensuring legislative reforms to tackle discrimination on the basis of disability. In the United Kingdom, disability groups were successful in shifting the terms of debate about disability from being perceived only as an individual impairment, to being understood as the interplay between a person's individual impairment and their interaction with society (Beresford 2002; Cook & Jonikas 2002). As an example, quadriplegia is an individual impairment, but it only becomes a disability if the specific nature of the impairment is not understood or catered for. For example, public buildings without wheelchair access limit both self-determination and social participation for a person with quadriplegia. Seen in this light, any attitude, institution, set of cultural beliefs, person or thing can be either enabling or disabling, or both.

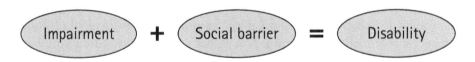

Figure 3.1 The social model of disability

Let's look at what this means for people with psychiatric disabilities by using the example of stereotypical cultural beliefs linking mental illness and dangerousness. This belief can have both individual and structural consequences. At the individual level, it may mean that a person's ordinary expressions of anger are seen as a symptom of illness (pathologising, attitude), limiting the ways in which the person is able to express themselves; or it may mean that others avoid the person out of fear, leading to the person feeling alienated and being isolated (behaviour). At a structural level, taking employment as an example, consequences might include increased discrimination, with employers less ready to hire people with psychiatric disabilities, leading to increased poverty and decreased well-being overall for this group of people. This type of social analysis is made possible only when we stop locating problems purely 'within' individuals.

CRITICAL THINKING

In what ways might having a diagnosis of mental illness be enabling/disabling?

Allies of recovery

By the late 1980s and early 1990s, the consumer/survivor movement had started to refine its messages. Strategically, if optimism about recovery was to replace negative assumptions about what people diagnosed with mental illness were capable of, the movement would need to find allies for its messages and concerns within the establishment. In the United States, the 'rehabilitation' sector proved to be fertile ground for the development and testing of recovery approaches and the promulgation of the idea that people can and do experience periods of crisis and distress while also living enriched and contributing lives.

Recovery was language adopted by consumer/survivors to reposition psychiatry's traditional approaches away from illness-saturated practices stemming from such beliefs as 'diseases' like schizophrenia are degenerative, so practitioners should not instil 'false hopes' in people about their capacities and interests (Mead & Copeland 2000). Recovery formed a platform from which to 'expose and contest a mental health system that disempowers, stigmatizes, constricts choice, and . . . offers no hope' (Masterson & Owen, 2006, p. 29). As a political strategy, there was always a danger that ideas about recovery might become trapped within the confines of the medical model, but the gain was a much greater likelihood of being able to shift the recovery agenda forward and start to influence policy and service delivery in ways that were true to the consumer/survivor movement. Activists argued that self-determination, empowerment, choice and the application of human rights, were fundamental to human well-being and therefore fundamental to recovery.

The narratives of people with lived experience began to be published. Consumer/survivors emphasised the subjective nature of the experience of mental distress—that the experience was different for each person, and that it could be meaningful, providing opportunities for valuable personal growth. These new depictions of recovery did not equate with achieving a prior state of health, or remission of symptoms. William Anthony's statement about what recovery is remains the most widely quoted:

A deeply personal, unique process of changing one's attitudes, values, feelings, goals, skills, and/or roles. It is a way of living a satisfying, hopeful, and contributing life even within the limitations caused by illness. Recovery involves the development of new meaning and purpose in one's life as one grows beyond the catastrophic effects of mental illness. (Anthony 1993, p. 527)

The sustained activism of consumer/survivors and their allies, along with the growing body of literature from people with lived experience of, and their engagement in, collaborative research was influential in the development of National US policy resulting in explicit recognition of recovery from 1999 onwards. By 2003 the US President's New Freedom Commission on Mental Health had recommended the transformation of mental health service systems to a recovery orientation.

It should be understood that while the United States and New Zealand have led the way in transforming service systems to a recovery orientation, and the United Kingdom, Scotland and Ireland are embarking on their journeys, countries such as Australia are just beginning to come to grips with how mental health service systems and practices can be founded on recovery principles—for example, with the recent development of a national framework for recovery practice and the development of the National Mental Health Commission Contributing Life Framework (see <www.mentalhealthcommission. gov.au>).

By now, you might be thinking, 'If recovery is an individual journey, directed by the person, doesn't that mean it can't be translated into practice and practitioners have no part to play?' It is true there is no single agreed-upon utilitarian definition of recovery (Pilgrim 2008). It is a hallmark of the recovery literature coming from service users that no single definition will capture the experience of recovery, for it is as unique as the person and the road to recovery they take. But we can articulate key concepts of a recovery approach. Self-determination, hope, empowerment and personal growth underpin a recovery framework, making it possible to identify service orientation, practices and policies that are consistent with a recovery approach, as well as those that are not.

The next section aligns key aspects of Australian mental health policy and standards with concepts fundamental to a lived experience recovery framework under the sub-headings of personhood, environment, services and practices.

PERSONHOOD

Most English-speaking countries now have mental health policies explicitly referencing recovery (Ramon et al. 2009), with many incorporating variants of Anthony's (1993) definition. Australian Commonwealth government policy defines recovery as:

A personal process of changing one's attitudes, values, feelings, goals, skills and /or roles. It involves the development of new meaning and purpose and a satisfying, hopeful and contributing life as the person grows beyond the effects of psychiatric disability. The process of recovery must be supported by individually identified essential services and resources. (Commonwealth of Australia, 2009 p. 31)

The narratives of people with lived experience are remarkably consistent in describing what is important to recovery. Research reviews of lived experience testimony about recovery show recurring themes such as the importance of hope, regaining autonomy and independence, finding purpose and meaning in life, re-establishing identity, developing self-respect, reconnection with the social world and learning to manage symptoms in one's own way (Ridgway 2001; Jacobson & Greenley 2001; Schrank & Slade 2007; Mead & Copeland 2000). These elements are vitally important to conceptions of recovery because, in many cases, people who have experienced distress and diverse beliefs have also experienced repeated trauma throughout their lives, lost confidence, been pressured into accepting services, treatments and explanations they may not have agreed to, been discouraged from taking risks, and been encouraged to think of themselves as not capable and in need of constant self-monitoring for signs of impending illness.

Hope

For many, hope is the starting point, for without it a future is unimaginable. Hope embraces the idea that change and personal growth are possible: 'hope emerges out of darkness. [It] can grow in nurturing environments that allow one to become rooted and secure.' (Deegan 1996, n.p.) Hope is a belief that others can hold for us when we cannot find it for ourselves. Building on hope comes the belief that regardless of diagnosis, everyone can recover (Masterson & Owen 2006). The metaphor of a journey is frequently used to describe the experience of recovery, in that what matters is not the destination, but rather the many roads taken:

> Recovery is a process, a way of life, an attitude, and a way of approaching the day's challenges. It is not a perfectly linear process. At times our course is erratic and we falter, slide back, regroup and start again . . . (Deegan 1988, p. 15)

Empowerment

Taking responsibility for one's own life, choices and decisions is vital to growth. These qualities are often referred to in the service user literature as 'empowerment'. As a corollary, for many, to hold on to the idea that recovery is about cure 'is an illusion that keeps people passive' (Boevink 2002, p. 3). Other key features of recovery articulated by the consumer/survivor movement include being treated as a person rather than a disease, and speaking for yourself rather than being devalued by others speaking for you (Pilgrim 2008).

Personal growth and meaning

Rather than returning to a prior state, recovery involves change, learning and growth: 'a deep searching and a questioning, a journey through unfamiliar feelings to embrace new concepts and a wider view of oneself' (Champ 1998, p. 59). 'I have learnt far more from my journey through mental illness than it has ever dared to take away from me' (Glover 2005, p. 2). For O'Hagan (2009), recovery is a philosophy that imbues the experience of madness with full human status and provides a pathway for life. Similarly, many narratives emphasise that the experiences people have had are meaningful and instructive, and that to have them dismissed as a product of illness has been unhelpful and alienating (Onken et al. 2002; Adame & Knudson 2008). For many, the role of spirituality in people's lives is also important for the task of finding meaning in their experience and for recovery (Onken et al. 2007).

ENVIRONMENT

Australian mental health policy recognises that recovery is dependent on social and material well-being:

> Access to clinical care needs to be complemented by access to a range of supported accommodation options, stable housing, and community support services focussed on employment, income support, education and social and family support. When one or more of these is not met, the person's recovery and their capacity to live in the community are jeopardised. (Commonwealth of Australia 2009, p. 18)

Personhood is an abstract notion if it does not include the social context within which a person lives. As with disability, it is helpful to think of recovery as occurring in the interaction between the person and their environment (Onken et al. 2007). Environmental factors include material resources such as having affordable, stable and safe housing, access to transport and medical care. Decision-making, choice and self-determination are only possible if there are opportunities for citizenship and membership in community life (Onken et al. 2002). Recovery is enhanced through being connected to one's community. This may be through employment, having a career, enrolling in studies or being involved in mental health advocacy, service or policy development (Onken et al. 2002). Social support and mutually satisfying relationships are important for everyone, but particularly for people who may have become isolated. Having friends, pets, someone to love and be loved by, family, peer support, access to formal services and staff are all important ways for people to connect (Onken et al. 2002). Increasingly, psychiatry is recognising the importance to recovery of the person's social environment and its role in the reclamation of social and personal identity (Topor et al. 2011). Considering each person who comes to the attention of mental health services as someone who loves and lives within their own community, who has a life and aspirations, supports and social networks, offsets the dangers of only seeing a person as ill. The concept of well-being is alternative language for expressing similar ideas:

> Well-being is about intrinsic human resilience, eagerness for growth, mindfulness, self-transcendence, social inclusion, participation and having access to full citizenship. Regardless of having a mental health problem or otherwise, well-being is everyone's goal. (Ning 2010, p. 113)

Social policy
In a broader sense, environment also includes social policy. For example, anti-discrimination law and public awareness campaigns can positively contribute to structural social change and to lessening feelings of shame or experiences of prejudice and discrimination at the individual level. Social inclusion policies can also be helpful in recognising the role that communities can play in valuing diversity and redressing social inequality for vulnerable and disadvantaged populations. Reducing barriers to full citizenship and social participation on the part of people with lived experience is critical to a recovery agenda. Empowering environments help to sustain recovery.

SERVICES
The Australian National Standards for Mental Health Services (NSMHS), by which mental health services are monitored and accredited, are explicit that services have an over-arching aim of 'facilitating sustained recovery' (Commonwealth of Australia 2010, p. 5). Services are required to support and promote recovery values in their policies and practices and to support the resourcefulness, individuality, strengths and abilities, self-determination and autonomy of service users and carers, and the connections people have within their communities. In accordance with the principles of recovery, mental health services need to become person centred rather than institution centred:

> Services in which all service users are prescribed medication, in which the term 'compliance' is used, in which the reasoning bias is present of [sic] attributing improvement to medication and deterioration to the person, and in which contact with and discussion about the service user revolves around medication issues, are not recovery-focussed services. (Slade, Amering & Oades 2008, p. 135)

CRITICAL THINKING
Research Dr Loren Mosher's Soteria project, an experimental alternative to traditional psychiatric care developed in the 1960s, at <www.madinamerica. com/2012/03/the-soteria-project>. What do you make of the results of the Soteria project?

In order to embed recovery approaches within its mental health services, Scotland has implemented a series of technologies designed to place the person at the centre of service delivery and monitor progress through the organisational change process (Smith-Merry, Freeman & Sturdy 2011). The first step was to derive a foundation for the translation of what recovery meant to Scottish service users by collecting their narratives. These were used to establish values and meanings of recovery, including what helped and hindered the local context. The project was widely publicised, and offshoots included a growth in the use of narrative practice and service users being encouraged to write their own narratives. The narrative project has been credited with helping to incorporate and reproduce recovery values as part of institutional knowledge.

In the United Kingdom, the Institute of Psychiatry is taking a different approach, engaged in a five-year research program, REFOCUS, which commenced in 2009. It was designed to investigate how mental health services can best support personal recovery. REFOCUS aims to help build an evidence base for personal recovery and the transformation of services, with the additional aim of informing mental health policy development. Elements of REFOCUS include coaching, goal striving, relationships between service users and providers, strengths, the role of values and stigma (Slade et al. 2011). A key feature of the model is the role that service users play in service delivery and in the associated research.

Strategies are needed to counteract any tendencies of services to drift away from recovery orientation. The international literature shows that peer support has the potential to drive through recovery-focused changes in service delivery (Smith-Merry, Freeman & Sturdy 2011; Repper 2011; Davidson et al. 2012).

Peer roles and service user led alternatives

Commonwealth policy recognises that providers of mental health services include 'consumer and carer consultants, and recovery and peer support workers' (Commonwealth of Australia 2009, p. 22). Formal peer-support roles within specialist and community-managed mental health services—although relatively new in the Australian landscape—are a rapidly growing workforce. Initiatives developed and provided by service users offering support based on the principles of mutual self-help are an essential feature of what should be available to people with lived experience.

In an integrative review, Doughty and Tse (2011) found that outcomes for clients of service user-led programs were just as positive as those for traditional services, notably in the areas of employment, housing and reduced hospitalisations. Additionally, it was found that involving service users in mental health service delivery provides benefits for both worker and the service, but that under-funding continues to limit potential gains.

Peer-developed practices

Australian mental health policy states that: 'In order to provide high quality care, services should consult consumers and carers as to what promotes recovery as well as relying on evidence-based best practice.' (Commonwealth of Australia 2009, p. 24) If practice is to reflect the value that each person's journey is unique, then much more than evidence-based medicine is required. Two examples of widely used peer-developed practices are Wellness Recovery Action Planning (WRAP) and intentional peer support. Peer-led voice hearing groups are discussed in a later section.

WRAP was developed by American service user Mary Ellen Copeland (see <www.mentalhealthrecovery.com>). It can be facilitated just with one individual or in a group. The individual reflects on what strategies they have used to stay well in the past, and creates a recovery plan that includes triggers, how to avoid them, identifying and responding to warning signs and planning for crisis. WRAP has the advantages of maintaining a focus on the person's own resources, and also potentially counter-acting service tendencies to drift away from personalised service delivery towards standardised clinical care.

Intentional peer support (IPS) is a practice developed by service user Shery Mead. It is grounded in the purposes of relational and social change, and uses mutual learning as its underlying value. The approach is a radical departure from other forms of peer support because it retains the value of mutual self-help, in which both parties in the relationship become aware of each other's experiences, values and world-views, and challenge each other to try new things. It is intentional because the relationship is the means through which new ways of seeing, thinking and doing are generated. In contrast, other peer roles are frequently based on role modelling recovery, or 'helping' the other person with their recovery. IPS is underpinned by the practice of learning to ask: 'What happened to you?' Rather than 'What's wrong'? in keeping with trauma-informed approaches.

CRITICAL THINKING
Visit the IPS website at <www.intentionalpeersupport.org>. How might you be able to use some of the IPS practices in working with service users?

INNOVATIVE APPROACHES
Open dialogue
Open dialogue is a form of community treatment originating in western Lapland, Finland. It is an integrated family and network approach aiming to treat people with psychotic symptoms in their own home, and brings together the person's own social network, relying on the involvement of a consistent team throughout contact—hence each team may work across both in-patient and community settings. All staff are given on-the-job training, becoming qualified psychotherapists. Open dialogue aims to promote a therapeutic process that mobilises the family/network's own psychological resources. Treatment meetings use dialogue to find new words and shared language for experiences that previously had no words to describe them. The approach has achieved dramatic success, helping people through extreme states while relying much less on medication and hospitalisation. It has even been suggested that the development of and fidelity to the open dialogue approach over two decades may have positively changed the overall culture of the basic population in relation to psychiatric treatment (Aaltonen, Seikkula & Lehtinen 2011).

Voice hearing
Voice hearing approaches began in the 1980s from the work of psychiatrists Marius Romme and Sandra Escher. Three tenets of the approach are that voice hearing is more prevalent in the population than previously thought; the content of voices is meaningful and often a reaction to life stresses, frequently linked to painful and traumatic experiences that have their origins in childhood; and voice hearing is best considered a dissociative experience and not a psychotic symptom. The principle behind the approach is that it is possible for a person to change the relationship they have with their voices, beginning from a position of acceptance of the voices, rather than denying their existence or seeking to dull or eradicate them. Clinicians are encouraged to begin with the Maastricht interview, designed to 'profile' the voices: When did they begin? How many are there? Do they have names? When did they first appear? What do they say? What tone do they use? How much control does the person have over them? (Corstens, Escher & Romme 2009).

Internationally, voice-hearing self-help groups influenced by the work of Romme and Escher have been established, in which experiences and strategies for dealing with voice hearing are shared. Techniques include listening to music, talking to the voices while holding a mobile phone to counter the social discomfort of appearing to be talking to oneself, meditation, contact with nature, complementary therapies, creative pursuits, brain gym exercises and other physical exercises. You can familiarise yourself with these techniques and the whereabouts of local self-help groups as part of the repertoire of resources you offer to service users. A comprehensive collection of self-help strategies can be found in Tamasin Knight's (2009) book, *Beyond Belief: Alternative ways of working with delusions, obsessions and unusual Experiences*.

RECOVERY PRACTICE AND YOU

While there exist many documents outlining mental health recovery-focused competencies for mental health workers, they do not necessarily elaborate on or make clear what constitutes recovery-focused practice and which competences might best assist people in their recovery (Lakeman 2010). To identify the most valued practices supportive of recovery, Lakeman conducted an online Delphi survey where experts by experience rated the importance of recovery competency statements. The research showed that listening to and respecting the person's viewpoint, conveying a belief that recovery is possible, and recognising, respecting and promoting the person's resources and capacity for recovery were the most highly valued practices.

Connection, disconnection, reconnection

Service users will value authenticity in relationships with you. They want to be recognised as individual people and to be approached with a 'spirit of unknowingness'; they also want you to get to know them as a person rather than be judged according to diagnosis or stereotypes (Shattell, Starr & Thomas 2007). To connect with others is a fundamental human need. However, real connections are mutual: they involve the ability to listen intently and to respond with honesty. Connecting with others involves being open-minded and curious about the other person. Even when a person is in the midst of a crisis or psychological emergency, it is usually possible to make some kind of connection, even if it is non-verbal, such as being a calm, silent presence with that person. Connection can be established through casual conversation—it does not have to be formally 'therapeutic'. There is a 'natural flow' in connection. Our 'gut' often tells us when it is time to disconnect, and we can always reconnect at a later time. Connection is something we offer freely to others, so if the offer is refused, this is not something to be taken personally. The ability to become aware of connection and disconnection in all our relationships is helpful.

Listening

Listening is an important part of connecting with people. Research investigating staff qualities that service users find helpful has shown that they accord great value to having conversations with practitioners where they are listened to and understood (Williams & Tufford 2012; Gilburt, Rose & Slade 2008). When people experience being listened to and understood, they are more likely to feel respected. Listeners who are open, non-judgmental and not patronising are able to develop communication that can lead to a person feeling supported and cared for.

Facilitation

Listening and making a connection with the person come before learning something about what the person is looking for in their contact with you, or their use of the service. In a recovery approach, the role of the practitioner shifts away from being the expert towards being a facilitator of the person's preferences, needs and aspirations. According to Topor and colleagues (2011), the goal should be to help service users face problems they may have, help them to generate their own solutions, and to discover and draw on their own expertise. Significantly, interventions aimed at supporting a person to manage their own life have a more robust evidence base than interventions aimed at reducing illness and its effects (Davidson et al. 2009). Facilitation also requires having good knowledge of services and supports in the community, being able to refer people on and being able to communicate information clearly, sharing your professional knowledge and expertise so that service users can be supported to make choices.

The following three questions are designed as useful 'mindset' prompts that you can use to help guide your thinking around connecting with the person. They are facilitative questions because they implicitly acknowledge and value the person's own expertise, and they do not presume a superior knowledge set over the person's own knowledge.

* What do you call the problem?
* What have you done in the past that has helped?
* Do you have any ideas about what I/we/this place might be able to do/not do that would be helpful? (loosely based on the work of medical anthropologist Arthur Kleinman)

The first question indicates you are aware that there are many ways to explain things; that you are interested in the particular language and ideas that the person uses; and that you do not have an interest in changing how the person understands what is happening for them. The second question demonstrates your belief in the person's capabilities and provides an opportunity for the person to draw on their own expertise. The last question acknowledges that each person has different ideas about what is or is not helpful, and invites the person to make requests.

Sitting with discomfort and uncertainty

Adopting recovery practice means developing the capacity to learn to sit with a degree of discomfort. It might be scary to acknowledge that you don't have all the answers, just as it might be scary to think of the service user as having knowledge and expertise—after all, they are sick, aren't they? What if what the person wants is impossible? What if I feel unsafe? What if I don't know how to help? What if they are in danger? It is important to accept the interplay of these types of feelings and anxieties and to have somewhere/ someone safe to explore them if need be. Should such feelings dictate how we act, there is a risk we may resort to using power over the person, denying both them and ourselves the opportunity to learn something or, horribly, treating the other person as not fully human.

Thinking critically about and reflecting upon what you see and hear around you is an important strategy for being able to analyse practice settings—for example, is people's dignity being upheld, and in what ways? Ask yourself: Is what I'm currently doing enabling this person's own preferences, needs and aspirations, or is it enabling the needs of the service? While in some instances the needs of the service will take precedence, it is important to become aware of the distinction between the two. When the needs of the service seem to be in ascendance, ask yourself why this is happening, whether it is really necessary and what can be done to swing the pendulum back the other way.

Getting support

We all make judgements about others, and we have our own moral positions and preferences. Becoming more aware of these is also very helpful because in knowing ourselves well we are better able to begin the process of getting to know another person. Being able to use the structures around you for support is integral to providing support to others. Preceptorship and clinical supervision are two important strategies for ensuring you have the support you need (see Chapter 15).

In summary, we find it helpful being around people who:

- believe in us, who believe that we will become 'who we are'
- want us to take charge of our lives
- can hold hope for us when we cannot
- want us to have real choices
- want us to make mistakes and take risks
- won't judge us or what we want from life
- won't hold us to an idea of 'normalcy'
- will direct us to helpful resources
- are optimistic about what they can offer
- are transparent about their limits.

THORNY ISSUES

One of the present challenges for recovery practice remains its implementation in legislated contexts. Service users who are involuntarily detained in hospital, or who are being treated involuntarily in the community, face incursions on their human rights because they cannot refuse mandated treatments. Thus the principle of self-determination, which lies at the heart of a recovery approach, is violated.

CRITICAL THINKING
Go to the New South Wales Council for Civil Liberties website at <www.nswccl. org.au/issues/mental_health.php>. Check the most recent figures for numbers of people compulsorily admitted to hospital in New South Wales. Do these figures surprise you? Why/why not?

In mental health, compulsory interventions are often delivered through force. The use of various forms of restraint and the administration of intramuscular injections after being held down and placed in seclusion are examples. Clearly, the consequences of such practices can be doubly negative in that a person's integrity and self-determination is violated and force itself is generally experienced as traumatising on a number of levels. That such experiences might not be regarded as forms of help is understandable. That providers who are engaged in such practices might not feel as though they are helping is also understandable. But these are current realities of working in legislated contexts. While Australian mental health policy is silent about these tensions, they have not been lost on practitioners who work within such constraints, and they are evident in the literature. To promote choice and empowerment on the one hand, but exercise control on the other, places providers in difficult situations (Cleary & Dowling 2009).

The framework for recovery that we have presented in this chapter cannot solve such tensions; however, it can remind us that whenever a person's rights, choices and freedoms are compromised, their self-determination is also compromised, and this is a human loss—regardless of the justification given for it. For example, in instances where a person is thought to be at risk of suicide, absconding or hurting others, acknowledging and counting the costs of any contemplated actions that will limit that person's self-determination and the potential impact of these losses for the person is very important. Similarly, when helping involves limiting another person's choices, rights and freedoms, there need to be safe spaces for practitioners to be able to count costs to themselves. A recovery framework allows us to analyse workplaces: do they provide easily accessed, effective reflective spaces and supports for staff?

Another significant challenge to recovery approaches within this context is the management of risk (Stickley & Wright 2011). Accepting the value that risk-taking is part of how we learn and part of what makes us who we are creates a tension within service cultures that are risk averse:

> Our only hope for accessing internal resources that have been buried by layers of imposed limitations is to be supported in making leaps of faith, redefining who we'd like to become, and taking risks that aren't calculated by someone else. (Mead & Copeland 2000, p. 321)

Again, while not providing all the answers, adopting a recovery framework does allow us to analyse the extent to which service responses foster or impede people's rights to the 'dignity of risk' inherent in self-determination.

Another challenge to recovery in legislated contexts is the dominance of medical frameworks that are based on the identification and treatment of illness. The way assessments are conducted, the types of care plans formulated and the criteria by which outcomes are measured may all emphasise deficits and problems, and will likely have less to do with recovery and more to do with external service obligations. There are also pressures for service users to adopt a medical view of their experiences from the initial receiving of a diagnosis through to the provision of psycho-education. Recovery approaches are not anti-medicine, but they are pro-choice. The recovery framework adopted here would allow us to examine the extent to which a service could tolerate or even celebrate alternative explanatory models, and the extent to which service users were able to make treatment choices.

CRITICAL THINKING
Visit the interactive decision-making guide at <http://decisionaid.ohri.ca/docs/das/ OPDG.pdf>. How might you use this tool in helping facilitate consumer choice?

ROLE OF LEGISLATIVE CHANGE
Mental health laws change periodically as a result of inquiries, changing social attitudes, international covenants and other reforms. Some of the tensions outlined in the above section may be ameliorated by forthcoming legislative reform. Concepts fundamental to recovery look likely to find expression in the new mental health laws of some Australian states and territories—for example, as a result of compliance with the United Nations Convention on the Rights of Persons with Disabilities (CRPD), to which Australia is a signatory. Article 1 of the CRPD states that its purpose is:

> to promote, protect and ensure the full and equal enjoyment of all human rights and fundamental freedoms by all persons with disabilities, and to promote respect for their inherent dignity.

We can see in this language the elevated status of citizenship and the importance of upholding the dignity and human rights of people with psychiatric disabilities, which is congruent with the consumer/survivor approach to recovery.

Supported decision-making
The CRPD also requires signatory states to ensure access for all persons with disabilities to decision-making support. Supported decision-making is an interdependent process recognising the role of friends, families and others in a person's network that may be part of decision-making:

> The premise of supported decision-making, as articulated by the disability community, is that everyone has the right to make their own decisions and to receive whatever support they require to do so. (Office of the Public Advocate, Victoria 2009, p. 9)

This is an important development because in legislated contexts the person has lost the authority to make their own treatment decisions. Supported decision-making takes us beyond the traditional idea that a person either does or does not have the capacity to make a decision, and requires that the person has access to good information and to a range of people who can address questions, which increases the likelihood that the person will be able to make an informed treatment decision. We can look forward to mental health legislation that better supports the self-determination of the person and better upholds their rights to make their own decisions about their life.

Advanced care planning: advance directives

Another useful tool in supporting autonomous choice in legislated contexts is an Advance directive (AD). This is a document that a person creates when they have legal capacity, which specifies treatment and other preferences and comes into effect if the person loses the capacity to make decisions or finds themselves in a situation where they cannot communicate their wishes. They are particularly useful if a person is hospitalised in an emergency. The information can be carried by the person electronically, and the service can keep a version with the person's file. The document may specify which treatments should or should not be administered, as well as setting out arrangements for such things as the care of children, who should be contacted in the event of an emergency, other health conditions the person has and any treatments they are taking for those, who would be welcomed/not welcomed as a visitor, and so on. Scotland's mental health legislation has provision for ADs. Currently in Australia, an AD is not legally binding, but they can be made stronger with the use of an advocate who can assist the service user to ensure that the person's voice and preferences are heard.

CONCLUSION

The project of transforming mental health services to a recovery orientation is an international one, and Australia is only on the cusp of its journey. Over the next several years, we can expect many challenges, and the development of many innovative practices and ways to measure the promise of recovery.

SERVICE USER AUTHORED STORIES AND RESOURCES

Deegan, P. (1996). 'Conspiracy of Hope' keynote presentation at the 1996 Mental Health Services conference, Brisbane. Viewed 20 February 2013, <www.patdeegan.com/pat-deegan/lectures/conspiracy-of-hope>.

Jeffs, S. (2009). *Flying with Paper Wings: reflections on living with madness*. Melbourne: Vulgar Press.

McLean, R. (2003). *Recovered, Not Cured: my journey through schizophrenia*. Sydney: Allen & Unwin.

National Empowerment Center Website (USA) contains a collection of service user-authored stories, articles, poems and many other useful resources. Viewed 20 February 2013, <www.power2u.org>.

Our Consumer Place is a Victorian resource centre run by mental health service users. The website contains service user narratives, websites, clips and other resources. See especially the excellent newsletters containing interviews with international leading lights of the consumer/survivor movement, and lots of homegrown articles/debate. Viewed 20 February 2013, <www.ourconsumerplace.com.au>.

Voices Vic was established in July 2009 to build a network of hearing voices groups across Victoria. It offers training and special events to mental health professionals, carers and voice hearers interested in the approach. Viewed 20 February 2013, <www.prahranmission.org.au/hearing_voices.htm>.

OTHER RESOURCES

The Tidal Model is a nurse-led model of care. Viewed 20 February 2013, <www.tidal-model.com>.

The International Network Toward Alternatives and Recovery (INTAR) believes the prevailing biomedical over-reliance on diagnoses, hospitals and medications has failed to respect the dignity and autonomy of the person in crisis, and that full recovery must be at the centre of ethical care. Viewed 20 February 2013, <http://intar.org>.

The Critical Psychiatry Network (CPN) is a group of practising psychiatrists based in the United Kingdom who share a critical attitude towards orthodox beliefs in psychiatry. There is also an Australian branch of the CPN accessible through the website. Viewed 20 February 2013, <hhttp://www.criticalpsychiatry.co.uk>.

The Intervoice Network is an international network for the training, education and research into hearing voices. Viewed 20 February 2013, <www.intervoiceonline.org>.

Beyond Meds has regularly updated links to blogs and other resources. Viewed 20 February 2013, <http://beyondmeds.com>.

Madness Radio. Viewed 20 February 2013, <www.madnessradio.net>.

Hornstein, G.A. (2009). *Agnes' Jacket: a psychologist's search for the meaning of madness*, Rodale Books, New York.

Romme, M. & Escher, S. (2012). *Psychosis as a Personal Crisis: an experience-based approach*. Abingdon: Routledge.

Romme, M., Escher, S., Dillon, J., Corstens, D. & Morris, M. (2009). *Living with Voices: 50 stories of recovery*, Ross-on-Wye: PCCS Books.

REFERENCES

Aaltonen, J., Seikkula, J. & Lehtinen, K. (2011). The comprehensive open-dialogue approach in Western Lapland: 1. The incidence of non-affective psychosis and prodromal states. *Psychosis: Psychological, Social and Integrative Approaches*, 3(3), 179–91.

Adame R.M. & Knudson, A.L. (2008). Recovery and the good life: how psychiatric survivors are revisioning the healing process. *Journal of Humanistic Psychology*, 48(2), 142–64.

Anthony, W.A. (1993). Recovery from mental illness: the guiding vision of the mental health service system in the 1990s. *Psychosocial Rehabilitation Journal*, 16(4), 11. Viewed 30 November 2012, <http://128.197.26.36/cpr/repository/articles/pdf/anthony1993.pdf>.

Beresford, P. (2002). Thinking about "mental health": towards a social model. *Journal of Mental Health*, 11(6), 581–4.

Boevink, W. (2002). Two sides of recovery. Viewed 30 November 2012, <http://akmhcweb.org/recovery/twosidesofrecovery.htm>.

Calabrese, J. & Corrigan, P. (2005). Beyond dementia praecox: findings from long-term follow-up studies of schizophrenia. In R.O. Ralph & P.W. Corrigan, *Recovery in Mental Illness: broadening our understanding of wellness*, Washington, DC: American Psychiatric Association.

Chamberlin, J. (1977). *On Our Own*, Boston: National Empowerment Centre.

—— (1990). The ex-patients' movement: where we've been and where we're going. *The Journal of Mind and Behaviour*, 11(3), 323–36.

Champ, S. (1998). A most precious thread. *Australia and New Zealand Journal of Mental Health Nursing*, 7, 54–9.

Clay, S. (ed.) (2005). *On Our Own, Together: peer programs for people with mental illness*, Nashville, TN: Vanderbilt University Press.

Cleary, A. & Dowling, M. (2009). Knowledge and attitudes of mental health professionals in Ireland to the concept of recovery in mental health: a questionnaire survey. *Journal of Psychiatric and Mental Health Nursing*, 16(6), 539–45.

Commonwealth of Australia (2009). *National Mental Health Policy 2008*. Viewed 30 November 2012, <www.health.gov.au/internet/main/publishing.nsf/content/532CBE92A8323E03CA25756E001203BF/$File/finpol08.pdf>.

—— (2010), *National Standards for Mental Health Services*. Viewed 30 November 2012, <www.health.gov.au/internet/main/publishing.nsf/content/DA71C0838BA6411BCA2577A0001AAC32/$File/servst10v2.pdf>.

Cook, J.A. & Jonikas, J.A. (2002). Self-determination among mental health consumers/survivors: using lessons from the past to guide the future. *Journal of Disability Policy Studies*, 13(2), 87–95.

Corstens, D., Escher, S. & Romme, M. (2009). Accepting and working with voices: the Maastricht approach. In *Psychosis, Trauma and Dissociation*. New York: John Wiley & Sons, pp. 319–32.

Crossley, N., (2006), *Contesting Psychiatry, Social Movements in Mental Health*, Routledge, New York, USA.

Davidson, L., Bellamy, C., Guy, K. & Miller, R. (2012), Mental Health Policy Paper: peer support among persons with severe mental illnesses—a review of evidence and experience, *World Psychiatry*, 11(2), 123–8.

Davidson, L., Chinman, M., Kloos, B., Weingarten, R., Stayner, D. & Tebes, J.K. (1999). Peer programs for people with mental illness: a review of the evidence. *Clinical Psychological Science and Practice*, 6(2), 165–87.

Davidson, L., Drake, R.E., Schmutte, T., Dinzeo, T. & Andres-Hyman, R. (2009). Oil and water or oil and vinegar? Evidence-based medicine meets recovery. *Community Mental Health Journal*, 45(5), 323–32.

Davidson, L. & Roe, D. (2007). 'Recovery from' and 'recovery in' serious mental illness: one strategy for lessening confusion plaguing recovery. *Journal of Mental Health*, 16(4), 459–70.

Deegan, P.E. (1988). Recovery: the lived experience of rehabilitation. *Psychosocial Rehabilitation Journal*, 11(4), 11–19.

—— (1996). *Recovery and the conspiracy of hope*. Paper presented at: 'There's a Person in Here': The Sixth Annual Mental Health Services Conference of Australia and New Zealand. Brisbane. Viewed 30 November 2012, <www.patdeegan.com/pat-deegan/lectures/conspiracy-of-hope>.

—— (2006). *The Legacy of Peer Support*. Viewed 30 November 2012, <www.patdeegan.com/blog/posts/legacy-peer-support>.

Doughty, C. & Tse, S. (2011). Can consumer-led mental health services be equally effective? An integrative review of CLMH services in high-income countries. *Community Mental Health Journal*, 47(3), 252–66.

Finn, L.D., Bishop, B.J. & Sparrow, N. (2009). Capturing dynamic processes of change in GROW mutual help groups for mental health. *American Journal of Community Psychology*, 44(3–4), 302–15.

Freire, P. (1970). *Pedagogy of the Oppressed*, 30th anniversary edn. New York: Continuum.

Gilburt, H., Rose, D. & Slade, M. (2008). The importance of relationships in mental health care: a qualitative study of service users' experiences of psychiatric hospital admission in the UK. *BMC Health Services Research*, 8: 92–104.

Glover, H. (2005). Recovery-based service delivery: are we ready to transform the words into a paradigm shift? *Australian e-Journal for the Advancement of Mental Health*, 4(3).

Hopper, K., Harrison, G., Janca, A. & Sartorius, N. (2007). Recovery from Schizophrenia: an international perspective. A report from the WHO Collaborative Project, the International Study of Schizophrenia. Oxford: Oxford University Press.

Jacobson, N. & Greenley, D. (2001). What is recovery? A conceptual model and explication, *Psychiatric Services*, 52(4), 482–5.

Knight, Tamasin (2009). *Beyond Belief: Alternative ways of working with delusions, obsessions and unusual experiences*, Berlin: Peter Lehman. Viewed 30 March 2013, <www.peter-lehmann-publishing.com/books/beyond-belief.pdf>.

Lakeman, R. (2010). Mental health recovery competencies for mental health workers: a Delphi study, *Journal of Mental Health*, 19(1), 55–67.

Lakeman, R., McGowan, P. & Walsh, J. (2007). Service users, authority, power and protest: a call for renewed activism, *Mental Health Practice*, 11(4), 12–16.

Masterson, S. & Owen, S. (2006). Mental health service user's social and individual empowerment: using theories of power to elucidate far-reaching strategies. *Journal of Mental Health*, 15(1), 19–34.

Mead, S. & Copeland, M.E. (2000). What recovery means to us: consumers' perspectives, *Community Mental Health Journal*, 36(3), 315–28.

Meadows, G., Farhall, J., Fossey, E., Grigg, M., McDermott, F. & Singh, B. (2012). *Mental Health in Australia* (3rd edn). Melbourne: Oxford University Press.

Ning, L. (2010), Building a 'user driven' mental health system. *Advances in Mental Health*, 9(2), 112–15.

Office of the Public Advocate, Victoria (2009). *Supported decision making: background and discussion paper.* Viewed 30 March 2013, <www.publicadvocate.vic.gov.au/research/132>.

O'Hagan, M. (2009). Recovery for mental health today. Viewed 30 January 2013, <www.maryohagan.com>.

Onken, S., Craig, C.M., Ridgway, P., Ralph, R.O. & Cook, J.A. (2007). An analysis of the definitions and elements of recovery: a review of the literature. *Psychiatric Rehabilitation Journal*, 31(1): 9–22.

Onken, S., Dumont, J.M., Ridgway, P., Dornan, D.H. & Ralph, R.O. (2002). *Mental Health Recovery: What helps and what hinders?* Washington, DC: National Technical Assistance Center for State Mental Health Planning. Viewed 20 February 2013, <www.mhcc.org.au/TICP/research-papers/NASMH-PD-NTAC-2002.pdf>.

Pilgrim, D. (2008). 'Recovery' and current mental health policy. *Chronic Illness*, 4(4), 295–304.

Ramon, S., Shera, W., Healy, B., Lachman, M. & Renouf, N. (2009). The rediscovered concept of recovery in mental illness: a multicountry comparison of policy and practice. *International Journal of Mental Health*, 38(2), 106–26.

Repper, J.T. (2011). A review of the literature on peer support in mental health services. *Journal of Mental Health*, 20(4), 392–411.

Ridgway, P. (2001). Re-storying psychiatric disability: learning from first person recovery narratives. *Psychiatric Rehabilitation Journal*, 24(4), 335–43.

Schrank, B. & Slade, M. (2007). Recovery in psychiatry. *Psychiatric Bulletin*, 31(9), 321–5.

Shattell, M.M., Starr, S.S. & Thomas, S.P. (2007). Take my hand, help me out: mental health service recipients' experience of the therapeutic relationship. *International Journal of Mental Health Nursing*, 16, 274–84.

Slade, M. (2009). *Personal Recovery and Mental Illness.* New York: Cambridge University Press.

Slade, M., Amering, M. & Oades, L. (2008). Recovery: an international perspective. *Epidemiologia e Psichiatria Sociale*, 17(2), 128–37. Viewed 20 November 2012, <http://docs.health.vic.gov.au/docs/doc/Recovery-oriented-practice-literature-review>.

Slade. M., Bird, V., Le Boutillier, C., Williams, J., McCrone, P., Leamy, M. (2011). REFOCUS trial: protocol for a cluster randomised controlled trial of a pro-recovery intervention within community based mental health teams, *BMC Psychiatry*, 11, 185.

Smith-Merry, J., Freeman, R., & Sturdy, S. (2011), Implementing recovery: an analysis of the key technologies in Scotland. *International Journal of Mental Health Systems,* 5(1), 11–22.

Stickley, T. & Wright, N. (2011). The British research evidence for recovery: papers published between 2006 and 2009 (inclusive). Part two: a review of the grey literature including book chapters and policy documents. *Journal of Psychiatric and Mental Health Nursing*, 18(4), 297–307.

Thomas, C., (1999). *Female forms: experiencing and understanding disability*. Open University Press, Buckingham, Philadelphia.

Topor, A., Borg, M., Di Girolamo, S. & Davidson, L. (2011). Not just an individual journey: social aspects of recovery. *International Journal of Social Psychiatry*, 57(1), 90–9.

Turton, P., Demetriou, A., Boland, W., Gillard, S., Kavuma, M., Mezey, G., Mountford, V.I., Turner, K., White, S., Zadeh, E. & Wright, C. (2011). One size fits all: or horses for courses? Recovery-based care in specialist mental health services. *Social Psychiatry & Psychiatric Epidemiology*, 46(2), 127–36.

Williams, C.C. & Tufford, L. (2012). Professional competencies for promoting recovery in mental illness. *Psychiatry: Interpersonal & Biological Processes*, 75(2), 190–201.

4

Mental health practice settings

Main points
- The delivery of a viable mental health service includes collaboration between a variety of disciplines working within a multidisciplinary framework.
- This service delivery involves the multidisciplinary team working in partnership with the service user, families/carers and non-government organisations.
- Nurses in mental health settings need to have an understanding of how policy impacts on practice.
- Mental health practice settings have developed in response to international trends, the lobbying of interest groups, changing ideology and policy.

Definitions
National Mental Health Strategies: A major reform process adopted by all governments beginning in 1992, when the first National Mental Health Strategy was endorsed. The strategy originally contained four documents: a national mental health policy, a national mental health plan, a mental health statement of rights and responsibilities, and a Medicare Agreement.

Mainstreaming: The provision of health services through a wide range of health-care agencies such as general hospitals, general practices and community services. Mental health services are delivered, managed and accessed as a central part of health-care service in the same manner as any other health-care service.

Early intervention: Interventions that target people who display early signs and symptoms of a mental health problem or mental illness, including early identification of people suffering from a first episode of a problem or disorder.

Case manager: A health professional who negotiates, integrates and coordinates the care of the person diagnosed with a mental health condition within health and welfare systems and who assists in coordinating care between government and non-government agencies.

INTRODUCTION

Until recently, the main setting for professional mental health care in Australia was large psychiatric hospitals or asylums. Since the mid-twentieth century, however, most developed countries have adopted policies of deinstitutionalisation, whereby the numbers of such hospitals have been reduced and the locus of care has shifted to community settings and smaller specialised mental health units. The pace of this change has been particularly fast in Australia, with dramatic reductions in the number of long-stay hospital beds and the rapid development of a range of community-based and specialist services. At the same time, a shift has occurred in the relationship between service users and service providers. A much greater emphasis is now placed on social inclusion, recovery and the protection of people's human rights than in the past.

The nature of mental health nursing has also changed, and the term 'psychiatric' is less likely to be used as a signifier for hospitals or in people's job titles. With the closure of the psychiatric hospitals, which typically had their own nursing schools, mental health nursing concepts have been assimilated into comprehensive nursing curricula, and statutory registration of the 'mental health nurse' has now been lost in Australia. Nurses with greatly varying levels of experience and education may work with people experiencing mental health problems. Those with specialist postgraduate qualifications and experience may apply to the Australian College of Mental Health Nurses to be credentialled and use the title 'Credentialled Mental Health Nurse'. Many such nurses work in specialist services. Nurses are often referred to as 'the backbone' of the health system, and this is particularly so within mental health services. In 2009, there were estimated to be over 15 000 nurses working principally in mental health, accounting for over 60 per cent of the professional mental health workforce (Australian Institute of Health and Welfare 2010).

This chapter will explore how government strategy has shaped the ways in which mental health services are delivered in Australia. A brief overview of some of the practice settings in which mental health nurses currently work will be presented. Finally, the impact of service delivery evolution for service users, carers and the health professionals who make up these communities will be discussed.

AUSTRALIAN NATIONAL MENTAL HEALTH STRATEGIES

Health-care policy may be defined as plans, decisions and actions to achieve particular health-care goals by governments, individuals or groups such as non-government organisations. Mental health-care policy in Australia encompasses:

- law—particularly pertaining to mental health, guardianship, privacy and human rights
- how health and welfare services are funded, and by whom
- the role of advocacy and interest groups in state and national planning
- agreements on what information is gathered and how or what outcomes are measured
- national statements, policies and agreements on how particular health issues might be addressed, such as chronic disease or how particular populations—such as children and youth—may best be served.

Figure 4.1, drawn from the National Mental Health Policy (Department of Health and Ageing 2009), illustrates some of the key policy areas, documents and agencies involved in the broad mental health policy environment in Australia. How services have evolved to take the unique form that they do has been a consequence of a combination of factors, such as general international trends relating to human rights and mental health treatment, political pressure, lobbying by particular groups and individuals, and to a lesser extent an analysis of research findings.

Australia was one of the first nations in the world to have a coherent and comprehensive mental health strategy, although this is a recent development. In keeping with international trends, deinstitutionalisation, the rise of community psychiatry and the mainstreaming of mental health services with general health services proceeded in the latter part of the twentieth century. By the mid-1960s, Australia's public mental health system had reached a peak of 30 000 beds, and when the first National Mental Health plan was commenced in 1992, approximately 8000 remained (Department of Health and Ageing 2007). According to the Department of Health and Ageing (2010), few alternative services were developed to replace the role of hospitals in this time. Target areas for the first National Mental Health Strategy in 1993 included the mainstreaming of mental health services, providing targeted services for special-needs groups (e.g. children and older people), early intervention and prevention, and developing partnerships in mental health provision.

In 1993, the Human Rights and Equal Opportunity Commission (HREOC) published a comprehensive and critical report following a national inquiry into mental health services, known as the Burdekin Report (Burdekin 1993). This report became an influential document in the subsequent evolution of mental health service provision in Australia. It achieved three important outcomes:

- People's lived experience of mental illness and 'the mental health system' were regarded for the first time as vitally important determinants of service reform and development.
- There was an increased focus on protecting and preserving people's human rights.
- The public mental health sector was exposed to a substantial and revealing critique.

CRITICAL THINKING
Access the website of the Australian Human Rights Commission (AHRC) at <www.hreoc.gov.au/disability_rights/inquiries/mental.htm> and read some of the report findings described in this chapter and transcripts of speeches. What appear to remain the main challenges in promoting people's human rights and what solutions do commentators recommend?

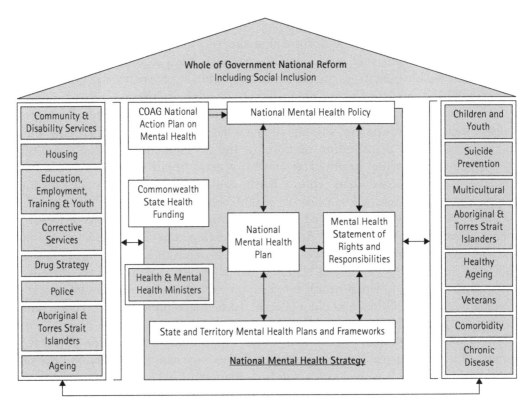

Figure 4.1 Mental health and the broader policy environment

Source: Reproduced from Department of Health and Ageing (2008).

In 2006, the Council of Australian Governments (COAG) responded to a series of reviews and inquiries on the response of government to mental illness in Australia and the success of the reforms to date. From this important forum, an agreement for a new national approach (action plan) for mental health was forged. The National Action Plan (COAG 2006) incorporated all Commonwealth, state and territory governments as well as non-government and private sectors. It aimed to support people in the management of mental illness by integrating services for service users, carers and families, focusing particularly on early intervention, improving access to services, improving the coordination of services and improving employment and social outcomes for service users. Importantly, this action plan was also accompanied by 'ring-fenced' resources for new initiatives. Spending amounted to over $5.6 billion by 2011 (COAG 2012). As illustrated in Figure 4.2, various indicators have been chosen in order to track progress in these areas.

In 2008, the National Mental Health Policy was formulated (Department of Health and Ageing 2008). It aimed to:

- promote the mental health and well-being of the Australian community and, where possible, prevent the development of mental health problems and mental illness
- reduce the impact of mental health problems and mental illness, including the effects of stigma on individuals, families and the community
- promote recovery from mental health problems and mental illness
- assure the rights of people with mental health problems and mental illness, and enable them to participate meaningfully in society.

This document expressed a vision of mental health services that enables recovery, prevents and detects mental health problems early and ensures access to effective and appropriate treatment to enable people to participate fully in community life.

Between 1993 and 2008, a series of National Mental Health Strategies were released as the Commonwealth government sought to guide state and territory mental health systems through the period of post-institutionalisation. Within the strategies, all state and territory governments remain responsible for financing, delivering and managing hospital and community-based mental health services. Some funding responsibilities remain at the Commonwealth level, however—for example, the Medical Benefits Scheme and Pharmaceutical Benefits Scheme, aged care services and returned services through the Department for Veterans' Affairs. Programs such as social security and disability benefits, community-support services, workforce training, re-entry and participation services, and housing services remain in the Commonwealth domain.

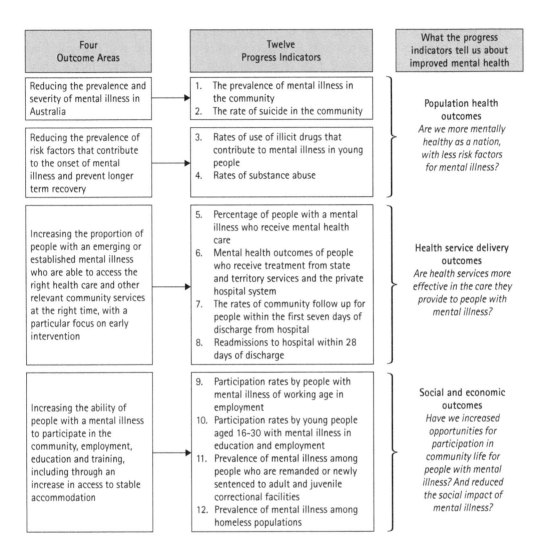

Figure 4.2 COAG Action Plan outcome areas and progress indicators

Source: COAG (2012, p. 14).

CRITICAL THINKING

Access the website of the Mental Health Council of Australia (National) at <www.mhca.org.au> and outline its key strategic breakthrough issues. How do these aims compare with the target areas of the National Mental Health Strategies above?

HOSPITAL–BASED CARE AND MAINSTREAMING

The biggest change resulting from the first national mental health strategy was the reduction of institutionally based mental health services and the development of 'mainstreamed' services. Essentially, it meant a change from the large institutions or psychiatric hospitals to a mixed health service combining general hospital services with in-patient acute mental health and community treatment and support services.

By 2008–09, there remained only 2069 beds in sixteen public psychiatric hospitals in Australia. However, a further 4527 beds were available in psychiatric units attached to general hospitals and 50 private hospitals provided a further 1844 beds (Australian Institute of Health and Welfare 2010). The relocation of acute in-patient services into general hospitals was also accompanied by a decrease in the number of days that service users typically spent in acute care services. However, shorter hospital stays such as a maximum of seven to ten days in acute care services are a worldwide phenomenon (Swadi & Bobier 2005), rather than simply being the result of the Australian government's strategies over the past few decades. The notion of providing care in the 'least restrictive environment', and changes to community care practices, are possibly the most important leading causes of shorter lengths of stay in acute care services.

Nevertheless, considerable resources continue to be invested in in-patient services. These provided care for over two million patient days in 2009–10 and in-patient services employed nearly 13 900 full-time equivalent staff, most of whom were nurses (Australian Institute of Health and Welfare 2010). Depressive episodes and schizophrenia are the most common diagnosis on discharge from specialised in-patient services, and nearly one-third of people are admitted involuntarily (Australian Institute of Health and Welfare 2010). People exhibiting signs of psychosis and those who may be deemed to pose a risk to themselves or others are most likely to be admitted to public hospitals. However, nurses working in acute mental health units are likely to encounter people with a range of mental health and social problems, and they require highly developed skills to work with people in crisis and with multiple and complex psycho-social problems. Nurses tend to be the only occupational group to have a continuous presence over 24 hours, and they play pivotal leadership roles in the running of in-patient units.

Australia also has private hospitals funded by individual contributions or private insurance schemes. The characteristics of people admitted to these hospitals are likely to be different from those admitted to the public system. Almost all people are admitted voluntarily, and fewer people with psychosis are likely to be admitted. A number of private hospitals also conduct out-patient services, and have specialist units catering for people with special needs such as those with eating disorders and drug and alcohol related problems.

While there are fewer 'long-stay' beds, states do continue to fund specialised mental health care, on an overnight basis, in a domestic-like environment. Residential mental health services may include rehabilitation, treatment or extended care. In 2009–10, there were nearly 4000 episodes of care, with most people staying for less than two weeks (Australian Institute of Health and Welfare 2010). Most people were diagnosed with a psychotic illness. Only a small number of people (fewer than 5 per cent) stay in specialist residential services for more than a year. Today, many more people are supported living in their home by non-government organisations (NGOs). These are organisations that are contracted by government departments or that win competitive bids to provide particular services such as employment assistance, recreational, 'lifestyle support' or residential services. People with an intellectual disability make up the majority of those who live in government-funded residential homes. However, many more people receive various levels and types of other disability support.

A positive consequence of the moving of acute in-patient services closer to the general hospital, often under shared governance structures, is the close proximity to medical care, monitoring, assessment, diagnostic services and medical treatment. This has contributed to a reduction in stigma associated with psychiatric hospitals and mental health services in general. Public anti-stigma campaigns, substantial investments in primary care and public health campaigns encouraging people to seek help for mental health problems are likely to have contributed to a shift in public attitudes towards mental illness. However, this might have also contributed to the medicalisation of many social problems not previously thought to be mental health problems, and ongoing tensions about who should be served by in-patient or specialist mental health services with their limited resources.

THE EMERGENCY DEPARTMENT AND CONSULTATION–LIAISON

For many people seeking mental health-related services, the general hospital emergency department is their initial point of contact with the care system. In 2008–09, there were around 172 000 emergency department occasions of service in which the principal diagnosis was mental health-related (Australian Institute of Health and Welfare 2010), and this greatly understates the number of people seeking help with mental health problems. Policies of deinstitutionalisation and mainstreaming have contributed to what has been estimated in some regions to be up to a tenfold increase in emergency department attendance (Kalucy, Thomas & King 2005).

Many hospitals have responded by locating specialist mental health staff in, or easily accessible to, emergency departments. While 80 per cent of emergency department mental health-related occasions of service were considered urgent, 60 per cent were resolved without the need for admission or referral (Australian Institute of Health and Welfare 2010). A mental health specialist is able to provide direct services and advice to service users, consultation or advice to other staff and streamline referrals or pathways to other services.

The concept of consultation–liaison teams or individual specialists providing consultation to colleagues in emergency departments or other branches of the health service has evolved into a common form of service provision over the last two decades. This is due to the recognition that problems with mental health often accompany, and greatly complicate, the care and treatment associated with many physical health problems. Sharrock et al. (2008) undertook a survey of consultation–liaison nurses and found that people worked across diverse settings providing advice or interventions when requested, but particularly in relation to people presenting with deliberate self-harm. Many were based solely in emergency departments, and utilised a crisis-intervention model of intervention.

Consultation–liaison services are often a feature of state-funded district health services and, like some other services, are generally developed in response to local need as state-funded health services have a degree of flexibility in the way allocated funds are spent. Thus some districts employ nurses or other specialist staff in court liaison roles, to assist people who might need to appear before courts and provide advice to judges and other court officers. Other specialist services such as those for older adults, children and youth, and forensic services, may provide primarily consultation, advice and referral services to professionals in other branches of the health service, or even specialist mental health services. More detailed information about consultation–liaison mental health nursing is provided in Chapter 16.

COMMUNITY MENTAL HEALTH

Most district mental health services in Australia provide a range of non-residential services, and the breadth of services provided has increased in line with policy trends. In 2009–10, some 6.5 million community mental health service contacts were reported for approximately 339 000 people (Australian Institute of Health and Welfare 2010). The traditional and still popular form of service delivery is for outpatient appointments, whereby people visit with a medical doctor, nurse or allied health professional at a community health facility. What are known as 'community mental health services' typically offer many other services, including crisis intervention, case management, day hospital, early intervention and psychotherapy services.

The dominant way of coordinating care by community mental health teams is via a system called case management. This involves problem-solving and coordinating services for a person to ensure continuity of services and to overcome system rigidity, fragmentation of services, misuse of facilities and inaccessibility. In practice, this translates to a nominated health professional (usually a nurse or allied health professional) being identified as the 'case manager' for an individual, and working with them in identifying needs, planning, coordinating the services provided by multiple agencies, and directly delivering and evaluating interventions. There are different forms of case management, which vary in the extent which the case manager provides linkage, brokerage, advocacy and service delivery functions.

Kantor and Miller (1988, quoted in Rosen & Teesson 2001, p. 732) describe different kinds of case-management models using the analogy of travel assistance:

- the travel agent model—where the professional just sits behind a desk offering advice
- the travel companion model—where someone goes with you but without any special expertise or training
- the travel guide model—where a person will not only be there and do things with you (rather than doing things to you), but also has appropriate training, experience and expertise to know the most scenic routes, how to take short-cuts without getting lost, how to reliably avoid the pitfalls, and how to arrive reliably at the desired destination.

In relation to the majority of people with mental health problems, the travel agent model of case management is probably sufficient, entailing the identification of needs and brokering of services based on that assessment. This approach is rarely helpful for people with the most complex needs, for whom more services by more people don't necessarily improve outcomes. In the late 1970s, a form of intensive case management was developed in the United States in order to better assist people discharged from long-term care. This model evolved into what is now known as Assertive Community Treatment (ACT) or Intensive Case Management (ICM). These are forms of case management that are carefully targeted to groups with particularly complex needs, in which specialist support services are largely provided by small teams of flexible, expert practitioners, largely in the person's environment rather than hospitals or mental health centres.

Hoult and colleagues (1981) are credited with being responsible for introducing a variation of ACT to Australia, and demonstrating the feasibility of providing assertive treatment by mobile community teams with the back-up of crisis services as a viable alternative to in-patient care without significantly increasing caregiver burden. There is strong evidence for the efficacy, effectiveness and cost-effectiveness of case management in psychiatry, particularly when it conforms to assertive community treatment models (Rosen & Teesson 2001). Many substantial reviews of ACT have been undertaken. The most recent Cochrane Review (Marshall & Lockwood 2000) concluded that, compared with standard community care, people allocated to ACT are more likely to remain in contact with services, less likely to be admitted to hospital and, when admitted, will spend less time in hospital. They are also more likely to be living independently, more likely to have found employment and more likely to be satisfied with the service they receive. A more recent review (1995–2005) suggests that:

> Assertive types of case management (including assertive community treatment and intensive case management) are more effective than standard case management in reducing total number of days spent in hospital, improving engagement, compliance, independent living and patient satisfaction. (Smith & Newton 2007, p. 2)

Today, most community mental health services offer a general case-management service for those people with complex needs, or those deemed to be at risk if not followed up. As illustrated in Figure 4.3, not everyone will benefit from intensive forms of case management. Assertive Community Treatment seems to work best when targeted at people who are heavy service users (Burns et al. 2007), and those with lower levels of complexity may only need to be linked to appropriate services. Teams that provide the more intensive forms of case management tend to focus on particular groups such as people who are in acute crisis (acute care teams), or they may target groups such as homeless people, intravenous drug users, people with forensic issues, those recently discharged from hospital or those considered actual or potential 'heavy service users'.

PRIMARY CARE

The National Mental Health and Well-being Survey (ABS 2007) estimates that 45 per cent of Australians aged between sixteen and 85 will have a mental disorder at some point in their lives, and one in five people will meet the criteria for a diagnosis of a mental disorder during any twelve-month period. Anxiety and mood disorders are by far the most prevalent and the majority of people receive assistance (if at all) in primary

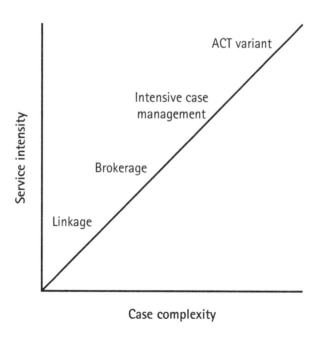

Figure 4.3 The form of case management most likely to be effective as a function of service intensity and case complexity

care. For example, of those people who met the criteria for an affective disorder, only 45 per cent used services to address their mental health and 80 per cent of these people saw a general practitioner.

How services are funded (among other issues) will ultimately affect which services are accessed. In Australia, the Medical Benefits Scheme (MBS) provides payment to medical doctors and some other professionals for particular interventions or services. A referral by a general practitioner is generally required to access other allied health services (which may also attract a rebate). As part of a package of reforms in 2006, COAG committed $507 million over five years to a program called 'Better Access', which enabled psychologists (and some social workers and occupational therapists) to receive MBS payments in order to see service users for up to twelve sessions in a year for 'evidence-based focused psychological strategies'. Such strategies target those people with high prevalence problems and have had some success in encouraging health professionals to deliver mental health services in rural areas (Bassilios et al. 2010, p. 999).

For those with the most complex needs, a finite number of sessions and focused interventions may not be optimally helpful. In 2007, the Mental Health Incentive Program was commenced, which provided incentives for general practitioners, Aboriginal health services and private psychiatrists to engage credentialled mental health services to work with people with complex mental health needs. This enabled mental health nurses to work with service users outside of state-funded health services. The employment relationships that nurses have had and the kind of work they have undertaken under this program have varied greatly, but it has at least provided a means by which nurses could be employed in primary-care settings. It has also provided service users with an alternative to the state-funded mental health services and a way for people to access longer term psychotherapy. An evaluation of the program suggests that the MHNIP has contributed to reductions in length of hospital stays and use of other services for at least some service users (Health Management Advisers 2012)

Good primary care is essential for people with mental health-related problems, as the majority of people with mental health problems also have physical health problems (ABS 2007). Over 1.8 million MBS-subsidised mental health service episodes were provided by general practitioners in 2009–10. The Australian Institute of Health and Welfare collates data on mental health-related services provided in Australia (see <http://mhsa.aihw.gov.au/services>), and this provides a snapshot of the kinds of services provided relating to mental health. In 2009–10, an estimated 11.45 per cent of GP encounters were mental health-related, with depression being the most common problem and medication prescription, supply or recommendation being the most common interventions. A mostly medication approach to depression (and indeed most mental health problems) is not in keeping with contemporary evidence-based guidelines, and considerable investment has been committed to increasing the skill of those in general practice at responding to common mental health problems and referring to others as appropriate. In recognition of the important role that GPs have in the care of the majority of people who present with mental health issues, many state-funded health services employ nurses in GP liaison roles in order to streamline care pathways and ensure a smooth transition between different service types.

CASE STUDY

Nicole has had several previous admissions to the acute care mental health unit, even though she is only nineteen years old. When at home with her parents and brothers, Nicole longed desperately for a place of her own. There was always some drama happening at home, someone fighting, yelling and unhappy. At her last discharge, Nicole remembered the promises made about trying to stay happy and trying to focus on her own well-being, but here she was again in acute care. The unit was fast becoming her second home and she could not help but be unhappy when she realised this.

Critical thinking

• How would you go about assisting Nicole with her current situation?
• What services do you think might be of help to Nicole?
• How many of these services are in your local area and how do people access them?

SPECIAL-NEEDS GROUPS

Special-needs groups are those who may have specific mental health needs, be at particular kinds of risk or have difficulty with access to services. Groups that have been recognised in public policy at various times as needing special consideration include:

• people in custody
• refugees and asylum seekers in detention
• veterans of war and their families
• older adults
• children and young adults
• Indigenous people
• people living in rural and remote areas
• people from culturally and linguistically diverse (CALD) backgrounds
• gay, lesbian, bisexual and trans-gender people.

Within these groups, there is a need to develop and maintain collaboration and partnerships. This is particularly important for people in rural and remote areas, and people from CALD backgrounds. Mental health nurses need to be able to work within a variety of diverse areas with special-needs groups, and also need to undertake qualifications and training in specialist areas of work.

For some groups, traditional or existing models of service delivery have been recognised as ineffective or inefficient. Concerted lobbying by individuals or groups has sometimes also served to crystallise political attention or interest on the needs of these groups. In Australia, the needs of youth (aged roughly twelve to 25) are one such example of how services have evolved due to political lobbying, as well as a consequence of sound argument and research. Child and youth mental health services generally offer a specialist service to people under the age of eighteen in line with the medical specialty of paediatrics. McGorry and colleagues (2007) have argued successfully that the needs of children are quite different from the needs of youth and that the prevalence of mental health problems are greater in adolescence and young adults than any other age group. Indeed, 75 per cent of major mental disorders develop before the age of 25 (Scott et al. 2009). If young people are provided with the scaffolding or support to negotiate young adulthood and address mental health problems then, this ought to lead to substantial savings in the future. They argue for improving community capacity to deal with mental health problems in young people through a range of initiatives, enhancing primary care services for youth and improving specialist youth-specific services (which they describe as the weakest link in the public mental health system). Consequently, Australia has committed large amounts of resources towards youth mental health initiatives.

Headspace is an example of a youth-specific mental health service. Over 40 of these organisations have been opened to date. Their day-to-day operation is funded through MBS and the aforementioned schemes. Headspaces typically employ a range of allied health professions, and they have less emphasis on diagnosis and more focus on problem-solving, support and reducing any impact or decline associated with mental health problems. Scott and colleagues (2009) do caution that the way these services fund their day-to-day operations seriously constrains genuinely innovative and collaborative care. For example, a freeze in the growth of the mental health nurse incentive program meant that no new Headspaces were able to employ nurses in this capacity since 2012. Further information can be found at <www.headspace.org.au>.

EARLY INTERVENTION AND PREVENTION

In Australia, the evolution of early intervention services has been driven by a combination of research, evidence and theory about the course of mental illness, concern about the sometimes traumatic impact of people's first encounter with the mental health system when in crisis, and lobbying by key figures in the industry. There have been a number of policies that incorporated the principle of early intervention. These included the National Mental Health Policy, the National Action Plan for Promotion, Prevention and Early Intervention for Mental Health, and Partners in Prevention—Mental Health and General Practice 2004.

Globally, the World Health Organization's (WHO) Department of Mental Health and Substance Abuse report on the prevention of mental disorders (WHO 2004) states that prevention is one of the most effective ways to reduce the negative impact of mental illness and improve population health. Key messages from this report include the following:

- Prevention of mental disorders is a public health priority.
- Prevention needs to be a multi-pronged effort.
- Effective prevention can reduce the risk of mental disorders.
- An evidence base is needed.
- Dissemination of effective programs should be widely available.
- Prevention needs to be culturally sensitive.
- Sufficient human and financial resources are necessary.
- Effective prevention needs inter-sectoral links.
- Prevention incorporates the protection of human rights. (WHO 2004)

Headspace provides one means of delivering interventions early. A number of early intervention and prevention programs have targeted early psychoses. One of the earliest and most well investigated in Australia was called EPPIC—the Early Psychosis and Prevention Intervention Centre. The EPPIC program was developed by McGorry and colleagues (McGorry et al. 1996), and aimed at reducing delays in access to treatment for young people with early psychosis. A range of interventions are thought to help prevent a major decline in a person's biological, social and psychological state that may occur after a psychotic episode in a young person's formative years (Barry & Jenkins 2007).

The EPPIC program consists of a comprehensive assessment of the individual; acute care in community and in-patient care; education concerning the person's illness (psycho-education); psychological interventions; substance use assessment; family work and carers' support and education; relapse prevention; and social, functional, education/vocational assessments and interventions. Relatively positive social and occupational outcomes have been reported for people who experienced a first episode of psychosis and were part of the program (Henry et al. 2010). Some form of early intervention program is provided by many health services in Australia, often in partnership with non-government organisations. These, and intensive responses to those with emerging problems or acute crisis, are hoped to reduce disruption to the person's life, family and networks, work and schooling, and ultimately reduce the need for hospitalisation or high doses of medication, as well as the risk of relapse. Further information can be found at <www.eppic.org.au>.

CRITICAL THINKING
Access the Headspace website at <www.headspace.org.au> and the selection of evidence summaries about what works in helping young people. The development of early intervention initiatives has been criticised in the past because of the perceived emphasis on identifying early signs of illness and initiating medication in order to prevent a worsening of illness. What do the evidence summaries say about how problems ought to be approached? What are suggested as the critical ingredients to successfully engage young people and support them in achieving positive mental health?

NEW WAYS OF ACCESSING CARE AND TREATMENT

Australia is a relatively sparsely populated country, with most of the population concentrated in or near the state capitals and the remainder dispersed across large distances in regional and remote areas. This creates challenges with regard to how to provide equitable access to services and care. It has long been recognised that the general health of people living in rural and remote communities in Australia is poorer than that of their city counterparts (Mathers 1994). This is due to a number of factors, including lack of appropriate services, distance from services, transport problems and fear of stigma associated with using mental health services. Strategies to date have also often looked at mental health in isolation from other important determinants of health. For example, the apparent poor mental health status of many Aboriginal people living in remote communities can only be understood by considering the broader issues relating to culture, identity, isolation and the impact of successive policies that have led people to become disempowered.

In 1997, the National Rural Health Alliance identified a series of strategies for working in rural and remote communities. Effective strategies relevant to community services workers who may be involved in implementing mental health promotion, prevention and early intervention include:

• local ownership and development of programs
• communication in a language and medium that the community understands
• goals that are developed with genuine consultation with the community
• programs that are based on fostering the capacity of the community to promote their own mental health
• supporting rural communities to enhance their sense of control. (Commonwealth Department of Health and Aged Care 2000, p. 91)

Other features of effective mental health promotion, prevention and early intervention strategies that could be implemented in rural and remote communities include:

• developing a sense of safety, connection and belonging

- providing emotional support, including through networks that support individuals and families
- providing a sense of control over decision-making
- building social capital in the communities, including through addressing economic, employment and education issues.

Enhancing the capacity of communities to identify and respond to their own needs is also fundamental to strengthening the capacity of rural and remote communities to be resilient to adversity (Commonwealth Department of Health and Aged Care 2000, p. 40).

Australia has led the world in the development of telemedicine to help with service provision due to the isolation of health workers, the lack of facilities close to hand and the expansion and advancement of technology. The potential use of telemedicine to improve access to rural and remote mental health care is also becoming more apparent (Lessing & Blignault 2001; McGinty et al. 2006). Videoconferencing has also been advantageous for improving family connections and professional activities for staff, including peer support, education and clinical supervision (Lessing & Blignault 2001).

The internet has shown promise as a conduit for accessing high-quality and helpful services. Indeed, for many people the internet will be the first place they look for information and help for a range of health problems, and increasingly people are able to find help. Internet-based psychotherapeutic interventions, particularly for high-prevalence problems, appear to be as helpful in reducing symptoms as face-to-face contact (Barak et al. 2008). Internet and other computerised treatments hold promise as potentially evidence-based treatments, but probably are best when augmented by the support of a skilled health professional (Andersson & Cuijpers 2009). The use of these internet-based programs is seen as useful for people in remote and rural areas, where there is a culture of independence and self-reliance, and where people want to use health care that they can access in their own time with some degree of autonomy (Griffiths & Christensen 2007). Increasingly, mental health service providers can expect to interact with service users via the internet and through online programs for particular problems.

CRITICAL THINKING

Identify and undertake an internet search on a mental health issue or problem. Consider how you might judge whether or not the information is accurate or from an authoritative source. Access the Beyond Blue website at <www.beyond blue.org.au> and review the information provided on the health problem.

You may also access the MoodGYM training program conducted by the Australian National University, which is an internet-based therapy program intended as a prevention program for depression. This site is also a good way to gain an understanding of and insight into Cognitive Behavioural Therapy. The MoodGYM website may be accessed directly at <www.moodgym.anu.edu.au>.

TRENDS IN SERVICE PROVISION

Mental health policy and strategy have been influenced by shifts and changes in ideology over the years. Mental health recovery, the development of self-help and international networks concerned with promoting mental health have accelerated the pace of change (see Chapter 3 for a discussion of mental health recovery). Demographic trends in the Australian population also mean that some practice areas will become increasingly important over time. For example, a consequence of the increased life expectancy of Australians is the need to provide for the mental health needs of older adults, and to provide specialist services for those people who develop dementia and other mental health problems associated with ageing. Australia has also seen a large rise in so called 'lifestyle diseases' associated with obesity and sedentary lifestyle, which inevitably contribute to mental health problems and complicate care and treatment for people with mental health problems.

There is a growing recognition of the intersection between adverse childhood experience, substance abuse, mental health and social problems (Breckenridge, Salter & Shaw 2012). The increased threshold to access or receive ongoing support from health and social services has meant that some people have 'fallen through the cracks', and people with mental health problems are often over-represented in other disadvantaged groups (such as homeless people) or present with highly complex needs.

Forensic mental health settings

While there has long been an interface between mental health and criminal justice systems, increasingly mental health services—at least at a regional level—offer a range of forensic services. In Australia, the most common understanding of forensic mental health practice is the assessment and treatment of people diagnosed with mental illness who have come into contact with the criminal justice system. Specialist forensic mental health nurses may practise in a range of adult settings, including police custody centres, prisons, courts, secure hospitals and the community, as well as juvenile justice settings. The nurse may be employed by a specialised forensic service or may be employed by a mainstream service such as a state Health Department.

The definition of a forensic service user is one who:

- has been found by a court of law to be unfit to be tried for a criminal offence, and is detained in a hospital, prison or other place
- is detained in a hospital after being transferred there from a prison
- has been found not guilty by a court of law because of mental illness.

Nurses require knowledge and skills that are additional to the basic mental health nursing preparation when working with people who have committed a criminal offence and have mental health problems. The forensic mental health nurse aims to understand the social, political, legal, ethical and practice context of care for this group of people, and integrates security into specific assessment and intervention skills to meet the therapeutic needs of clients. In general, the skills required include:

- effective skills, interest and experience in multidisciplinary health team work
- excellent communication skills, including verbal and written reporting
- an ongoing commitment to self-learning and development
- the ability to manage emergency situations and be competent in conducting health assessments
- the ability to work independently and in a team
- the ability to advocate for the mental health needs of people diagnosed with a mental illness in criminal justice environments.

Mental health nurses and multidisciplinary forensic teams work closely with other services to attempt to negotiate treatment, the provision of basic needs and the requirements of the criminal justice system for people who are involved in both systems. This is just one example of a need to work in partnership in a highly collaborative, interdependent way with a range of services.

Collaborative care / 'joined-up' service delivery

A significant change to mental health-care delivery, which began in the first National Mental Health Strategy and has continued throughout each National Mental Health Strategy, is partnerships within service development, delivery and reform. This refers to the goal of achieving a coordinated system of care incorporating the needs of service users, carers and service delivery personnel. It includes the development, improvement and establishment of strategic alliances in:

- networks
- other departments such as social services, housing and police services
- general practitioner initiatives
- non-government services.

CRITICAL THINKING

People with a mental illness too often revolve through prisons, with periods of incarceration interspersed with spells in the community (Butler et al. 2006). Prison does represent an opportunity for intervention and treatment, and in some cases may be the only time certain individuals are in contact with treatment services. Notwithstanding this, it is unlikely that prison is the best therapeutic environment for those suffering from a mental illness. (Butler et al. 2006)

Critical thinking

- What do you consider are the important issues raised in this quote?
- How might prison provide an opportunity for treatment?
- Based on your reading so far, what would you consider the best therapeutic environment for people diagnosed with a mental health problem?

These alliances should incorporate specific stakeholders such as service users, carers and service delivery personnel. Engebretson and Wind Wardell (1997, p. 38) describe partnership as 'a relationship resembling a legal partnership and usually involving close co-operation between parties having specified and joint rights and responsibilities as in a common enterprise'. Partnerships require ongoing collaboration in order to succeed. Collaboration in a mental health context refers to identifying who the stakeholders are that work together towards shared goals. Stakeholders include service users, families/carers, mental health workers, managers, government and non-government agencies, emergency services, including police, ambulance officers and the staff of emergency departments in general hospitals.

Non-government agencies or organisations (NGOs) can provide a vital role in mental health care, including broad advocacy and networking (e.g. New South Wales Association for Mental Health), services specifically for schizophrenia (e.g. Schizophrenia Fellowship) and specific care provisions for people with schizophrenia (e.g. rehabilitation, housing and living skills). Nurses have important roles working within non-government organisations, and facilitating access to and collaborating with them. Community-support services, including housing, home help, recreation, family support, employment and education, are essential elements in improving the quality of life of people with a mental illness.

CRITICAL THINKING

The Mental Health Council of Australia (MHCA) is a national non-government organisation that claims to represent and promote better mental health outcomes in Australia. The Council was established in 1997 with the main directive of gaining better mental health outcomes. Access the MHCA website at <www.mhca.org.au>.

Which organisations are represented by the MHCA? How does the MHCA facilitate collaboration? What have been the major achievements of the MHCA?

Access the website of the Australian Mental Health Consumer Network (National) at <www.nmhccf.org.au> and discuss how this network promotes working in partnership.

CONCLUSION

This chapter has highlighted some of the forces that have shaped contemporary mental health practice settings and the ways in which services are delivered in the context of government policy. Services have developed partly in line with international trends, which have seen a shift from and focus on institutional care towards mainstreaming and providing care in various forms in the community. An increased emphasis on protecting people's rights was made explicit in the Mental Health Statement of 1991, which stated that people with long-term and enduring mental health problems have rights that are 'equal to other citizens to health care, income maintenance, education, employment, housing, transport, legal services, equitable health and other insurance and leisure appropriate to one's age' (Commonwealth of Australia 2000, p. 1). In practice, this has meant that, to every extent possible, the aim has been to not separate out mental health from the delivery of other health and welfare services. However, negotiating the complex health and welfare system is difficult, and forms of case management have been developed to help people access and coordinate the services they need.

Deinstitutionalisation and mainstreaming are only part of the story of Australia's mental health policy and reform. Coalitions and partnerships of interest groups have worked together to undertake research, lobby for research and shape policy so as to change the emphasis and ways in which care is provided within existing service structures, and by creating new services unheard of only decades ago. This has required an unprecedented level of cooperation between stakeholders, including service users and traditional service providers. Perhaps an even more fundamental change has been a shift in the relationship between service user and service provider, and the challenge of the adoption of mental health recovery as a central tenet of policy.

REFERENCES

Andersson, G. & Cuijpers, P. (2009). Internet-based and other computerized psychological treatments for adult depression: a meta-analysis. *Cognitive Behaviour Therapy*, 38(4), 196–205.

Australian Bureau of Statistics (ABS) (2007). National Survey of Mental Health and Wellbeing: summary of results. Canberra: ABS.

Australian Institute of Health and Welfare (2010). *Mental Health Workforce*. Viewed 12 March 2012, <http://mhsa.aihw.gov.au/resources/workforce>.

Barak, A., Hen, L., Boniel-Nissim, M. & Shapira, N.A. (2008). A comprehensive review and a meta-analysis of the effectiveness of internet-based psychotherapeutic interventions. *Journal of Technology in Human Services*, 26(2–4), 109–60.

Barry, M. & Jenkins, J. (2007). *Implementing Mental Health Promotion*. Sydney: Churchill Livingston Elsevier.

Bassilios, B., Pirkis, J., Fletcher, J., Burgess, P., Gurrin, L., King, K., Kohn, F. & Blashki, G. (2010). The complementarity of two major Australian primary mental health care initiatives. *Australian and New Zealand Journal of Psychiatry*, 44(11), 997–1004.

Breckenridge, J., Salter, M. & Shaw, E. (2012). Use and abuse: understanding the intersections of childhood abuse, alcohol and drug use and mental health. *Mental Health and Substance Use*, 5(4), 314–27.

Burdekin, B. (1993). Human Rights and Mental Illness: Report of the National Inquiry into the Human Rights of People with Mental Illness. Canberra: Human Rights and Equal Opportunity Commission.

Burns, T., Catty, J., Dash, M., Roberts, C., Lockwood, A. & Marshall, M. (2007). Use of intensive case management to reduce time in hospital in people with severe mental illness: systematic review and meta-regression. *British Medical Journal*, 335(7615), 336.

Butler, T., Andrews, G., Allnutt, S., Sakashita, C., Smith, N.E. and Basson, J. (2006), Mental disorders in Australian prisoners: a comparison with a community sample. *Australian and New Zealand Journal of Psychiatry, 40,* 272–6.

Commonwealth Department of Health and Aged Care (2000). *Promotion, Prevention and Early Intervention for Mental Health: a monograph.* Canberra: Commonwealth Department of Health and Aged Care.

Commonwealth of Australia (2000). *Mental Health Statement of Rights and Responsibilities.* Canberra: Australian Government Publishing Service.

Council of Australian Governments (COAG) (2006). *National Action Plan on Mental Health 2006–2011.* Canberra: COAG.

—— (2012). COAG *National Action Plan on Mental Health: progress report (2009–10).* Canberra: COAG. Viewed 20 February 2013, <www.coag.gov.au/node/441>.

Department of Health and Ageing (2007). *National Mental Health Report 2007.* Canberra: Commonwealth of Australia.

—— (2008). *National Mental Health Policy 2008.* Canberra: Commonwealth of Australia.

—— (2009). *National Mental Health Policy 2009.* Canberra: Commonwealth of Australia.

—— (2010). *National Mental Health Policy 2010.* Canberra: Commonwealth of Australia.

Engebretson, J. & Wind Wardell, D. (1997). The essence of partnership in research. *Journal of Professional Nursing*, 13(1), 38–47.

Griffiths, K.M. & Christensen, H. (2007). Internet-based mental health programs: a powerful tool in the rural medical kit. *Australian Journal of Rural Health*, 15(2), 81–7.

Health Management Advisers (2012). Evaluation of the Mental Health Nurse Inventive Program. Department of Health and Ageing. Viewed 24 December 2012, <www.health.gov.au/internet/main/publishing.nsf/content/mental-pubs-e-evalnurs>.

Henry, L.P., Amminger, G.P., Harris, M.G., Yuen, H.P., Harrigan, S.M., Prosser, A.L. et al. (2010). The EPPIC follow-up study of first-episode psychosis: longer-term clinical and functional outcome 7 years after index admission. *The Journal of Clinical Psychiatry*, 71(6), 716–28.

Hoult, J., Reynolds, I., Charbonneau-Powis, M., Coles, P. & Briggs, J. (1981). A controlled study of psychiatric hospital versus community treatment: the effect on relatives. *Australian and New Zealand Journal of Psychiatry*, 15(4), 323–8.

Kalucy, R., Thomas, L. & King, D. (2005). Changing demand for mental health services in the emergency department of a public hospital. *Australian and New Zealand Journal of Psychiatry*, 39, 74–80.

Kanter, J. (1989). Clinical case management: definition, principles, components. *Hospital & Community Psychiatry*, 40(4), 361–8.

Lessing, K. & Blignault, I. (2001). Mental health telemedicine programmes in Australia. *Journal of Telemedicine & Telecare*, 7(6), 317–23.

Marshall, M. & Lockwood, A. (2000). Assertive community treatment for people with severe mental disorders. *Cochrane Database Systemic Review*, 2, CD001089.

Mathers, C. (1994). *Health Differentials Among Adult Australians Aged 25–64 Years.* Canberra: Australian Institute of Health and Welfare.

McGinty, K.L., Atezaz Saeed, S., Simmons, S. & Yildirim, Y. (2006). Telepsychiatry and e-mental health services: potential for improving access to mental health care. *Psychiatry Quarterly*, 77(4), 335–42.

McGorry, P.D., Edwards, J., Milhalopoulos, C., Harrigan, S.M., Jackson, H.J. (1996). EPPIC: An evolving system of early detection and optimal management. *Schizophrenia Bulletin*, 22, 305–26.

McGorry, P.D., Purcell, R., Hickie, I.B. & Jorm, A.F. (2007). Investing in youth mental health is a best buy. *Medical Journal of Australia*, 187(7), 5.

Rosen, A. & Teesson, M. (2001). Does case management work? The evidence and the abuse of evidence-based medicine. *Australian and New Zealand Journal of Psychiatry*, 35(6), 731–46.

Scott, E., Naismith, S., Whitwell, B., Hamilton, B., Chudleigh, C. & Hickie, I. (2009). Delivering youth-specific mental health services: the advantages of a collaborative, multi-disciplinary system. *Australasian Psychiatry: Bulletin of Royal Australian and New Zealand College of Psychiatrists,* 17(3), 189–94.

Sharrock, J., Bryant, J., McNamara, P., Forster, J.D & Happell, B. (2008). Exploratory study of mental health consultation-liaison nursing in Australia: Part 1—demographics and role characteristics. *International Journal of Mental Health Nursing*, 17(3), 180–8.

Smith, L. & Newton, R. (2007). Systematic review of case management. *Australian & New Zealand Journal of Psychiatry*, 41(1), 2–9.

Swadi, H. & Bobier, C. (2005). Hospital admissions in adolescents with acute psychiatric disorder: How long should it be? *Australasian Psychiatry*, 13(2), 165–8.

World Health Organization (WHO) Department of Mental Health and Substance Abuse (2004). *Prevention of Mental Disorders: effective interventions and policy options summary report*. Geneva: WHO.

5

Legal, ethical and professional issues in mental health nursing

Main points
- In addition to the legal and ethical issues of the broader nursing profession, there are specific issues relevant to mental health nursing.
- Each state and territory of Australia has a *Mental Health Act*, which sets out the legal requirements and framework for mental health service provision.
- The potential for treatment being given against the will of the person concerned creates significant ethical issues for nurses.
- The practice of mental health nursing is expected to conform to professional standards.

Definitions
Ethics: The philosophical consideration of what makes specific actions morally correct.

Legislation: An Act of parliament that provides legal regulation for specific activities or behaviours. It may specify what can be done, what cannot be done or a combination of both.

INTRODUCTION
There are similarities between mental health nursing and other specialties with respect to legal, ethical and professional issues. For example, from a legal perspective, the mental health nurse is subject to the same regulation as a nurse employed in an intensive care unit in relation to practices such as the administration of medication. However, the

underlying assumptions of mental health services mean there are also some significant differences in the legal and ethical aspects of practice. The mental health field is the only area of nursing with a specific Act of parliament that pertains to and regulates many of its practices.

This chapter will provide an overview of professional, legal and ethical issues that relate specifically to mental health nursing, including:

- the *Mental Health Act*
- ethical issues in mental health nursing
- professional regulation.

MENTAL HEALTH NURSING AND THE LAW

Most Western countries have mental health laws operating within in-patient mental health services and extending into the community. Contemporary mental health care and treatment are based on a fundamental assumption that people with a mental illness may not realise that they need treatment and that, in certain given circumstances, health services have the right to impose treatment in the identified 'best interests' of the person. This assumption led to the development of legislation to deal specifically with mental health care. However, mental health legislation is the subject of ongoing international debate for a number of reasons, including the legal and ethical position of people treated involuntarily under mental health laws who are competent (Molodynski, Rugkasa & Burns 2010) and whether Acts should include 'dangerousness' criteria, or should focus solely on a person's well-being (Ryan 2011). Separate mental health laws are critiqued because they attack human rights, perpetuate prejudice and stigma, form an association of mental illness with dangerousness, and cause the marginalisation of people with mental illness (Ryan 2011).

Each state and territory of Australia has a *Mental Health Act* designed as a legal framework for the care and treatment of people diagnosed with a mental illness. While differences can be observed between the legislation of specific jurisdictions, there are fundamental similarities between the Acts, which tend to be organised according to the following areas:

- definitions of mental illness and other conditions that justify treatment under the Act
- the required process for admission, detention and treatment within mental health services
- the types of treatment available according to the Act
- the rights of people treated according to the Act
- processes for review and appeal. (Staunton & Chiarella 2013)

The website <www.austlii.edu.au> has links to each state and territory's mental health legislation. Just select the relevant state or territory and follow the links.

It is not possible to provide an extensive description of the Act for each state and territory of Australia, and you are advised to familiarise yourself with the Act for your specific jurisdiction during your course of study. However, a brief overview of the major sections of legislation will be presented.

DEFINITIONS: MENTAL ILLNESS AND MENTAL DISORDER

Legal definition is an important part of any legislation, to clearly show who is and is not regulated by the Act. All *Mental Health Acts* now include a definition of mental illness, although the extent to which they clearly convey the meaning of this term can be disputed. For example, Victoria defines mental illness as 'A medical condition that is characterised by a significant disturbance of thought, perception or memory'.

The South Australian definition is simply 'any illness or disorder of the mind'. Ultimately, this leaves the power with psychiatrists and medical practitioners to determine whether or not a person has a mental illness. Conversely, the New South Wales definition is more directive:

Mental illness means a condition which seriously impairs, either temporarily or permanently, the mental functioning of a person and is characterised by the presence in the person of any one or more of the following symptoms:

(a) Delusions;
(b) Hallucinations;
(c) Serious disorder of thought form;
(d) A severe disturbance of mood;
(e) Sustained or repeated irrational behaviour indicating the presence of any one or more of the symptoms referred to in paragraphs (a)–(d).

CRITICAL THINKING

Consult the definition of mental illness pertaining to your state or territory and consider the following questions.

- How clearly do you think this definition would enable medical practitioners to determine whether or not a person has a mental illness?
- Do you think it is possible for diagnosis of mental illness to be completely accurate?
- How and why do you think diagnosing mental illness might differ from diagnosing a physical illness?
- What differences can you see between a psychiatric definition of mental illness and a legal one?

The New South Wales Act distinguishes between *mental illness* and a *mentally ill person*. This reflects the change in focus to a more human rights-based approach to legislation. The fact that a person has a mental illness is considered insufficient grounds to enforce treatment within a mental health service. There needs to be a view that mental health treatment, care or *control* is necessary for the protection of the person or others.

CRITICAL THINKING

Consult your state or territory *Mental Health Act*.

- What criteria must be met before a person can be admitted on an involuntary basis? Do you think these criteria are fair and just? Consider why or why not.
- How do the rights and responsibilities of the person relate to the rights and responsibilities of others (such as family/friends and health professionals)?

Similar stipulations are made in the Acts of other jurisdictions. The Victorian legislation also requires that the person is in need of care and treatment that can be provided by the mental health service. This criterion is significant because it requires active treatment to be part of the admission. It is not justifiable to contain or isolate a person from the broader community on the basis of an apparent mental illness alone.

Most *Mental Health Acts* also include characteristics or conditions that, on their own, are not reason for admission to and detention in a mental health service. These vary between jurisdictions and include:

- anti-social behaviour or personality
- intellectual disability
- intoxication (drugs or alcohol)
- sexual promiscuity
- specific political opinion or belief
- religious opinion or belief
- sexual preference or sexual orientation
- immoral conduct
- illegal conduct.

This clarification is intended to protect people against involuntary detention for simply being different or behaving in a manner that is not socially acceptable.

It is important to note that these are not exclusion criteria—for example, a person with an anti-social personality *can* be admitted if they also have an illness that meets the criteria for admission. Anti-social personality *cannot* be the only reason for admission.

Section 15 of the New South Wales Act also includes a definition for a *mentally disordered person*:

A person (whether or not the person is suffering from a mental illness) is a mentally disordered person if the person's behaviour for the time being is so irrational as to justify a conclusion of reasonable grounds that temporary care, treatment or control of the person is necessary.

(a) For the person's own protection from serious physical harm; or
(b) For the protection of others from serious physical harm.

CRITICAL THINKING
Consult your state or territory *Mental Health Act.*

*   What criteria are included as not representing a mental illness?
*   Do you think these exclusions are fair and reasonable?
*   What consequences do you think there would be if these characteristics or behaviours were considered to be evidence of mental illness?

The Act does not attempt to describe what is meant by irrational behaviour and therefore is open to individual interpretation and judgement.

CASE STUDY
The police are called to a disturbance at 2.00 a.m. one Sunday morning. A young man named Damien is found sitting on his roof screaming at the 'bastards' who are out to get him; he is dressed in jungle greens. The neighbours describe him as a usually quiet and polite young man. Damien's girlfriend arrives and informs police she ended their relationship the previous afternoon.

Critical thinking

*   Do you think it would be fair and reasonable to detain Damian in a mental health service?
*   Would your answer be different if he showed signs of intoxication?
*   Do you think there is likely to be a common understanding of irrational behaviour?
*   Have you ever been accused of behaving irrationally when you consider your behaviour was appropriate and reasonable in the circumstances?

ADMISSION, DETENTION AND TREATMENT
Voluntary admission

All state and territory Acts make provision for voluntary admission into psychiatric hospitals or mental health services. A voluntary patient (as this term is the one used in legislation, it will be used in place of 'service user' in the description of legislation) requests or agrees to the hospital admission and may be discharged on request.

However, some Acts (including Victoria) allow a person to be refused admission as a voluntary patient if there is no reason to be confident the person will benefit from care and treatment as an in-patient. If the patient is not happy with this decision, he or she can appeal it.

Involuntary admission

Some Australian mental health legislation (see the Acts of New South Wales, Queensland and Victoria) now stipulates the importance of providing care and treatment within the *least restrictive environment*. According to this philosophy, involuntary admission should be considered as a last resort. For example, the New South Wales Act states:

> A person must not be admitted to, or detained in or continue to be detained in, a hospital under this Part unless the medical superintendent is of the opinion that no other care of a less restrictive kind is appropriate and reasonably available to the person. (section 20)

This approach is consistent with the philosophy underpinning the deinstitutionalisation movement, reflecting the view that the community should constitute the primary location for mental health care.

CRITICAL THINKING
Consult your state or territory *Mental Health Act*.

- Does it make reference to the least restrictive environment?
- What do you understand by the term 'least restrictive environment'?
- How important do you think this might be for people experiencing mental illness?

Mental Health Acts make provision for persons to *request* an assessment of a person they consider may be experiencing a mental illness, and for whom involuntary admission and detention are considered necessary. In theory, any person can make a request; however, it is usually someone in close proximity, such as a friend, family member, work colleague or neighbour.

Admission or recommendation requires authorisation by a medical practitioner who (following examination) considers the person to have a mental illness requiring immediate treatment for the safety and protection of themselves or others.

In situations where a medical practitioner is not readily available, or the circumstances are considered urgent, the Acts allow for authorised persons such as police and ambulance officers, mental health nurses and other mental health professionals to transport a person they consider to meet the criteria for involuntary detention within that jurisdiction to an authorised mental health service for assessment.

CRITICAL THINKING

Consult your state or territory *Mental Health Act* and note the following:

*   procedure for involuntary detention
*   process for request
*   process for recommendation
*   process for admission in emergency situations or where a medical practitioner is unavailable.

Authorisation and review of involuntary admission

After admission, the involuntary patient must be seen by an authorised psychiatrist within 24 hours. The psychiatrist examines the patient to decide whether the person meets the criteria. If the criteria are met, the patient is detained; otherwise, they are discharged.

All Acts include a process for review of and appeal against involuntary detention. For example, in South Australia, continued detention can only be authorised for an additional 21 days. If continued detention is still considered necessary, two psychiatrists must independently examine the person and confirm that continued detention is necessary and warranted (section 12(6)).

COMMUNITY TREATMENT ORDERS

A community treatment order (CTO) implies that a person can live in the community while remaining an involuntary patient in the eyes of the law. This usually occurs when a person is considered well enough to be discharged but still needs ongoing supervision. This is usually because the treating team believes that the person will not continue treatment unless it is enforced.

The CTO will include specific conditions that may relate to:

- adherence to prescribed medication
- attendance at a community mental health clinic
- where the person may live.

CASE STUDY

Paul is a community mental health nurse. He has been the case manager for Teresa for nearly six months; he began this role shortly after her discharge from the local in-patient unit. Teresa lives in a small unit with her mother; she has a part-time job and says she is 'pretty happy with life'. Her mother contacted Paul because she was worried about her daughter. Teresa has become angry and hostile towards her mother, accusing her of trying to poison her. When Paul visits, Teresa has barricaded herself in her bedroom. She refuses to come out. Paul attempts to persuade her without success. She begins to throw her belongings at the walls and threatens to kill anyone who comes near her. Paul contacts the Crisis, Assessment and Treatment Team. Teresa is assessed by the duty doctor and is recommended for admission to the in-patient unit as an involuntary patient under the *Mental Health Act.*

Critical thinking

Refer to your state or territory *Mental Health Act* to answer the following questions.

- Do you think Teresa meets the criteria for involuntary admission?
- What is the legal process for Teresa following admission?

CRITICAL THINKING

Consult your state or territory *Mental Health Act* and note the following regarding CTOs:

- indications for a CTO
- conditions that can be included
- length of order and process for renewal
- process for appeal
- the process when a person does not meet the conditions of the CTO.

> What benefits and/or disadvantages can you see for the person themselves, their family and friends and/or health professionals if a person receives involuntary treatment in the community?

CTOs generally remain effective for up to twelve months; however, a process for renewal exists if this is considered necessary.

PATIENT RIGHTS

Mental health legislation in Australia claims to be based on human rights, particularly for those people receiving treatment against their will. The rights of patients vary between jurisdictions, but the law generally insists that persons must be made aware of their rights. Often this information must be provided in writing. Patient rights include:

- legal representation
- a second psychiatric opinion
- right of appeal
- information about community visitors or official visitors (discussed below) and the right to make contact with them
- access to a list of community visitors
- access to a copy of the *Mental Health Act* and other relevant legislation.

CRITICAL THINKING
Refer to the section on patient rights in your state or territory *Mental Health Act.*

- Do you consider these rights fair and reasonable?
- Are there any other rights you think should be included?

MENTAL HEALTH REVIEW BODY

This body is known as the Mental Health Review Board in Victoria and the Mental Health Review Tribunal in New South Wales and Queensland. Essentially, it is an independent body established to review and hear appeals against involuntary detention in mental health services.

These bodies generally undertake reviews of people detained involuntarily beyond a specified period of time (the timeframe varies between states and territories). Persons detained as involuntary patients can appeal to this body to have their involuntary status overturned. Board/tribunal members include legal practitioners, psychiatrists and other persons considered to have suitable qualifications and/or experience (including nurses). The board/tribunal is much less formal than a court.

The aim is to create a more personal and comfortable environment for the patient. To help the members make decisions, they may seek the opinions of people who know the patient well, including nurses.

During your clinical placement in a public mental health service, there may be a board/tribunal hearing. If the patient concerned is agreeable, you may ask permission to attend as an observer.

CRITICAL THINKING
Consult your state or territory *Mental Health Act*.

- Does it refer to a mental health review body?
- What is the role of that body?
- What is its membership?

COMMUNITY OR OFFICIAL VISITORS
Some jurisdictions make provision for the appointment of persons known as community or official visitors. These officials are entitled to visit approved treatment facilities and make reports to state parliament. They have a broad brief, which enables them to comment on the adequacy of:

- access to and treatment provided by services
- standard of facilities
- information provided about rights of individuals accessing services
- complaint procedures
- actions by staff that contravene the Act
- other matters considered important and relevant.

Information about community visitors in Victoria can be found at
<www.publicadvocate.vic.gov.au/Services/Community-Visitors.html>.

TREATMENT UNDER *THE MENTAL HEALTH ACT*
When a person is legally detained in a mental health service, appropriately qualified mental health professionals can administer medical and psycho-social interventions according to their clinical judgement. However, two forms of treatment also require

a formal legal process to be followed. These are electro-convulsive therapy and psycho-surgery.

CRITICAL THINKING

- Refer to your state or territory *Mental Health Act* to find out whether it makes provisions for community/official visitors.
- If it does, do an internet search to find out more about their role and how they can be accessed.

Electro-convulsive therapy

Electro-convulsive therapy (ECT) is defined in Chapter 9. It can be administered where it is considered to be of clinical advantage to the service user. However, current Australian legislation provides firm guidelines for the use of this treatment, including informed consent.

Informed consent

Irrespective of whether the person has been admitted voluntarily or involuntarily, they must only consent to ECT after receiving:

- a full description of the procedure, the expected benefits and possible side-effects using language that can be understood by the person
- detailed information about alternative treatments
- full information regarding rights, including the right to withdraw consent at any stage and the right to seek legal and medical advice
- the opportunity to ask questions and to have them answered fully and honestly.

Consent must be given by the service user in writing on the legally prescribed form.

The various Acts make provisions for situations where an involuntary patient is considered incapable of consenting to treatment or refuses to do so. For example:

- In New South Wales, two medical practitioners (at least one being a psychiatrist) must certify as to clinical importance of the treatment. Treatment must be authorised as necessary by the Mental Health Tribunal.
- In Victoria, the authorised psychiatrist can authorise ECT if he or she considers it of clinical value or necessity. The authorised psychiatrist must make all reasonable efforts to ensure the person's guardian or primary carer has been notified.
- In South Australia, consent may be provided by a parent or guardian, or by the Guardianship Board.

- In Queensland, the ACT, Northern Territory and Western Australia, consent can be given by the Mental Health Tribunal/Mental Health Review Board.

Psycho-surgery

Most Acts include a specific definition of psycho-surgery, which refers to surgery or the use of intracerebral electrodes on the brain 'primarily for the purpose of altering the thoughts, emotions or behaviour of that person' (*Mental Health Act*, Victoria, section 54(1)). More information about psycho-surgery and its uses is provided in Chapter 9.

The legal regulations for the administration of psycho-surgery are even more stringent than those for ECT. In addition to consent from the person, consent from the Psycho-surgery Review Board (however named by the individual states and territories) is required following application.

CRITICAL THINKING

Consult your state or territory *Mental Health Act* and familiarise yourself with the process and procedures for the administration of ECT or psycho-surgery.

RESTRAINT AND SECLUSION

Authorising restraint and seclusion

Restraint and seclusion should normally be authorised by a medical practitioner; however, in the case of an emergency, authorisation can be given by the senior registered nurse or authorised mental health professional. In these instances, a medical practitioner or authorised psychiatrist must be notified without delay.

Physical restraint

Restraint is defined in section 121 of the Western Australian *Mental Health Act* as: 'preventing the free movement of the person's body or a limb by mechanical means, other than by the use of a medical or surgical appliance for the proper treatment of a physical disease or injury'.

Most jurisdictions have provision for the administration of some form of physical restraint. Generally, the process requires formal reporting on the use of restraint, which may include:

- the form of mechanical restraint
- reasons for using restraint
- the person who approved or authorised the use of restraint

- the person who applied the restraint
- the length of time the restraint was used.

Seclusion

Seclusion is defined in the *Mental Health Act* of Victoria (section 82) as 'the sole confinement of a person at any hour of the day or night in a room of which the doors and windows are locked from the outside'. In Victoria, seclusion must be formally reported in a manner similar to that of restraint.

There are certain legislative rights granted to persons placed in seclusion, which include that they be:

- observed and reviewed at specific intervals of time—usually every fifteen minutes (in some cases, it is specified that this must be by a registered nurse)
- provided with 'appropriate' bedding and clothing
- provided with food and drink at appropriate times (i.e. mealtimes)
- provided with access to toilet facilities
- medically examined at regular prescribed intervals.

CRITICAL THINKING

- What do you think is meant by 'appropriate' bedding and clothing?
- What would be appropriate for you?
- What factors might influence nurses' decision-making about what bedding and clothing might be appropriate?

Restraint or seclusion practised outside the conditions set down in legislation represents an offence against the specific Act of parliament, and penalties apply. For further information about penalties, consult your state or territory *Mental Health Act*.

LEGISLATIVE REFORM

Mental health laws are reviewed periodically as a result of inquiries, changing social attitudes, international covenants and other reforms. Tasmania, the Australian Capital Territory, Queensland, Western Australia and Victoria are reviewing their *Mental Health Acts*, in part to ensure compliance with obligations under the United Nations Convention on the Rights of Persons with Disabilities (2006), to which Australia became a signatory in 2008. The Convention emphasises the rights of all persons to make decisions and requires signatory states to ensure access for all persons with disabilities to decision-making support. Proposed changes to Victoria's *Mental Health Act* seek to embed supported decision-making actioned through the presumption of decision-making capacity, the use of advance statements and a 'nominated persons' scheme. There will be new criteria for involuntary assessment and treatment. Other reform objectives include establishing a recovery-oriented framework, minimising the duration of involuntary treatment, increasing protections for the rights of service users through advocacy and a second opinion process. New oversight mechanisms include the establishment of a Mental Health Complaints Commissioner.

MENTAL HEALTH NURSING AND ETHICS
What is ethics?
Ethics refers to a branch of philosophical inquiry that encourages people to:

> question why they considered a particular act right or wrong, what the reasons (justifications) are for their judgements, and whether their judgements are correct. (Johnstone 2008, p. 13)

Ethical principles
Staunton and Chiarella (2013) describe five main ethical principles:

1. Concern for the well-being of all individuals and of society.
2. Embodies ideals—that is, 'what should be done' is valued over 'what can be done'. World peace, for example, represents an ethical stance, despite the numerous and significant barriers that mean this goal is unlikely to be achieved in the foreseeable future.
3. Uses moral reasoning to determine what is appropriate or inappropriate in specific situations.
4. Are applied universally and equally, to all persons at all times.
5. Ethics is considered to be of ultimate importance—more so than the law or other influences such as politics. Ethical decisions should also prevail over individual interests. For example, those who believe in the right of individuals to die with dignity might consider assisting a person with a terminal illness to end their life to be ethically correct despite the fact that the law stipulates that such a practice is illegal. Under these circumstances, the individual would probably consider the law to be unethical.

Bioethics
This is the term used to describe the exploration of ethical issues specifically related to medical or health care. It includes four main ethical principles that should guide medical and health-care practice: autonomy, beneficence, non-maleficence and justice.

Autonomy

This refers to the individual's right to self-determination. In health care, this gives rise to the concept of informed consent, which respects the right of individuals to determine whether or not they wish to have specific interventions or treatments. This principle overrides professional opinion, meaning that medical and nursing staff may strongly believe a particular course of action is best for the person, but ultimately the decision lies with that individual.

Autonomy has limits—for instance, when the autonomous acts of a person negatively affect the rights of others. This concept has implications for ethics in relation to mental health, and will be explored later in this chapter.

Beneficence

In simple terms, this means 'above all, do good'. In health care, it is assumed that professionals will act in ways that will provide benefits to service users of health services. However, as the example of Anastasia (see case study below) shows, there can be conflict between what the health professional thinks is best for the service user and what the service user wants for themself. This means that at times there can be conflict between autonomy and beneficence.

CASE STUDY

Anastasia is a 43-year-old woman recently diagnosed with advanced breast cancer. Medical staff have advised her that a radical mastectomy would be likely to increase her life expectancy for at least twelve months. After extensive research, Anastasia believes her quality of life is likely to be very poor and refuses the surgery. Anastasia's family is very distressed and asks the doctor to 'do something' to make her change her mind.

According to the ethical principle of autonomy, Anastasia's decision must be respected, despite the views of her family and her medical team that surgery would be a preferred option. However, if Anastasia had been involuntarily detained in a mental health facility for treatment of severe and persistent depression, a psychiatrist would be able to consent on her behalf to a course of ECT, for example—even if Anastasia did not consent to this treatment.

Critical thinking

- What do you think about these differences?
- Do you think there are circumstances when a person should be forced to have treatment? If so, how would you decide when the rights of an individual should be respected and when they should not?

Non-maleficence

'Above all, do no harm.' In health-care terms, this is related to our duty of care. As nurses, we have a duty to ensure that service users of health services are not harmed as a result of the care and treatment they receive or do not receive.

Beneficence and non-maleficence may appear to refer to the same thing—that is, by doing good, we are avoiding harm. Often this may be the case, but sometimes there is conflict between the two. While beneficence focuses on the benefits, non-maleficence focuses on the risks and how they can be avoided.

Justice

In terms of ethics, justice has two specific meanings. First, it refers to what is right or fair, and suggests that all people should be treated equally. In health-care terms, this would mean people should be given equal access to treatment and information about that treatment.

CASE STUDY

Janice is a 36-year-old woman with a thirteen-year history of bipolar affective disorder. During the depressive stages of her illness, Janice frequently has suicidal thoughts, and has made several attempts to take her own life. Her husband contacts the family doctor after finding that Janice has stockpiled her medication, revised her will and given a number of her treasured possessions to close friends and family members. She is extremely withdrawn and refuses to eat. On exam-ination, the doctor confirms the diagnosis of depression and recommends that she be hospitalised. Janice protests strongly; she claims she hates being 'in a psych hospital', that she would rather die than be there.

This situation illustrates a conflict between 'doing good' and 'doing no harm'. Clearly, if Janice is admitted as an involuntary patient this will 'do harm' to her by denying her the right to exercise self-determination regarding the decision to be treated in hospital. On the other hand, the motives of her husband, the family doctor and the staff of the mental health service would appear to be to 'do good', and to let her continue to remain at home may result in a greater harm—even death.

The term 'equality' is sometimes mistaken for sameness, meaning that people should be treated the same. However, individuals differ in terms of needs, education, knowledge base and cultural heritage, to name just a few, and these differences need to be considered and respected in order to provide *equal* access to treatment and information.

Second, the concept of *distributive justice* refers to the allocation of resources. In terms of health care, this suggests that people should have equal access to care, irrespective of a number of factors—including their specific health issue.

You may already be aware, through your formal studies or your clinical experience, that some areas of health care receive higher levels of funding than others. Traditionally, mental health has not been one of these. For example, until recently only 7 per cent of the Australian health-care budget was allocated to mental health services, despite the fact that approximately 20 per cent of the population experiences a mental illness and that depression is expected to become the second highest contributor to total disease burden by the year 2020 (Hayman-White, Sgro & Happell 2006).

Bioethics and health care

The above description of the four main ethical principles shows just how complex ethics and health care can become. The four principles can regularly be in conflict in many situations. The nurse or other health-care professional can feel conflicted between what they feel is right or best and many other factors, including the wishes of the service user, the wishes of the family, the decisions of other members of the health-care team (particularly doctors), hospital policy and legislative requirements. This situation is known as an ethical dilemma, which Johnstone (2010, p. 102) defines as 'a situation requiring choice between what seem to be two equally desirable or undesirable alternatives'.

CRITICAL THINKING

- Why do you think mental health receives less funding than services provided for physical health or injury?
- What factors do you think are likely to influence how funding allocations are decided?

CASE STUDY

Pam is working as a community nurse. She believes in an individual's right to die with dignity, and strongly supports the introduction of euthanasia laws. She is caring for David, an 83-year-old man diagnosed with a terminal illness. He is in considerable discomfort and is expected to die within a matter of weeks. Both he and his family have asked Pam to assist him to bring on the end of his life. They are all very distressed by what they see as unnecessary discomfort involved in waiting for the inevitable.

Critical thinking

- Consider this situation according to the four principles of ethics:
  a. autonomy
  b. beneficence
  c. non-maleficence
  d. justice.
- List your views on ways to encourage each of these.
- Consider the situation from Pam's point of view. How do you think she would assess the situation against the four principles?
- Are your views on the desired outcome the same as or different from Pam's?

If your views are different, this illustrates the complex nature of ethics, particularly as it relates to health care. The principles can be interpreted differently depending on individual views.

In the example above, each of the four principles could have quite different interpretations. The following presents some thoughts on how David's situation might be viewed from an ethical standpoint.

Autonomy

The evidence presented above suggests that David and his family have made an autonomous decision that David would prefer, and benefit from, interventions to end his life. However, opponents may suggest that David's pain and his family's inability to cope with his suffering mean they are not capable of making an autonomous decision.

Beneficence

To Pam, and those who support her views, the ability to hasten the end of David's life would clearly 'do good', as it would bring relief from suffering for him and his family. Those opposed to euthanasia would likely consider such an act as 'doing harm', based on the view that life is sacrosanct and must be preserved at all costs.

Non-maleficence

While it might be seen that ending life equates to 'doing harm', Pam would likely argue that a greater harm (that of suffering and pain) would result from inaction. Others would argue that ending life is causing harm, and there is no greater harm that can be caused.

Justice

Pam would probably argue that it is right, fair and *just* that David be allowed to hasten his death, and that he have the right to make that decision. An alternative view may be that this is not a decision David is entitled to make, and that justice is served through the preservation of life.

Pam's decision
Pam's views and beliefs clearly lead her to the conclusion that from an ethical perspective David should be able to hasten his death. However, legally and professionally she would be prohibited from doing so. Irrespective of individual beliefs, providing the assistance asked for could result in a charge of murder and would almost certainly result in the cancellation of Pam's nursing registration. Therefore, Pam is likely to be torn between the desire to help David and his family and the legal and professional ramifications of such a decision.

ETHICAL PRINCIPLES AND MENTAL HEALTH NURSING PRACTICE
The major difference in the application of ethical principles within the mental health field concerns the principle of autonomy. Consider the case of Janice introduced earlier in this chapter. Janice has refused to go to a psychiatric in-patient unit of her own free will. She has indicated that she wishes to be left alone. If Janice were experiencing any form of illness other than mental illness, this decision would likely be respected. However, because she has a mental illness, Janice is not considered capable of autonomous decision-making to the same extent as a person without a mental illness. Her capacity to make informed decisions is considered to be impaired during acute stages of her mental illness. Ethically, these legally governed practices in mental health are justified on the basis of the belief that people experiencing acute symptoms of a mental illness may have an impaired ability to make decisions. The legal power that overrides the individual's autonomy to make decisions is called 'substitute' or 'proxy' decision-making.

SUPPORTED DECISION-MAKING
An alternative form of decision-making that seeks to uphold autonomy is 'supported decision-making'. A supported decision-making model assumes that the important decisions we make are often made interdependently, with the help and support of our personal networks like friends and relatives. Under this model, it is not assumed that the person is unable to make any and all decisions; rather, effort goes into establishing what the person wishes with the aim of retaining legal capacity.

Some principles of supported decision-making are:

- All individuals of legal age are persons before the law, and have a right to self-determination and respect for their autonomy, irrespective of disability.
- All adults are entitled to the presumption of capacity, irrespective of disability and to the decision-making supports necessary to exercise capacity.
- Decisions made interdependently with family, friends and trusted others chosen by the individual will be recognised and legally validated.

CRITICAL THINKING

Take a look at the interactive Ottawa personal decision-making guide at <http://decisionaid.ohri.ca/docs/das/OPDG.pdf>. How might you be able to use this tool to support service user decision-making?

Earlier in this chapter, you were introduced to the *Mental Health Acts* of the Australian states and territories. These Acts all refer to entitlements and practices that can restrict the autonomy and freedom of individuals to a far greater extent than any other form of health-related legislation. People can be brought into hospital against their will, receive treatments they do not want and be subject to enforced treatment even after they leave hospital. Whatever your views as to whether involuntary treatment and hospitalisation might be necessary, the fact remains that freedoms and rights are lost in this process. Being mindful of these losses is important.

The decisions Janice wishes to make at this time might be quite different from those she would make if she were not experiencing acute symptoms. An examination of Janice's medical history may reveal that she responds well to treatment with antidepressants and develops a more positive attitude towards life and expresses gratitude that she was hospitalised before she had the opportunity to take her life.

Table 5.1 presents an overview of Janice's situation from her own perspective and from that of mental health professionals.

CRITICAL THINKING

- How would you manage the tension between Janice's wishes and those of the mental health professionals as stated above? What other options might there be apart from hospitalisation?
- In your view, does Janice meet the criteria for involuntary admission? What would be going through your mind if you were required to make this decision?
- What do you think the impact of prior experience of involuntary admission/involuntary treatment might be on how Janice feels about going to hospital again?
- What do you see as the main differences (if any) between Janice's situation and that of David?

Table 5.1 Individual and professional views of ethical principles in mental health

Ethical principle	Janice's views	Mental health professionals' views	Human rights considerations
Autonomy	There is nothing wrong with me. I want to stay at home.	Janice is extremely depressed and does not have the capacity to make decisions in her best interests.	The right to determine one's own health decisions
Beneficence	To 'do good', you should leave me alone and let me do what I want.	To 'do good', we must ignore Janice's stated wishes. We are confident that she will feel more positive after treatment.	The right to choose between different treatment options
Non-maleficence	If you admit me to hospital, you will 'do harm'.	If we do not admit Janice, we will cause greater harm by allowing her physical condition to deteriorate and running the risk that she will attempt suicide.	The right to freedom of movement
Justice	I have the same right as anyone else to make my own decisions. Other people can't be forced to go to hospital if they don't want to.	While Janice is not able to make the best decisions for her health, we must make them for her to ensure she has the same access to necessary health care as everyone else.	The right to refuse treatment

MENTAL HEALTH NURSING AND PROFESSIONAL REGULATION

You may be aware of the Royal College of Nursing Australia, the professional body for nursing. The specialist field of mental health nursing has its own professional body, the Australian College of Mental Health Nurses (ACMHN). The aim of the ACMHN is to represent the professional interests of nurses employed within the mental health field. Further information about the ACMHN can be found at <www.acmhn.org>.

The ACMHN espouses the Standards of Practice for Mental Health Nursing developed by the former body, the Australian and New Zealand College of Mental Health Nurses (ANZCMHN 2010). The standards are designed to guide mental health nursing practice. However, it is important to note that professional standards do not have legal authority, they do not prescribe behaviour and a nurse cannot be penalised for not meeting them. Rather, standards operate as a set of principles that a professional body believes *should* determine acceptable practice. In a sense, this is like the statement *love thy neighbour*, which is intended to encourage people to be respectful and considerate of one another. It is not against the law to refuse to speak to your neighbour, but it might be regarded as against the principles of being a good citizen.

The Standards of Practice for Mental Health Nursing (2010) require that mental health nurses:

1. acknowledge diversity in culture, values and belief systems and ensure that their practice is non-discriminatory
2. establish collaborative partnerships that facilitate and support people with mental health issues to participate in all aspects of their care
3. develop a therapeutic relationship that is respectful of the individual's choices, experiences and circumstances. This involves building on strengths, holding hope and enhancing resilience to promote recovery.
4. collaboratively plan and provide ethically based care consistent with the mental, physical, spiritual, emotional, social and cultural needs of the individual
5. value the contributions of other agencies and stakeholders in the collaborative provision of holistic, evidence-based care and in ensuring comprehensive service provision for people with mental health issues
6. actively pursue opportunities to reduce stigma and promote social inclusion and community participation for all people with mental health issues
7. demonstrate evidence-based practice and actively promote practice innovation through lifelong education, research, professional development, clinical supervision and reflective practice
8. practise, incorporate and reflect common law requirements, relevant statutes and the nursing profession's code of conduct and ethics. The mental health nurse integrates international, national, local and state policies and guidelines with professional standards and competencies.
9. hold specialist qualifications and demonstrate advanced specialist knowledge, skills and practice.

While few would argue with the sentiment of these standards, they are not particularly prescriptive in relation to the skills, knowledge or competencies considered essential for effective and safe mental health nursing practice.

The National Practice Standards for the Mental Health Workforce (of which mental health nurses form a large group) (Department of Health and Ageing 2010) present fifteen standards with associated knowledge, skills and attitudes that are considered essential for the professional groups working in mental health services (nursing, occupational therapy, psychology, psychiatry and social work). These standards are intended to complement, not replace, the specific standards for each professional group.

NATIONAL PRACTICE STANDARDS FOR THE MENTAL HEALTH WORKFORCE

Mental health professionals:

1. promote optimal quality of life for people with a mental health problem and mental disorders
2. focus on service users and the achievement of positive outcomes for them
3. recognise service users', family members' and/or carers' unique physical, emotional, social, cultural and spiritual dimensions, and work with them to develop their own supports in the community
4. learn about and value the lived experiences of service users, family members and/or carers
5. recognise and value the healing potential in the relationship between service users and service providers, and carers and service providers
6. recognise the human rights of people with mental disorders as proclaimed by the UN Principles on the Protection of People with Mental Illness and the Australian Health Ministers' Mental Health Statement of Rights and Responsibilities
7. wherever possible, provide equitable access to appropriate mental health services when and where they are needed, and notify service managers of any gaps in service delivery
8. encourage decision-making by individuals about their treatment and care
9. recognise and support the rights of the child with a parent with a mental health problem and/or mental disorder to appropriate information, care and protection
10. maintain an in-depth knowledge of support services in the community, and develop partnerships with other organisations and service providers to ensure continuity of care
11. involve service users, family members, carers and the local community in mental health service planning, development, implementation and evaluation
12. are aware of and implement best practice and continual quality-improvement processes
13. ensure clinical practice is driven by the evidence base where this exists
14. provide comprehensive, coordinated and individual care that considers all aspects of an individual's recovery
15. participate in professional development activities and reflect these learnings in practice.

CRITICAL THINKING

- What are the essential similarities and differences between these two sets of standards?
- Do you think there should be one set of standards for all mental health professions, or are nursing-specific standards important?

PRACTISING AS A MENTAL HEALTH NURSE

As mentioned in Chapter 1, there is no requirement for specific qualifications or expertise to be mandatory for practice as a mental health nurse. Like many other specialty areas in nursing, postgraduate qualifications in mental health are encouraged but not required. Therefore, we now have a mix of skills and knowledge among nurses working in mental health, and it may not be easy to distinguish between those who have specialist qualifications and those who do not.

The ACMHN has developed a system of credentialling to recognise those who have completed postgraduate qualifications and have otherwise made a commitment to mental health nursing on a professional level. In order to be recognised by the ACMHN as a mental health nurse (and be entitled to use the post-nominals MHN), for those members of the college who choose to do so, a nurse needs to have postgraduate or specialist qualifications in mental health nursing. Other criteria, such as engagement in professional development activities (attendance at conferences, short training courses, clinical supervision) and commitment to the profession (active participation in professional organisations, writing for publication, running training programs), must also be met.

Once credentialled, the MHN needs to demonstrate ongoing commitment and contribution to the profession by showing that they have engaged in enough professional activities to receive the required number of points every three years. Further information about credentialling can be found on the college website at <www.acmhn.org>.

CONCLUSION

The health, safety and welfare of people accessing health services is of primary importance. Because of this, the nursing profession (like other health professions) is highly regulated by specific legislation and influenced by professional standards of practice. Nurses are also influenced by their own set of values and ethical viewpoints. While these are some of the factors that make nursing a fascinating and fulfilling area of practice, they can also create confusion, uncertainty and sometimes discomfort, when nurses find themselves torn between what is expected of them professionally and legally and what they believe to be the right thing to do.

This is particularly so in the case of mental health nursing, where the principle of autonomy is so often called into question and nurses are required to do things to people that often they don't want done. This can be particularly challenging because most people want to become nurses to 'help people'. Hopefully this chapter won't deter you from considering mental health nursing as an area in which to practise, but will help you to appreciate the complexity of this specialist environment.

REFERENCES

Australian and New Zealand College of Mental Health Nurses (ANZCMHN) (2010). *Standards of Practice for Mental Health Nursing*. Canberra: ANZCMHN. Viewed 20 March 2013, <www.acmhn.org/publications/standards-of-practice.html>.

Department of Health and Ageing (2010). *National Standards for Mental Health Services*. Canberra: Commonwealth of Australia. Viewed 20 February 2013, <www.health.gov.au/internet/publications/publishing.nsf/Content/mental-pubs-n-servst10-toc>.

Hayman-White, K., Sgro, S. & Happell, B. (2006). Mental health in Australia: The ideal vs financial reality. *Australian e-Journal for the Advancement of Mental Health*, 5(1), 1–7. Viewed 20 June 2007, <www.auseinet.com/journal/vol5iss1/hayman-white.pdf>.

Johnstone, M.J. (2008). *Bioethics: a nursing perspective* (5th edn). Sydney: Churchill Livingstone.

Molodynski, A., Rugkasa, J. & Burns, T. (2010). Coercion and compulsion in community mental health care, *British Medical Bulletin*, 95: 105–19.

Ryan, C. (2011). One Flu Over the Cuckoo's Nest: comparing legislated coercive treatment for mental illness with that for other illness, *Journal of Bioethical Inquiry*, 8(1), 87–93.

Staunton, P.J. & Chiarella, M. (2013). *Nursing and the Law* (5th edn). Sydney: Elsevier.

PART II

DEFINING AND UNDERSTANDING MENTAL HEALTH PROBLEMS

6

Diagnosing mental illness

Main points

- There are a number of theoretical explanations for mental illness, and no universal agreement regarding causation.
- The identification and diagnosis of mental illness is particularly challenging, as mental illness cannot be observed directly in the same manner as physical illness.
- Complex diagnostic systems have been developed to assist psychiatrists to diagnose mental illness in the absence of clear biological markers.

Definitions

Diagnosis: The determination of the nature and circumstances of an illness or other condition through an examination process.

Labelling: The theory that when a person is given a socially negative label (like being diagnosed as 'mentally ill'), it has the power to 'spoil' identity.

Prejudice: Assumptions or negative judgements made by one person about another person/people that are usually based on stereotypes.

Discrimination: Words, actions, policies, processes, laws, etc. that are based on entrenched notions of inferiority and superiority, often in relation to people's age, gender, class, ethnicity or sexual orientation. Discrimination excludes people from enjoying full citizenship.

INTRODUCTION

To begin this chapter, we ask you to visualise two scenarios that you might experience in your clinical practice, and then to think about the questions that follow. In this chapter, we explore and critique the concept of diagnosis. By now you will be familiar with diagnoses and how they are used in the health-care system. It would be difficult to imagine a hospital or other health-care service functioning without them. Although diagnoses are central to health care and nursing practice, we encourage you to consider them critically and laterally in terms of what they tell you about a person and, more importantly, their limitations. Think about the differences in making diagnoses and planning care for them in the mental health field as opposed to other areas of health care.

SCENARIO 1

You are working in a medical unit on an afternoon shift. When you come in, you see that the staff are very busy—it has been 'one of those days'. Handover is very rushed and plagued with frequent interruptions. There is only time to tell you about the last patient, for whom you will be the primary nurse: 'She is 47 and has been diagnosed with chronic obstructive airways disease.'

Critical thinking

- What is your first reaction?
- What are your images of how the patient will appear when you meet her?
- How will you plan her care?
- What underlying knowledge and principles are guiding your decisions?

SCENARIO 2

You are working in a psychiatric unit on an afternoon shift. When you come in, you see that the staff are very busy—it has been 'one of those days'. Handover is very rushed and plagued with frequent interruptions. There is only time to tell you about the last patient, for whom you will be the primary nurse: 'She is 47 and has been diagnosed with schizophrenia.'

Critical thinking

- What is your first reaction?
- What are your images of how the patient will appear when you meet her?
- How will you plan her care?
- What underlying knowledge and principles are guiding your decisions?

The concept of diagnosis is inherent in the medical model (discussed in Chapter 2). Nevertheless, the classing of particular behavioural patterns commonly associated with mental illness as being abnormal, and seeking to treat the behaviours (at times against the individual's will) in order to restore what professionals (most notably psychiatrists) define as 'normality' has been the subject of criticism (Galasiński & Opaliński 2012).

For example, until 1973, homosexuality was listed as a mental illness in the *Diagnostic and Statistical Manual of Mental Disorders* (DSM) (American Psychiatric Association 2000). This meant that a person could be considered to have a mental illness or disorder purely because their sexual preference was not considered normal or healthy. These assumptions give rise to labelling, which may lead further to prejudice and discrimination.

CRITICAL THINKING

After completing the above exercise, it is useful to reflect on the similarity or differences in your reaction to the two scenarios. The following questions might help to guide your thinking:

- What is the effect of hearing a diagnosis on your thoughts and expectations about a patient?
- Is this thinking different for a physical and a psychiatric diagnosis? If so, in what way?
- What do these differences (if any) mean for the usefulness of diagnoses for physical and psychiatric conditions respectively?

In this chapter, we will explore psychiatric diagnosis from multiple perspectives, including service user, carer, medical and sociological approaches. More specifically, we will address:

- theories of causality of mental illness
- classification of mental illness
- diagnostic systems and processes
- diagnosing mental illness
- labelling theory
- prejudice and discrimination
- implications for nursing.

CAUSATION OF MENTAL ILLNESS

Over time, a number of theories have been developed to explain what causes mental illness. Today, there remains no universally accepted agreement about causation. However, broadly speaking, theories of causation fit into one of three broad categories:

1. the medical model or disease approach
2. psychological theories
3. sociological theories.

THE MEDICAL MODEL OR DISEASE APPROACH

Central to the medical model is the belief that mental illness is in fact an illness, in which distinct patterns of symptoms are observed as the direct result of an altered physical state (Sadock, Sadock & Ruiz 2009). Mental illness is therefore an illness in the same way as a physical disorder such as influenza or cancer. Considerable research activity in the mental health field has focused on determining the precise physical abnormalities that ultimately result in the development of a mental illness. Broadly, it is argued that the development of a mental illness occurs as a result of one of three main factors, discussed below.

Hereditary or genetic factors

Over a long time period, mental health research has sought evidence to demonstrate that mental illness is a genetically determined disorder—that is, it runs in families. Studies using identical twins are considered the most effective, as they allow the research to be conducted with people who have identical genetic makeup. An examination of twin studies found that where one twin developed schizophrenia, the other also did in 47 per cent of cases (Sadock, Sadock & Ruiz 2009). These figures are generally considerably higher than those found with non-identical twins, further strengthening the genetic argument.

Critics of the genetic explanation argue that because there is not a 100 per cent concordance between identical twins, it cannot be a genetically determined disorder. Supporters have subsequently contended that genetics are influencing rather than determining factors. As influencing factors, they place persons with a familial history of mental illness at greater risk. However, other psycho-social factors are likely to determine whether or not this predisposition becomes a reality.

It is also argued that certain results have occurred by chance rather than accurately reflecting a genetic trend. The environmental argument is also used. Just as monozygotic twins are identical in genes, their sameness means they are likely to have as close to the same environmental conditions, and that this—rather than hereditary influences— explains higher rates of concordance.

Organic changes to the brain through illness or injury

The development of a mental illness can occur as a result of injury (i.e. head injury) or illness (e.g. Parkinson's Disease). The emphasis is to treat the underlying cause as a primary focus and the symptoms of mental illness as a secondary focus.

Altered physiological functioning (e.g. nervous system disorders)

In a notable example, the dopamine hypothesis has been advanced as an explanation for the development of schizophrenia (Howes et al. 2012). Schizophrenia is believed to result from an increase in the neurotransmitter dopamine. The validity of this theory is strengthened by the effectiveness of anti-psychotic medication, which tends to block the dopamine receptors and subsequently decrease the activity of the excess dopamine. That is, dopamine inhibitors reduce the symptoms of schizophrenia, which logically leads to the conclusion that excessive dopamine is the cause of schizophrenia. However, it has also been argued that excessive dopamine is a response to the real cause of schizophrenia, which could just as easily be a psychological or sociological factor. Take, for example, the hormone adrenaline. An increase in adrenaline occurs when people experience heightened levels of fear or anxiety. It is likely that people who experience anxiety disorders would have higher levels of adrenaline than those who do not. If we followed the dopamine argument, it might be hypothesised that anxiety disorders are caused by excessive adrenaline rather than as a response to fear.

PSYCHOLOGICAL THEORIES

Psycho-social theories arise from the view that personality influences behaviour (see Chapter 2). Just as physical status can range from healthy to unhealthy, psychologists refer to a range in personalities from the healthy or normal state to the unhealthy or abnormal. A so-called 'normal' personality generally is equated with living a happy and fulfilling life, having the capacity to maintain effective social, personal and occupational relationships and, overall, a sense that one fits in with the broader environment.

Personalities described as abnormal or deviant, on the other hand, generally are associated with people who do not fit in as a result of their behaviours and actions. This abnormality tends to be observed as delinquent, anti-social, criminal behaviour, or can be manifested through the symptoms of mental illness.

There exists a diversity of psychological theories of human behaviour, some of which you may have studied in psychology. This section provides a brief overview of some of the major psychological theories and how they are used to explain the existence of mental illness, including psychoanalytic theory, behavioural psychology, cognitive psychology and humanistic psychology.

Psychoanalytic theory

Sigmund Freud led the development of psychoanalytic theory. Although he has been the subject of considerable criticism, Freud revolutionised the study of human beings and behaviour by describing the psyche as comprising the id, the ego and the superego, referred to overall as the unconscious. Freud's work implied that people could have thoughts and emotions of which they were unaware, but that could profoundly influence their conscious thoughts and behaviour. Unconscious thoughts generally are those that make us feel uncomfortable or ashamed.

In order to protect our conscious minds, Freud theorised that all people utilise a number of unconscious defence mechanisms. These mechanisms conceal unwanted thoughts and urges, or provide an explanation for them while protecting the conscious mind from the real cause or issue—and from intolerable levels of anxiety that these processes can induce. However, there is a limit to the effectiveness of the defence mechanisms, and they go on in turn to also influence thought and human action.

One psychoanalytical explanation for mental illness is the inability of the defence mechanism to protect the unconscious from unacceptable thoughts. This disharmony leads to the development of the symptoms of mental illness, such as psychosis, anxiety or depression.

Behavioural psychology

Some of you may have heard of Pavlov's dog. Pavlov conducted an experiment where he would ring a bell at the time of feeding his dog. Initially, the dog would begin to salivate at the sight of the food. After some time, the ringing of the bell was itself sufficient to cause the dog to salivate. This process, known as 'classical conditioning', demonstrated a direct relationship between the stimulus (bell) and the response (salivation).

CRITICAL THINKING

Imagine that you fail an assignment in your course. It is an assignment into which you have put a lot of work. Overall, you have been getting good marks and this result comes as a huge shock. You might react to this in a number of ways. For example, you may consider that the course is too hard for you and other assignments have been marked too easily; feel you produced high-quality work but misunderstood the question; or believe that the academic who marked your assignment doesn't like you and marked you down because of that. You may be able to add further possibilities to this list.

* What defence mechanisms are at work here?
* How does the way we view a situation affect how we then deal with it?

Table 6.1 Overview of the defence mechanisms

Defence mechanism	Definition
Repression	Experiences or thoughts that a person cannot cope with are removed from conscious thought—for example, a child who witnesses the murder of a parent.
Regression	The person moves back to earlier stages of development to respond to a problem—for example, throwing tantrums when not being taken seriously in a social interaction.
Denial	There is no acknowledgement that something has occurred—for example, a recently separated woman believes her husband will return to her.
Sublimation	Unacceptable thoughts are channelled into more socially acceptable activities—for example, the boy who has thoughts of harming his sister achieves expression through art.
Rationalisation	A socially acceptable explanation is given for a less acceptable action—for example, 'I didn't complete my assignment on time because the topic was really boring'.
Intellectualisation	The person removes their feelings from the occurrence—for example, 'I don't care that Sally won't go out with me. I didn't really like her anyway'.
Displacement	Feelings towards a person or situation are directed towards a more acceptable target—for example, a man who is belittled by his boss says nothing, but goes home and yells at his wife because the dinner is cold.
Projection	One's own emotions or feelings are attributed to someone else—for example, a boss who feels uncomfortable with her own skill level accuses a subordinate of being incompetent.
Reaction formation	A person develops a personality trait opposite to the one the person is trying to hide—for example, a father who has physically harmed his children joins a children's rights group.

While the same scenario could not be expected with humans, B.F. Skinner considered that people behaved in particular ways in response to reinforcers. Where reinforcers are positive, people are likely to continue the behaviour that produces them, while negative reinforcers are more likely to encourage the person to stop that behaviour. This process is known as 'operant conditioning'. B.F. Skinner believed that these basic principles could be used both to explain and alter undesirable or pathological behaviour (Santrock 2009). In terms of explanation, a person who has developed a mental illness may have done so because they behaved in ways considered abnormal or inappropriate but were rewarded for doing so.

As stated, B.F. Skinner believed operant conditioning could also be used to alter behaviour. Subsequently, the behavioural theories tend to focus on altering the stimulus in order to change behaviour. Various critiques have been mounted against Skinner's behaviourism, mainly because humans are much more complex than rats or dogs and it is problematic to think of human being and action as mere 'behaviour'.

In the case of Nathan (see case study below), Skinner would advise the parents and significant others not to respond to his injurious practices. Rewards should be provided when Nathan responds appropriately to the situation—for example, when he plays sport with his colleagues or mends the back fence for his partner.

CASE STUDY

As a young child, Nathan did not have any aptitude for or interest in sport and practical hobbies. Whenever he was expected to play sport, he would deliberately hurt himself. His parents would coddle him, and not only didn't he have to play sport, but he usually received a present. Once he attended school, Nathan found it harder to impress teachers in the same way, so his self-harming behaviour intensified. He would deliberately cut himself quite deeply on the arms or legs and cry in pain. If teachers attempted to force Nathan to contribute in any way, he would tell his parents. His parents would heap sympathy on Nathan and would contact the school principal. As Nathan continued through high school and into the workforce, he would use self-injury as a means to avoid activities he did not like. Over time, this affected his study, employment and relationships. After the breakdown of a two-year relationship, Nathan went to saw a psychiatrist and was diagnosed with avoidant personality disorder.

Critical thinking

Reflect on Nathan's situation and consider the concept of operant conditioning.

- What was the stimulus?
- What was the response?
- How has the stimulus led to the response?
- How might you alter the stimulus to alter the response?

Cognitive psychology

Where the behavioural model focuses on external factors as the primary influence on behaviour, the cognitive model focuses on the internal processes. People are viewed as more actively involved in determining their behaviours and opinions. They take in information from external stimuli, but they subsequently interpret the information in a particular way. The way in which the person interprets information will then determine how they behave.

The cognitive therapist works on the assumption that behaviour will not change for any period of time unless thinking changes. The cognitive therapist will therefore encourage the client to examine and challenge irrational or unhelpful thought patterns.

Humanistic psychology

Humanistic psychology conceptualises humans as whole beings, and for that reason is a theoretical model that is well suited to nursing, with a strong emphasis on holistic care (see Maslow's hierarchy of needs in Chapter 2). This model poses three main categories of need, moving from the basic physiological needs for survival, through psychological needs for belonging and self-esteem, to self-actualisation where the person is able to achieve their true potential for creativity and development. In order to achieve self-actualisation, physical and psychological needs must first be adequately met. Mental illness would be seen as a consequence of unmet need in the psychological stages. A positive and supportive environment would therefore form a major component of any approach to care and treatment.

SOCIOLOGICAL MODELS

Sociological models focus on the impact of broader societal factors on the individual. In relation to mental illness, factors such as gender, age, education level, occupation, socio-political history, socio-economic status and geographical location have been found to influence the prevalence of specific diagnoses of mental illness. For example, anxiety disorders are considered more common for women while substance abuse disorders are more commonly found in men.

CRITICAL THINKING
Why do you think that women more often experience anxiety while men more commonly abuse substances?

THE BIO–PSYCHO–SOCIAL MODEL

The medical, psychological and sociological models have all been the subject of considerable critique, particularly as they do not explain why some people develop a mental illness and others do not. For example, none of the twin studies has demonstrated a 100 per cent concordance between identical twins. Similar criticisms are made of psychological models (Santrock 2009). Take, for example, the case of Nathan discussed above. Many children may experience a similar upbringing, but react in completely different ways. Sociological models are no better able to provide a definitive explanation. While gender might be seen to be an influence, it is not a determinant: not all women develop anxiety disorders.

However, most of us would identify some merit in all of these approaches. This thinking has led to the popularity of the bio-psycho-social model, which recognises the influence of a multitude of factors on each unique individual (see Chapter 2). Logically, these factors should also be considered in appreciating each individual's response to mental illness and in planning their care and treatment.

CLASSIFICATION OF MENTAL ILLNESS
Why classify mental illness?
Classification of mental illness is of particular benefit to the medical model approach to care and treatment. Psychiatrists argue that the classification and diagnosis of mental illness are essential for ensuring the provision of optimal care and treatment. However, its usefulness extends beyond the care of specific individuals. It provides a framework for the collection of statistical information that can be analysed to increase our understanding of aspects of mental illness, such as prevalence, aetiology and course of illness.

Critics of the medical model suggest that classification of mental illness legitimises psychiatry as a medical specialty (Read, Mosher & Bentall 2004). It replaces diagnostic tests and examinations by categorising groups of behaviours as symptoms of specific conditions. In the absence of physical markers of disease, diagnosis of mental illness involves subjective judgements about whether or not characteristics or behaviours are 'acceptable'. These circumstances mean that medical model psychiatry is far from scientific, and accounts for the variety of diagnoses with which one person might be labelled during their 'psychiatric career'.

Classification systems
There are two main systems for the classification of mental illness:

1. *International Classification of Diseases and Health Related Disorders* version 10 (ICD-10). This is a World Health Organization (WHO) publication. It also includes physical disorders.
2. *Diagnostic and Statistical Manual of Mental Disorders* (DSM-IV-TR). This is produced by the American Psychiatric Association, and refers specifically to classification of mental illness.

History
The ICD did not include mental illnesses until the production of version 6 in 1950. However, the American Psychiatric Association was dissatisfied with the classification of mental illness by ICD and introduced the first version of the DSM in 1952.

Subsequent revisions of DSM have related to revisions of ICD. DSM-IV-TR is now fully compatible with ICD-10. This helps to ensure uniformity in diagnosis and statistical information between individuals and across countries.

DSM-V
The most recent edition was released in May 2013. It has been nearly fourteen years in the making—further evidence that portraying behaviour and actions as indicative of mental illness is a problematic exercise. The main differences expected in the new volume include:

- *Changes to diagnostic categories.* For example, 'autism spectrum disorders' will be used as an umbrella for the following illnesses: autistic disorders, Asperger's Syndrome, childhood disintegrative disorder and pervasive developmental disorder (not otherwise specified).
- *Changes to the name of disorders.* For example, gender incongruence has become gender dysphoria.
- *The creation of a new category of 'behavioural addictions'.* Gambling is currently the only disorder.
- The inclusion of scale to more accurately identify those most at risk of suicide.
- *Changes in language*—for example, from 'mental retardation' to 'intellectual disability' to reflect contemporary terminology.
- A stronger focus on how gender, age and ethnicity may influence the identification and diagnosis of mental illness.

Updated information can be found at <www.dsm5.org>.

DSM-IV-TR
This is the classification system most commonly used in most states and territories of Australia. The information in DSM includes:

- diagnostic features (including diagnostic criteria)
- brief descriptions of sub-types
- recording procedures—numerical codes collected for statistical purposes
- associated features, including:
  - clinical features (these are common but not essential for a diagnosis to be made)
  - laboratory findings: diagnostic and those commonly associated with the condition but not diagnostic
- complications of disorder (e.g. substance abuse)
- physical examination and general medical findings (significant but not essential to diagnosis):
  - culture, age and gender features
  - prevalence

   – course of illness
   – familial pattern
   – possible differential diagnoses.

WORKING THROUGH THE *DIAGNOSTIC MANUAL*

Disorders are grouped into sixteen main classes according to common features:

1. disorders usually first diagnosed in infancy, childhood or adolescence
2. delirium, dementia, amnesic and other cognitive disorders
3. mental disorders due to a general medical condition not elsewhere classified
4. substance-related disorders
5. schizophrenia and other psychotic disorders
6. mood disorders
7. anxiety disorders
8. somatoform disorders
9. factitious disorders
10. dissociative disorders
11. sexual and gender identity disorders
12. eating disorders
13. sleep disorders
14. impulse-control disorders not elsewhere classified
15. adjustment disorders
16. personality disorders.

SEVERITY OF DISORDER

As is the case with physical disorders, mental illness is considered to vary in its severity according to certain factors. Generally, conditions range from mild to severe:

- *Mild*: Few (if any) more symptoms than those required for diagnosis. Minimal impairment to social or occupational functioning.
- *Moderate*: Symptoms and impairment ranked between mild and severe.
- *Severe*: Many symptoms in addition to those required for diagnosis. Severe impairment to social and/or occupational functioning.

Furthermore, the illness can be considered to be:

- *In partial remission*: Full criteria for diagnosis was previously met, but only some signs or symptoms are currently evident.
- *In full remission or recovered*: No signs and symptoms currently present, but still clinically relevant to note the disorder. Describing the state as in full remission instead of recovered depends on:

- the usual course of the illness for that individual person
- length of time since last episode
- total duration of disorder
- need for ongoing monitoring or prophylactic treatment.

MULTI-AXIAL ASSESSMENT

DSM-IV-TR divides information relevant to clinical diagnosis into five axes. The aim of multi-axial assessment is to facilitate thorough, comprehensive and systematic evaluation of the person's condition, ensuring that all aspects of the person's health, well-being and functioning are considered, rather than simply focusing on psychiatric symptomatology:

Axes 1–3

- Axis 1: Clinical disorders
- Axis 2: Personality disorders
- Axis 3: General medical conditions

These include conditions relevant to the cause or management of the person's mental illness. For example:

- complications of pregnancy or childbirth that might increase the risk of postpartum psychosis
- medical conditions that might be exacerbated by treatment of certain mental illness (e.g. diabetes).

Axis 4 Psychological and environmental problems

This axis includes:

- problems that may have contributed to the development or exacerbation of mental illness (e.g. traumatic event, sexual abuse)
- problems developing as a result of the mental disorder (e.g. isolation, loneliness)
- problems to be considered in terms of the person's individual management plan, such as:
    - housing and financial problems
    - legal problems
    - employment or educational problems
    - problems with family and primary support group relationships
    - views about any prior experiences with mental health services.

Axis 5 Global assessment of functioning

This is measured with the Global Assessment of Functioning (GAF) scale. Initially, this scale is used to determine a treatment plan. It is then generally used to determine the effect of treatment.

The GAF is scored from 1 to 100:

- A score between 1 and 10 suggests a persistent danger that the person will severely hurt themself or others, or a persistent inability to maintain minimal personal hygiene, or a serious suicidal act with clear expectation of death.
- At the other end, a score between 91 and 100 indicates 'superior' functioning in a wide range of activities; the person is able to cope effectively with life's problems. No symptoms of mental illness are evident. However, not many of us are ever likely to attain this—a score of approximately 65 would be accepted as a level of functioning within the community.

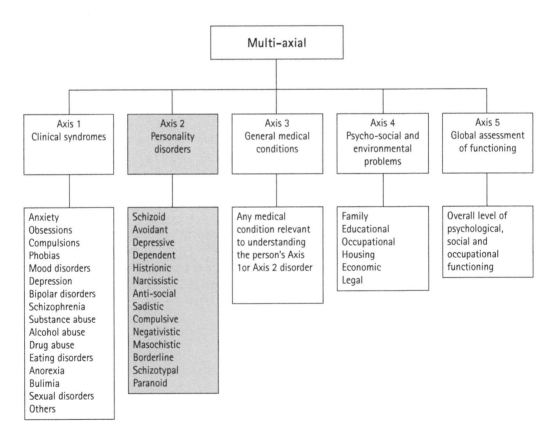

Figure 6.1 Multi-axial assessment

Source: Adapted from Millon & Davis (2000, p. 6).

USING MULTI-AXIAL ASSESSMENT

CLINICAL EXAMPLE: TERRY

Terry is a 37-year-old man. He is currently unemployed and has not had secure employment for four years since losing his job as a sales manager. Terry had difficulty finding a new job and increasingly became withdrawn, spending significant periods alone. After six months of job-seeking, he stopped actively looking for work, stating there was no point as he was no longer good enough to get a job, although on one occasion he told his wife he was becoming demoralised by attending interviews but not being selected (which he later denied). Terry's wife left him two years ago because she felt 'nothing I do or say makes any difference and I feel like I'm living with a corpse who breathes'. Their divorce had become final three months earlier, putting an end to Terry's hope that she would eventually return to him. Terry now lives in a small flat, does not have a phone and continually finds excuses not to accept invitations from friends and family, and now he rarely receives them. Since his divorce, Terry has not been attending to his personal hygiene, he has experienced a loss of appetite and he rarely eats more than one meal per day. Terry is feeling that his life has no purpose, and experiences recurring suicidal thoughts; he has begun to think about how he would end his life.

Terry's clinical assessment

- Axis 1:   Major depressive disorder
- Axis 2:   Avoidant personality disorder
- Axis 3:   Nil diagnosed
- Axis 4:   Divorced (recently), unemployed
- Axis 5:   Score 26

Comments: Remains isolated, preoccupied with suicidal thoughts.

Critical thinking

Consider Terry's situation and diagnoses.

- To what extent do you think that being unemployed and recently divorced might explain feelings of depression, suicidality and wanting to avoid interacting with other people?
- How do you think Terry might react to a diagnosis of major depression and avoidant personality disorder?
- If you, or a person close to you, were in this position, what do you think you would consider to be most helpful?
- How might you encourage Terry to focus on his strengths in order to feel more positive about his future?

CLINICAL EXAMPLE: JANINE

Janine is a 23-year-old unemployed single female. She was referred to mental health services by her parents after being expelled from university. Janine's parents described her as a bright and happy child. She loved school and was considered a model student by her teachers. After completing high school, Janine was accepted to study law at university. In her first year, she did very well academically; however, she did not socialise much and became increasingly withdrawn and isolated. After her first year, Janine's academic performance declined steadily. She was referred to the university counselling service, where she first expressed her concern that people were talking about her. She remained enrolled at university, although she rarely attended classes and did not complete the required work. When she was finally expelled from university due to unsatisfactory progress, she claimed she had been victimised for being different and stopped communicating with her family. On examination, it was found that Janine had a medical condition that had resulted in significant hearing loss; it was likely that this had occurred gradually over a number of years.

Janine's clinical assessment

- Axis 1:   Nil diagnosed
- Axis 2:   Paranoid personality disorder
- Axis 3:   Severe hearing impairment
- Axis 4:   Academic problems, unemployed
- Axis 5:   Score 39

Comments: Tends to be isolated, avoids people.

Critical thinking

Consider Janine's situation and diagnoses:

- Have you ever had a significant hearing impairment? If so, reflect for a moment on how this affected your interactions with others. If not, think about how you interact with people with hearing problems—for example, are you less likely to talk to them if they continually ask you to repeat yourself?
- What impact do you think a severe hearing impairment might have on a person's mental state?
- What impact might the severe hearing impairment have on academic achievement and other aspects of global functioning?
- Would medical treatment be likely to resolve Janine's problems?
- How might you encourage Janine to recognise and build upon her strengths?

Think about the two preceding examples. From the information presented, are you confident that the two people have a mental illness? What factors are influencing your decisions?

MULTIPLE DIAGNOSES

Just as a person can be diagnosed with a physical disorder and a mental illness, so a person can receive more than one diagnosis of mental illness. In the case of a mental illness and a substance abuse disorder, this is frequently referred to as dual diagnosis, or dual disability in the case of mental illness and intellectual disability.

In these instances, the primary diagnosis is listed first. This generally refers to the condition that is considered to be most in need of treatment (American Psychiatric Association 2000). Subsequent diagnoses are listed in order of the focus of attention and treatment. For example:

- Principal diagnosis: Schizophrenia
- Other diagnoses: Alcohol abuse
                          Intellectual disability

Provisional diagnoses

As the name suggests, a provisional diagnosis is used when there is not enough information currently available for a definitive diagnosis, but there are reasonable grounds to presume this diagnosis will be made.

DIAGNOSING MENTAL ILLNESS

As stated earlier in this chapter, the symptoms of mental illness cannot be observed through laboratory testing. The only way for a psychiatrist to determine whether a person has a mental illness according to DSM-IV-TR is to conduct a psychiatric interview. Like the diagnosis of physical conditions, it is based on signs and symptoms. Symptoms are determined by asking a series of questions to elicit information. This process is generally structured and sequential, and includes the following:

- *Reason for referral*—including who made the referral and for what reasons. The extent to which the individual being assessed was willingly involved in the referral is determined.
- *Current situation*—such as marital status, employment status, accommodation.
- *Presenting problem*—as described by the individual. This is where the person describes the circumstances leading to the assessment from their own perspective.
- *History of presenting problem*—this refers to the attempt to determine when the signs and symptoms of the illness first became apparent. Where the onset is abrupt

and sudden, this can be relatively simple to determine, but it is significantly more difficult when the illness has developed slowly over months or even years.

- *Family history*—this section attempts to capture an extensive picture of the family of origin, and consists of two main parts: first, the existence or otherwise of living family members and the quality of the relationship with them; and second, a history of medical and/or psychiatric illness, with particular interest in determining genetic risk factors for mental illness.
- *Personal history*—a thorough history is sought, including education, employment, marriage and relationships, sexual history, children, legal history and previous physical and psychiatric illness. (Adapted from Epstein et al. 2012, pp. 345–7).

Similar information is often sought from family members and significant others.

In addition, the clinician will observe the behaviour of the individual, particularly following the completion of the mental state assessment (see Chapter 5). Here the clinician observes factors such as the appearance and behaviour of the person to determine whether or not they meet the diagnostic criteria for a mental illness. Because the presence of a mental illness cannot be observed visually in the same way that, for example, a bone fracture can, diagnosis is made on the basis of the clinician's judgement.

LIMITATIONS OF DSM

There is, and has historically been, great fear surrounding the concept of madness (Lakeman 2006). Moreover, to experience unusual thoughts can be very frightening and confusing; it is not straightforward. While a bone break might follow a predictable path from the time it is treated to the time it has mended, in real life no two people with the same psychiatric diagnosis will experience it the same way. In addition, while diagnoses indicate what treatments will be tried, individuals will respond very differently.

The criticisms posed by anti-psychiatry can be either connected to the treatments imposed by psychiatry—or what is seen as the 'myth of mental illness', where psychiatry is seen to be 'posing' as a medical science. Indeed, during the 1960s there was a strong movement known as 'anti-psychiatry' that disputed the very notion of mental illness. One of the pioneers of this movement, Thomas Szasz, argued that the concept of mental illness could not be substantiated unless it could be identified and verified scientifically—like physical diseases. Szasz viewed mental illness as a term used to describe behaviour which is disturbing to the individual or to the community around them. The diagnosis is being used primarily as a system of social control (Szasz 1974). In short, Szasz did not acknowledge any use for the discipline of psychiatry: unacceptable behaviour should be either tolerated or dealt with through legal means. The deprivation of freedom and intent to change behaviour that occurred as part of psychiatric treatment was viewed as immoral (Szasz 1974).

The desire of African American slaves to flee captivity was once considered a mental illness, Drapetomania (Wikipedia n.d.). Recommended treatment was amputation of the toes and whipping. With our modern 'eye', we can clearly see this for the institutionalised racism it is. However, what about a 'treatment' for extreme sadness that relies on electric shock—the scientific explanation for the apparent efficacy of which is not fully known? Can we imagine looking back in a hundred years' time with a different social view of this treatment, which is often given without the consent of the individual receiving it?

It has been relatively easy to attack psychiatry on this level—there are as yet no 'proven' organic causes for mental illness. It is also clear that prejudicial social reactions towards people who have been diagnosed with mental illness can have an impact on all opportunities in life, such as employment, housing, education and health care, and that discrimination can be a factor in people's lives with which they must deal on top of any problems of living they may face.

Recent public health promotion campaigns have focused on the idea that mental illness is just like any other illness, and can be treated effectively with medications. The concept behind these campaigns was to try to combat the social discrimination (stigma) that often accompanies a psychiatric label. In truth, though, 'mental illness' is not 'just like any other illness'—if for no other reason than that most illnesses do not attract social stigma, but rather typically engender a sympathetic response. Indeed, it has been argued that such public campaigns would be more effective if they were to avoid the use of illness/disease terminology and instead target discrimination (Read, Mosher & Bentall 2004). If you can appreciate the ways in which social discrimination plays a significant part in the lives of many people diagnosed with mental illness, this will stand you in good stead.

LABELLING

A psychological research study conducted by David Rosenhan in the 1970s showed that when eight ordinary people, termed 'pseudo patients', presented to a psychiatric hospital complaining of hearing voices, all were assessed, diagnosed and treated as though they had a mental disorder. Even though each 'pseudo patient' was to cease reporting hearing voices upon admission, all were held as in-patients, on average for nineteen days (Rosenhan 1973). The criticism frequently levelled at psychiatry is that it is imprecise, and this experiment not only highlighted this but also highlighted how, once somebody is diagnosed, all behaviour tends to become viewed as an associated pathology. Labelling theory contends that once a person has been given a psychiatric label, all other behaviours are viewed through this lens. The service user literature abounds with clear understanding of how this happens and what it feels like. The following poem highlights this:

YOU AND ME

by Debbie Sesula

If you're overly excited
You're happy
If I'm overly excited
I'm manic.
If you imagine the phone ringing
You're stressed out
If I imagine the phone ringing
I'm psychotic.
If you're crying and sleeping all day
You're sad and need time out
If I'm crying and sleeping all day
I'm depressed and need to get up.
If you're afraid to leave your house at night
You're cautious
If I'm afraid to leave my house at night
I'm paranoid.
If you speak your mind and express your opinions
You're assertive
If I speak my mind and express my opinions
I'm aggressive.
If you don't like something and mention it
You're being honest
If I don't like something and mention it
I'm being difficult.
If you get angry
You're considered upset
If I get angry
I'm considered dangerous.
If you over-react to something
You're sensitive
If I over-react to something
I'm out of control.
If you don't want to be around others
You're taking care of yourself and relaxing
If I don't want to be around others
I'm isolating myself and avoiding.

> If you talk to strangers
> You're being friendly
> If I talk to strangers
> I'm being inappropriate.
> For all of the above you're not told to take a
> pill or are hospitalized, but I am!
>
> (Sesula n.d.)

It is likely we have all experienced being labelled and having our behaviour inter-preted as reflecting the label given. One example commonly experienced by women relates to premenstrual tension (PMT). It is not uncommon for the behaviour of a female to be dismissed on the basis of PMT, and this is used as an excuse not to have to take it seriously. Not only can this suggest that the thoughts and/or actions of women experiencing PMT do not need to be considered, but female readers will almost certainly be able to recount instances of being accused of having PMT even when they do not—and the accuser would have no way of knowing their current menstrual patterns in any case.

An example for male readers relates to your choice of profession. It is likely that you have been criticised for choosing nursing as a career, and possible that you have been accused of being gay. Whether or not you are gay, this amounts to labelling. It reflects a stereotypical view that suggests that masculinity and the caring aspects of nursing are incompatible, and therefore men who choose to be nurses must be gay. It also implies that gay men choose to be nurses because they are gay, rather than any other factors that might have attracted them to nursing. In short, it is based on the assumption that what we are influences what we do.

One of the dangers of relying on a classification system to analyse observable behaviour is that it is not of itself beneficial—it says nothing about what it might feel like for the person, or what might best be done to help that person on an individual level. There is growing interest in understanding the role that trauma plays in the lives of people who are diagnosed with mental illness. This is something that can be under-stood and worked on with an individual. An approach to care that takes account of the nature of trauma in people's lives is very useful. Such an approach can include an appreciation of any trauma associated with people's prior or current experiences of receiving psychiatric care, particularly if people have or are being treated without consent.

CRITICAL THINKING

Consider a situation where you have been labelled, and subsequently treated according to that label.

- How did you feel about this?
- How did it affect your relationship with the person(s) who gave the label?
- Did the experience alter your behaviour in any way?
- What have you learnt from this experience that might influence your nursing practice?
- To what extent are we labelling traumatic experiences as a sickness?

It is also useful to try to appreciate what life is like for someone who might hear voices, or who sees things that you cannot see. Rather than being fearful, it can be helpful to try to find out how the person feels about what they are experiencing. They may themselves be confused or frightened, but they might not be—it is good not to assume, but rather to try to find out directly from the person how they feel.

WHAT DOES THIS MEAN FOR THE PRACTITIONER?

Whether or not psychiatry is a 'real' science is open to debate. Because mental health nursing is about caring for people when they are most in need, what matters most is your ability to be approachable, and to respond to service users with compassion and without fear or judgement. Drawing on the attributes that make you a good spouse, friend, parent, son or daughter will be just as useful to you in mental health nursing as your clinical knowledge.

Classification systems are intended as a guide only, and are always expected to be used within the context of clinical judgement. However, classification systems have been criticised for pathologising certain types of behaviour that are not considered acceptable to the broader community. In light of discussions of anti-psychiatry earlier in this chapter, the development of classification systems may be viewed as psychiatry's quest to develop 'objective' markers to signify the existence of a mental illness. However, the challenge to be considered is the extent to which behaviour that might be considered odd or unusual can be seen as symptomatic of mental illness.

PREJUDICE

Prejudice describes assumptions or negative judgements made about a person/people that are usually based on stereotypes. 'The mad professor', 'the eccentric aunt', 'the axe-wielding psychopath', 'the grumpy old man' are some well-known archetypal descriptions. The feelings and attitudes we have about people are inevitably influenced by what we believe. Sometimes we are not even certain where our beliefs come from, but some are gained from mass media, or from our cultural context, or from knowing one person and making generalisations from that. It is important that we try not to be influenced by stereotypical thinking, and that we examine where such ideas come from. Try the short quiz below.

For instance, the idea that most service users must be violent and dangerous is a belief that obviously has an impact on social thinking, on law-making and on the professions that might be involved with people diagnosed with mental illness; most importantly, though, it has an impact on the person whom it describes. All prejudice can have internal and external ramifications. To be thought of as dangerous might make it more difficult to try to form friendships (internal effect). If an employer is driven by a belief that people diagnosed with mental illness are dangerous, the employer is unlikely to employ that person (external effect).

When somebody comes under the provisions of mental health legislation, they are not considered competent to make decisions about their own health and well-being. Service users often report being treated like children, and this can be a direct consequence of being thought of as incompetent.

IMPLICATIONS FOR NURSING PRACTICE

If, as a nurse, you come to believe in the service user's incompetence as an all-encompassing and lasting state, this will become a prejudicial attitude affecting how you think about and treat that person. There is a danger, too, that the service user also will view themself as wholly incompetent. This has deep consequences for the person's sense of agency in the world, and their sense of hope and optimism. Prejudice is often hidden—even from ourselves—and it can take courage to face up to knowledge that we don't want to own up to. This is another reason why it is so important in mental health care to be able to reflect on one's own practice.

QUIZ
Which of the following statements are true?

1. People diagnosed with mental illnesses are more likely to be violent than other people.
2. People diagnosed with mental illnesses have general health conditions on a par with Indigenous Australians.
3. An estimated 50–70 per cent of women who come to the attention of mental health services have a background of sexual/physical abuse.
4. People diagnosed with mental illness are likely to have a low IQ.

5. Mental illness is not something from which people are likely to recover.
6. Schizophrenia means having a split personality.
7. People who are depressed need to be dealt with firmly, so they can snap out of it and get on with their life.

(For the answers to this quiz, see the end of the chapter.)

DISCRIMINATION

Discrimination results from prejudice at the individual, structural, institutional and socio-political levels. At an individual level, discrimination can affect people diagnosed with mental illness in key areas of life, such as access to housing, access to the jobs market, access to good physical health care and access to training and education opportunities.

Discrimination can be experienced by the individual in a direct or indirect way. Direct discrimination would be where a person is treated less favourably because of their disability. An example of indirect discrimination towards somebody diagnosed with a mental illness would be where an employer does not make the reasonable adjustments to the workplace that the employee would need in order to carry out their role. On the face of it, the expectations that the employer has are equal for everyone; however, in reality somebody with a disability could not be expected to perform at their best without reasonable adjustments to the workplace.

Discrimination can also occur at the level of our institutions and laws. For instance, using a human rights framework, it is possible to argue that our mental health legislation is discriminatory against people with a diagnosis of mental illness, because it does not support the right to refuse medical treatment—which all other citizens are entitled to do.

CASE STUDY

Jenny is a 22-year-old woman who believes in reincarnation through ancestral lines. Indeed, she is convinced that she is in fact her great-grandmother reincarnated. Through a process of guided meditation, she learns that her great-grandmother was physically abused by a male relative and, although Jenny has not had the same experience, she carries the scars of her great-grandmother: she has the same fears and the same difficulties in establishing and maintaining relationships with men. Jenny is seeking spiritual counselling as the only means to ensure these problems are resolved, because she believes that if they are not they will be passed on to future generations of females indefinitely.

> **CRITICAL THINKING**
>
> - Do you think that Jenny has a mental illness?
> - Do you think she should be encouraged, or even forced to seek treatment?
> - What other explanations might you offer for her beliefs and experiences?
> - Would your responses be different if Jenny was part of a recognised religious or spiritual group whose members shared these beliefs?
> - Who do you think is best placed to determine what is best for Jenny?

CULTURAL CONSIDERATIONS

Attempts to classify mental illness as universal phenomena are rightly criticised for failing to reflect cultural sensitivities (Cox 2009, 2010). As we know, there are many and diverse cultural backgrounds, each of which is followed to varying degrees by those who may identify with it. Even the most sensitive and conscientious health professional could not possibly be expected to be familiar with all of them. It is for this very pragmatic reason that this text adopts the approach of cultural safety, which does not require nurses to be experts in any other culture apart from their own. What is expected is that nurses treat clients according to their needs and in a way which does not deny, devalue or put them down. Rather, nursing professionals are required to respect the cultural identity of a client as the client expresses and experiences it, not according to some static stereotypical view of a culture that a nurse might have learnt about.

For example, what is considered acceptable in one cultural context might well be defined as a symptom of a mental illness by the culture of medical-model psychiatry. For example, some Christian Australians might practise exorcism to dispel the evil spirit that they view as causing the very signs and symptoms that medical-model psychiatry will attempt to dispel with anti-psychotic medication. Such activities as exorcism might be interpreted as further evidence of psychoses in psychiatry.

The recognition of diverse cultural contexts and experiences, and their impact on an individual's beliefs and behaviours, has been acknowledged in the *National Standards for the Mental Health Workforce* (Department of Health and Ageing 2010). In accordance with these standards, mental health professionals are expected to acknowledge diversity on a number of levels, including culture. While nurses cannot be expected to know the intricate details of the norms and values of the many cultural groups that currently reside in Australia, they can nevertheless be culturally self-aware and sensitive to the fact that cultural differences are both real and legitimate (see Chapter 14). Importantly, seemingly odd behaviour should not automatically be interpreted as symptomatic of mental illness. Readers are referred to Chapter 14 for an extended discussion of cultural safety, case examples and activities.

CONCLUSION

There remains a lack of clear agreement about the causes of mental illness, or even whether mental illness exists. The fact that mental illness cannot be observed in the same manner as a physical disorder has led to the development of classification systems to aid the diagnosis of mental illnesses. However, classification systems rely on clinician interpretation and judgement about what is and isn't 'normal' or 'acceptable' behaviour. Prejudice, discrimination and the labelling of people as 'mentally ill' so that everything about the person is viewed through a pathological lens are unnecessary social factors that can contribute directly to a person's difficulties.

ANSWERS TO QUIZ

1. The answer is false. In fact, people diagnosed with mental illness are more likely to be the victims of violence. If you wanted to select a section of the population that is statistically more likely to be perpetrators of violence, it would be young males who have consumed alcohol.
2. The answer is true.
3. The answer is true.
4. The answer is false.
5. The answer is false.
6. The answer is false. The image of 'Dr Jekyll and Mr Hyde' was popularised in fiction and film, and bears no relation to modern classifications of symptoms experienced by people with a diagnosis of schizophrenia.
7. The answer is false. Clinical 'depression' describes something more profound than a state where the individual is able to exercise control over what they are feeling and the way in which they deal with it.

REFERENCES

American Psychiatric Association (2000). *Diagnostic and Statistical Manual of Mental Disorders: DSM-IV-TR* (4th edn text revision). Washington DC: APA.

Cox, L. (2009). Queensland Aborigines, multiple realities and the social sources of suffering: psychiatry and moral regions of being. *Oceania*, 79(2), 97–120.

—— (2010). Queensland Aborigines, multiple realities and the social sources of suffering: psychiatry and moral regions of being, Part 2. *Oceania*, 80, 3.

Department of Health and Ageing (2010). *National Practice Standards for the Mental Health Workforce.* Canberra: Commonwealth of Australia.

Epstein, M., Fossey, E., Leggatt, M., Meadows, G. & Minas, H. (2012). Assessment: essential skills in. In G. Meadows, B. Singh & M. Grigg (eds), *Mental Health in Australia: collaborative community practice* (3rd edn). Melbourne: Oxford University Press, pp. 342–93.

Galasiński, D. & Opaliński, K. (2012). Psychiatrists' accounts of insight. *Qualitative Health Research*, 22(11), 1460–67.

Howes, O.D., Kambeitz, J., Kim, E., Stahl, D., Slifstein, M. & Abi-Dargham, A. et al. (2012). The nature of dopamine dysfunction in schizophrenia and what this means for treatment: meta-analysis of imaging studies. *Archives of General Psychiatry*, <archgenpsychiatry.2012.2169 v2011>.

Lakeman, R. (2006). An anxious profession in an age of fear. *Journal of Psychiatric and Mental Health Nursing*, 13, 395–400.

Millon, R. & Davis, R. (2000). *Personality Disorders in Modern Life*. New York: John Wiley.

Read, J., Mosher, L.R. & Bentall, R.P. (eds) (2004). *Models of madness: psychological, social and biological approaches to schizophrenia*. Hove: Brunner-Routledge.

Rosenhan, D. (1973). On being sane in insane places. *Science*, 179, 250–8.

Sadock, B.J., Sadock, V.A. & Ruiz, P. (eds) (2009). *Kaplan and Sadock's Comprehensive Textbook of Psychiatry* (9th edn). Philadelphia, PA: Lippincott Williams & Wilkins.

Santrock, J. (2009). *Life-span Development* (9th edn). Sydney: McGraw Hill.

Sesula, D. (n.d.). 'You and Me', poem. National Empowerment Centre. Viewed 20 March 2013, <www.power2u.org>.

Szasz, T.S. (1974). *The Myth of Mental Illness: foundations of a theory of personal conduct*. London: Harper and Row.

Wikipedia (n.d.). Drapomania. Viewed 2 January 2013, <http://en.wikipedia.org/wiki/Drapetomania>.

7

Symptomatology in mental health

Main points
- Symptoms are subjectively experienced indicators of ill-health or distress.
- A range of symptoms are associated with mental health problems, which can be grouped according to cognition, mood, personality, anxiety and behaviour.
- Almost all symptoms may be experienced in the absence of any diagnosable illness, and may be experienced by any individual in specific circumstances, and therefore caution is required before assuming a symptom is an indicator of illness.
- Symptoms can provide a useful focus of intervention. Nurses have an important role to help people make sense of and cope with symptoms.

Definitions
Affect: The external representation of a person's internal emotional state or mood as observed by others.

Mood: A subjective or internal state of feeling or emotion.

Delusions: Fixed, false beliefs not amenable to change in light of conflicting evidence.

Hallucinations: Perception-like experiences that occur without an external stimulus.

Psychosis: A syndrome or cluster of symptoms characterised by distortions in reality. Psychosis can include delusions, hallucinations, disorganised thinking (speech), grossly disorganised behaviour, and negative symptoms.

Thought disorder: Disturbances of thought (usually inferred from a person's speech) where the expression, flow and form of thoughts is disrupted.

INTRODUCTION

In most mental health textbooks, you will see a chapter or chapters detailing the specific mental disorders that can be classified according to the diagnostic systems. We have chosen a different approach here. Rather than discussing mental health problems according to specific diagnoses, in this text we focus on the symptoms a person may experience. This approach recognises that notions of mental 'health' and 'illness' are socially constructed rather than being absolute 'truths'. Our approach maintains that the subjective nature of mental distress is an essential element to be explored and understood. As Geekie (2004) has recognised, service users' experiences of their mental health problems (and indeed their experiences of being in care) have been marginalised within a system that focuses on understanding and diagnosing 'the problem'. We also aim to emphasise the *nurse's* role in understanding and caring for the person in mental distress through concentrating on the person's symptoms rather than the labels and diagnostic categories that have been ascribed to them.

The term 'symptom' is used very loosely to connote some kind of deviation of usual psychological or physiological functioning, and is indicative of the existence of something else, such as an underlying disease or illness. A symptom typically is subjectively experienced—in contrast to a 'sign', which is noticed by others. For example, consider a time when you felt anxious or afraid. There is a good probability that you experienced physical symptoms such as an increase in heart rate, a dry mouth or 'butterflies' in the stomach. You may have experienced psychological symptoms such as irrational thoughts or a compulsion to escape from the situation. All these (and many more) might be considered symptoms of anxiety, an entirely normal and common experience. Anxiety (the term for a particular cluster of symptoms) often accompanies or impacts on other symptoms. For example, people who experience hallucinations may be anxious or fearful, and helping the person to reduce the intensity of anxiety symptoms will be helpful in enabling them to process the experience. Anxiety symptoms may also vary in both their intensity and the extent to which they may cause problems. Clearly, a little bit of anxiety can assist a person to focus, learn or problem solve, but anxiety that is excessive or prolonged may be disabling. Any of the specific experiences associated with anxiety might also be symptoms of other underlying problems. For example, an elevated heart rate may be associated with many health problems, some of which may be serious or life threatening. However, in themselves many experiences that may be symptoms in one context may be entirely normal and explicable in another.

Most entities that commonly are called mental illness or disorders should properly be called syndromes. Syndromes are clusters of symptoms that sometimes appear to go together. A disease, in contrast, is a cluster of symptoms with a known or a presumed common aetiology. The boundaries between the syndromes that may be called mental illness tend to be fairly amorphous and subject to change. What counts as a particular disorder at a point in time can be quite arbitrary. Thus a person may present with more or less the same symptoms but be diagnosed with different 'illnesses' over time (although quite often biomedical treatment is similar and focuses on symptom alleviation). Symptoms provide a unit that is more easily understood than a syndrome, and thus a clearer target for interventions. Most interventions (including pharmacotherapy) target the reduction of particular symptoms (they do not tend to treat disorders, illnesses or whole syndromes), and nursing interventions ought to be focused on making sense of, helping people cope with, and even alleviate symptoms.

While focusing on symptoms such as obsessions, compulsions, perceptual disturbances and problems of cognition or mood regulation may be appealing, it is worth noting that this reductionist approach has the potential to shift our attention away from seeing the humanity of the other person—the service user (Walsh & Moss 2007). It is possible that attending to the symptoms of mental health problems could reinforce a view of the person as essentially flawed or having deficits, and symptoms as being without meaning. It is essential to view the person as having strengths and resources, and being open to the idea that symptoms are imbued with significance and meaning. So, as you read through the symptoms in this chapter, it will be important to stop from time to time and remind yourself that these are experienced by the person within the context of their overall physical, mental, emotional and spiritual self.

Symptoms do not occur in isolation from each other, or from other aspects of the person's self (such as their physical health), or from the context (that is, the environment/setting) within which the person functions. Indeed, most symptoms of mental illness—including hearing voices (Stip & Letourneau 2009)—are commonly experienced in the general population; few of those experiencing this phenomenon reflect definitive signs of pathology, and the majority of people successfully cope with symptoms without recourse to help from mental health professionals. Nurses should meet the person experiencing symptoms with a desire to understand where they come from, why they are manifesting as they do and what they mean to the individual. As Shanley and Jubb-Shanley (2007) point out, not all symptoms, cause the person distress or pose a coping challenge. These authors propose that a fundamental purpose of nursing is to engage with people as partners in coping with their experience. This ought to raise particular questions that the reader should keep in mind when reviewing lists of symptoms or working with a person experiencing a symptom:

- What does this symptom represent?
- What does it mean to the person?
- What about this symptom causes distress or disruption?
- Does the person want the experience to go away or be modified in some way to reduce distress?
- What is the relationship between this symptom and others the person may be experiencing?
- How does the symptom challenge the person's capacity to cope?
- What coping recourses or skills does the person possess that might be mobilised to deal with this experience?

In this chapter, we will explore the more common symptoms that service users may report. In order to assist your understanding, they have been discussed and grouped according to a particular type of symptom or feature. However, because symptoms of mental health problems don't occur in isolation from each other, there are also case studies scattered throughout the chapter that draw together a number of symptoms so that you can see how they might impact on the person as a whole.

CASE STUDY

Joanne is a 24-year-old woman who has become increasingly withdrawn from her family and friends over the past four or five weeks. She spends a lot of time in her room playing loud music and talking loudly to herself in an agitated way. She has become increasingly suspicious of her family, and thinks they are trying to harm her by putting poison in her food, so she keeps her door locked and refuses to accept food from them, making sandwiches for herself in the kitchen late at night when everyone else is asleep. Her sleep pattern has also changed, and she sleeps for long periods during the day and is up late into the night. She has stopped showering as often as usual, and has started looking dishevelled and wearing unusual combinations of clothing. When Joanne does talk to anyone, her speech is rambling and it is hard to understand what she is saying as there are so many ideas jumbled together. Joanne also believes the military are coming to take her away to interrogate her, so she has nailed up wood across her windows to stop them getting in to her room, and has taped over the air vents on the walls and put towels under the door to stop them from gassing her out of her room.

Critical thinking

• If you or a family member/friend were to experience the kinds of symptoms Joanne has, how would you feel about you/them being diagnosed with a disorder such as schizophrenia?
• What potential benefits and disadvantages do you see in having diagnostic labels for mental health problems?
• What potential benefits and disadvantages do you see for nurses and service users in working together in terms of symptoms rather than diagnoses?
• What questions might you wish to ask about Joanne's experience?

We could approach the above case study in a number of ways. From a conventional psychiatric approach, we might look at Joanne's behaviour according to a diagnostic manual and identify that she seems to have a number of symptoms that may justify a diagnosis of paranoid schizophrenia or substance-induced psychosis. We could also simply approach this situation from the perspective of her symptoms—that is, Joanne appears to be experiencing auditory hallucinations (a cognitive/perceptual symptom); she seems to be having difficulty communicating with others due to a loosening of association or connection between her thoughts (a cognitive symptom); she appears to have persecutory delusions or beliefs that others are trying to harm her (a cognitive symptom); and these symptoms appear to be distressing to her, as she is agitated, has withdrawn from others (behavioural symptoms), has made attempts to cope with some aspects of the experience (for example, playing loud music to drown out the voices) and has tried to protect herself (makes her own sandwiches, nailed the windows, locked her door, taped the air vents and put towels under the door).

As nurses looking to provide comprehensive care for Joanne, we might also want to note the change in her sleep pattern, personal hygiene and grooming, and explore how her symptoms have affected her relationships with family, friends and work/study colleagues. We might want to find out whether this is the first time she has had these symptoms, and whether she has stopped going to work or stopped studying because of them. As the nurse or other members of the team get to know Joanne and her family, they ought to draw on their evolving understanding and professional knowledge to develop a formulation of the problem, or an explanation/interpretation of what is going on—and, importantly, what might be done to help (Crowe, Carlyle & Farmar, 2008).

There are many ways to explain symptoms. They may be a consequence of trauma, genetics, current stressors, unconscious processes, or drug and alcohol use. Nurses and teams are likely to find it useful to consider what biological, psychological or social/cultural factors may have predisposed the person to experience the symptom, precipitated the emergence of the symptom, perpetuated or contributed to the ongoing manifestation of the symptom or be acting as a protective factor in relation to deterioration or exacerbation of the symptom or problem (Davies 2003). It may be helpful to draw up a grid and consider each one of these factors in turn (see Table 7.1). Thinking about problems in this way will likely prompt you to ask further questions or attempt to elicit further information. It might be that Joanne experienced developmental trauma (social) or has a strong family history (biological) of mental health problems that may predispose her to having these experiences. Often an event such as illicit drug use (biological), a loss of a relationship (social/cultural) or the experience of anxiety or stress (psychological) may precipitate the emergence of symptoms. Joanne's methods of coping (isolation and other defensive measures) may in some way be perpetuating the symptoms. Joanne also has some significant assets in terms of good functioning prior to this crisis (psychological) and perhaps a supportive family (psychological), which may be protective factors. As you read through the descriptions of various symptoms, consider what bio-psycho-social or even spiritual factors might contribute to the symptom or syndrome.

Table 7.1 A bio-psycho-social problem formulation

	Biological	**Psychological**	**Social/cultural**
Predisposing factors			
Precipitating factors			
Perpetuating factors			
Protective factors			

SYMPTOMS RELATING TO COGNITION AND PERCEPTION

'Cognition' is a commonly used term in mental health, and refers to thought processes. It includes memory, concentration, thought form (how the person thinks) and thought content (what they are thinking). 'Perception' refers to a person's ability to perceive stimuli according to their senses (also referred to as sensory perception)—that is, sight, hearing, touch, taste and smell. Disturbances to cognition and perception are common symptoms in a number of major mental health problems. Table 7.2 describes diagnosis in which cognitive and/or perceptual disturbances are major features. These share some common symptoms but are thought to reflect very different aetiologies and have quite different prognosis. It is exceptionally important that signs of delirium are recognised as delirium constitutes a medical emergency and a need to discover and correct what is causing it (for example, infection, drug reaction, dehydration or metabolic disturbance) while keeping the person safe. The diagnosis of schizophrenia of any type requires the presence of some symptoms for months. Dementia may initially present with innocuous non-specific symptoms that may be misdiagnosed as part of other syndromes such as depression.

COGNITIVE DISTURBANCES

Cognitive disturbances include:

- *Delusions:* These are beliefs held with a great deal of conviction despite external evidence to the contrary, and despite others of the same culture not sharing these beliefs. These are sometimes categorised in terms of content (e.g. grandeur, persecution, somatic, nihilistic, of influence). The intensity of the conviction with which beliefs are held may vary over time.
- *Disordered thought:* The person's flow and form of thoughts may be disrupted. Problems with stream of thought include flight of ideas, perseveration (inappropriate repetition of thoughts) or retardation (slowing). Problems with form of thought include loosening of association, thought blocking, concrete thinking. A person may experience agnosia (or difficulties recognising objects, persons, sounds or shapes).

Table 7.2 Mental health problems with cognitive and perceptual symptoms as a major feature

Diagnosis	Features
Schizophrenia	The schizophrenias are syndromes that are characterised by psychotic symptoms. The person's thinking may appear illogical or disorganised. Positive symptoms include those that may reflect over-activity or excess in usual function such as pressured speech, hallucinations and delusions. Negative symptoms are those that appear to reflect deficits in functioning, and may include social withdrawal, poverty of thought and speech, apathy and blunted emotional expression or affect. According to ICD-10, the major sub-types of schizophrenia are paranoid, hebephrenic, residual, simple, undifferentiated and catatonic.
Schizo-affective disorder	This is a variation of the syndrome of schizophrenia in which people may also experience predominant mood symptoms, including mania or depression.
Dementia	A cognitive disorder involving progressive cognitive decline. Significant and usually irreversible changes in thought, memory, behaviour and personality occur, and over time the person becomes unable to care for themself and to live independently. New learning becomes increasingly difficult, and the ability to manage complex tasks, process information and the use of language are markedly diminished. Major forms of dementia that reflect different causes include Alzheimer's, vascular, alcohol-related (Korsakoff's), Lewy body dementia and Pick's disease.
Delirium	A cognitive disorder where the primary symptom is acute confusion. Includes a disturbance in cognition, attention and/or consciousness, and changes to perception, which occur over a relatively short time period of a few hours to days. These disturbances are usually related to a metabolic disturbance, physical health problem, intoxication or withdrawal from substances. Fluctuations in cognition and/or consciousness often occur during a 24-hour period and the person may be incomprehensible, engage in harmful behaviour and appear disorientated. Delirium usually resolves once the underlying cause has been removed and/or treated.

Source: Adapted from American Psychiatric Association (2006); Insel & Badger (2002); Treatment Protocol Project (2000).

- *Speech and language disturbances:* These are closely related to problems of disordered thought and include various kinds of aphasia or difficulties with comprehension and formulation of language.
- *Disturbances in executive functioning:* These impact high-level mental functions, including the ability to conceptualise or make abstractions, to plan, organise and learn from mistakes.
- *Cognitive deficits:* This is a broad term used to describe impairments in areas of functioning such as memory problems, learning difficulties and problems relating to attention and concentration.

In terms of cognitive disturbances, assessment of mental state usually distinguishes between the person's form and content of thought.

SYMPTOMS RELATING TO FORM OF THOUGHT

Form of thought generally refers to how thoughts and cognitive process are organised. It includes the amount of thought, the rate at which the person is thinking, and the flow or continuity of ideas they are expressing. Common types of thought form disturbances include disordered thoughts or connections between thoughts, where the person has difficulty sticking to the point or topic. For example:

- *Loose association*: This is a global term referring to an apparent disconnection or loosening of connections between one thought and the next. These include:
  - *Derailment*: The person appears to 'jump track' in their conversation.
  - *Tangential speech:* A train of thought and response that misses the question asked and drifts off the topic.
  - *Circumstantial speech:* The person is incidental and irrelevant with details, and the conversation appears to drift away from the topic but ultimately gets to the point.
- *Clang association:* The frequent use of puns or rhymes or other words with similar sounds.
  - *Flight of ideas:* There are many ideas and the person cannot keep up with the rapid flow, resulting in fragmented or incoherent speech with many changes in topic.
  - *Word salad:* A rare and extreme example of loosening of association in which each word or phrase appears to be entirely disconnected, and there appears to be no coherence or meaning to the listener.
- *Perseveration*: Repetition of the same words/ideas.
- *Echolalia*: Repetition of other people's words or phrases.
- *Neologisms:* The use of words that don't exist, or are constructed by the person and have particular idiosyncratic meaning to them.
- *Thought blocking*: A sudden interruption to the flow of thought or speech.
- *Poverty of thought*: The person has a restricted or minimal amount of thoughts, and therefore their speech is often minimal.

SYMPTOMS RELATING TO CONTENT OF THOUGHT

As the name implies, thought content refers to what the person is thinking, and includes disturbances of content such as delusions, ideas of reference, thoughts of suicide or homicide, obsessions, phobias and preoccupations.

Delusions and over-valued ideas

Delusions are considered false beliefs that are held to be true despite exposure to evidence that contradicts them, and despite others of the person's cultural background not sharing those beliefs. Delusions are considered common symptoms of a number of major mental health problems, including schizophrenia, bipolar disorder, depression with psychotic features, schizo-affective disorder and dementia. They may be common in the general population if thought about as a problem of conviction. Delusions are beliefs that are held with a great deal of certainty or conviction, whereas an over-valued idea is a false or exaggerated belief held with somewhat less conviction. Think about times when you've believed in something with a great deal of certainty but later discovered that the fact as you understood it was not true (perhaps a belief in Santa Claus or the Easter Bunny). With beliefs that we know to be true, we tend to engage in particular kinds of cognitive filtering—for example, we notice things that confirm our belief and often dismiss evidence that runs counter to that belief. Hence, as the seed of a belief takes hold, we can become more convinced of the truth of it—particularly if we are not exposed to countervailing viewpoints.

Nelson (2005) argues that there are two broad roots for processing information, which are implicated not only in how we respond and interact with the world generally but also in the formation of delusional ideas. When faced with a stimulus, we have in common with other animals a lower order or 'sub-cortical' response that is rapid, automatic, causes us to jump to conclusions and might be said to reflect a 'better-safe-than-sorry' approach to a threat. This sub-cortical response enables us to act quickly with a strong sense of conviction (even if we are wrong), in the interest of preserving our safety or that of others. For example, when driving we might see something in the road that we conclude to be an animal and break or swerve. The response is almost automatic, accompanied by strong feelings as well as thoughts, and not dependent on having all the facts. The development of delusional beliefs involves a process of 'jumping to conclusions' (Garety et al. 2011) and may involve this sub-cortical route of information processing. Delusional beliefs tend to be experienced as almost without thought—that is, they are simply taken for granted facts or givens.

In contrast, the cortical response engages higher order brain functions, is slower, more rational and weighs up available information, leading to a 'considered' response that is useful in all kinds of occupations and aspects of everyday life, which calls for a careful approach to decision-making (Nelson 2005). Working with people experiencing the propensity for jumping to premature conclusions or delusions might entail attempting to strengthen this slower, more considered way of responding. Thus interventions and practices such as mindfulness (Oliver 2012) show promise in helping people overcome a propensity towards delusional thinking. Such practices and coaching may help people to disentangle the strong emotion associated with the idea from the idea itself. For example, rather than knowing that something bad is about to happen, one is able to identify the strong feeling ('I feel . . .') but consider what they know to be more reasonable ('. . . but I really know'). Delusions or over-valued ideas are sometimes described or categorised in terms of content (see Table 7.3).

Table 7.3 Types of delusion

Delusion	Features
Grandiose	False and exaggerated beliefs where the person considers themself to be extremely important and/or famous and/or to have significant power or knowledge.
Ideas of control (also known as delusions of control or influence)	Belief that others, or an external force(s), are controlling the person's thoughts, feelings or actions. Includes feelings of passivity or being at the will or control of external forces.
Ideas of reference (also known as delusions of reference)	The incorrect interpretation of casual incidents and external events relating directly to the person. Commonly, people may believe that others are talking about them or that a news story relates to something they have done; or the beliefs may be secondary to the experience of hallucinatory or illusionary experiences, whereby they are addressed directly through various kinds of media.
Nihilistic	Belief that a part or parts of the self, others, external objects or the world at large do not exist. For instance, the person believes his or her stomach is dead.
Paranoid	An unfounded or exaggerated distrust of others. The person may be suspicious of those around them.
Persecutory	Beliefs of being conspired against or harmed by others. Includes the person thinking that others are spying on them, that they are trying to kill them, cheat them or harass them, or that they are being obstructed in trying to achieve their goals. The most common type of delusion.
Religious	Beliefs with a central religious theme. Often includes reference to deities, 'god', the devil, etc.
Somatic	Where the person believes parts of their body are problematic or diseased in some way and/or their physical appearance is altered, or unusual physical sensations are experienced.
Thought broadcasting	The person believes his or her thoughts are being broadcast or made known so that others can hear them thinking. This can be, for example, via telepathy, newspaper articles and radio broadcasts.
Thought insertion	The person believes some of their thoughts are not their own, and others are able to insert thoughts into their mind, even against their will.

Delusions can be isolated or fragmented. Some people will develop well-organised or highly systematised delusions. These systems of belief may be so broad and complex that they are used to explain much that happens to the person. Again, cognitive processes that are entirely normal—for example, noticing evidence that is in accord with pre-existing beliefs—may play a role in the evolution from a discrete delusional idea to a system of delusional ideas. Often, too, there is a theme to delusional beliefs, and this can be religious, grandiose, persecutory or paranoid in nature. As with much of our thinking, the themes or content of delusions tend to be congruent with our predominant emotional state. Indeed, feelings and thoughts coexist in a complex interplay. People who may be profoundly depressed are more likely to have delusions relating to guilt or paranoia, whereas someone with an expansive mood is more likely to have grandiose themes. One relatively uncommon form of delusion that is shared by others is known as *folie à deux* (literally meaning 'madness between two'). This is most often seen when a family member or friend who is close to the person comes to believe his or her delusion/s. Arnone, Patel and Tan (2006) note that in *folie à deux*, it is not uncommon for the family member or friend sharing the delusion/s to have a mental health problem themselves, although this is not always the case.

Perceptual disturbances

Common perceptual disturbances include:

- *Hallucinations*: Sensory perceptions that occur in the absence of external or objective stimuli.
- *Misinterpretations*: An inaccurate interpretation of a sensory experience. For example, a person sees their brother walking towards them with a large bag and concludes that the bag contains a gun.
- *Illusions*: An alteration or distortion of sensory perception. For example, in the dark at night, a coat hanging on a door is perceived to be a person.

Other forms of perceptual disturbance include 'derealisation' and 'depersonalisation'. Depersonalisation is where the person feels separated from, or out of touch with, their physical body. Derealisation refers to the person feeling cut off or detached from their external environment, which may be perceived as less significant or changed in character. These two symptoms are often seen in states of anxiety, intoxication with some drugs, psychosis, and in response to trauma. People who engage in self-harm often report a feeling of 'dissociation' or a disconnection between their usual thoughts, feelings and perceptions when they harm themselves.

Any sensory pathway may be subject to a hallucinatory or illusionary disturbance or misinterpretation, and hallucinations may be characterised according to the sensory pathway involved:

- *Auditory*—for example, hearing voices telling the person they are the devil.
- *Visual*—for example, seeing elephants flying around the backyard.
- *Olfactory*—for example, smelling gas coming out of the air vents in a room.
- *Gustatory*—for example, tasting poison in the mouth.
- *Tactile*—for example, feeling insects crawling under the skin.
- *Kinesthetic*—for example, feeling as if the body is flying through space.

Hallucinatory or illusionary experiences have been found to be relatively common in the general population, but can be more common in mental illness in which delusional explanations may sometimes be formed to explain them. Most people will experience vivid dreamlike hallucinations when going to sleep (known as hypnagogic hallucinations) or upon waking (hypnopompic hallucinations) at some time. Auditory hallucinations appear to be particularly common in people experiencing mental health problems such as bipolar disorder, depression and schizophrenia, whereas tactile hallucinations and illusionary experiences are common in alcohol or drug withdrawal. There is a growing recognition that hallucinations such as voices are meaningful, and the content, perceived identity and features of voices ought to be explored (Romme & Escher 2000).

Hallucinatory experiences can be frightening, particularly when people first experience them. People may be distressed by the content of voices, but also particular features such as the intrusiveness of them. The term 'command hallucination' is used to describe voices that instruct people to behave in particular ways. Most people don't act on the instruction of dangerous voices, but it is important to assess whether or not an individual experiences these kind of voices, and to understand the factors that might contribute to people acting on harmful instructions. The identity (whether the voice represents a known or powerful figure) and perceptions of the voices intent (whether benevolent or malevolent) appear influential in whether or not people are distressed and how they cope with voices (Birchwood & Chadwick, 1997). Aspects of people's personality (such as whether they are impulsive) and other beliefs such as the social acceptability of particular actions may influence whether or not people do what the voices instruct (Beck-Sander, Birchwood & Chadwick 1997).

Experiencing hallucinations

The Hearing Voices Network has collated an impressive collection of stories of people who hear voices and ways in which individuals cope with them. Romme et al. (2009) collected 50 stories from voice hearers that traced how the voices evolved and how people recovered. There appears to be a huge variation in how voices are experienced. Below are some brief extracts from an account by Sue Clarkson (in Romme et al. 2009, pp. 314–15) in which she discusses how her voice hearing evolved:

> I was five years old. The voice was kind, caring and comforting. I was being sexually abused at the time. The relationship with my voices has always been related to suppressed

emotions and the identity of my human spirit. Whenever I have been through traumatic experiences in my life, the voices have always seemed stronger, yet they have
led me through a time of personal growth and understanding of myself on a deeper
level . . . The voices have made me commit violence; they have evoked strong feelings
of suicide; they have depressed me; they have created changes to my lifestyle and my
negative thinking . . . They completely took over—I felt like a puppet . . . I learned
how to gain control by having set times when they could talk with me . . . I believe
my voices are suppressed emotions that are denied within myself . . . My coping strategies are . . . most of all to strive towards self-respect, self-worth and, more importantly,
self-acceptance.

Sue's experience is consistent with research suggesting that many voice hearers have
a history of childhood trauma (Read et al. 2005). Recovery, as Romme and colleagues
(2009, p. 97) explain, is always described in combination with changing the relationship with the voices, and medication alone never helped people to recover. However,
some people perceived that medication helped to reduce the intensity or frequency of
their voices, as Karina (in Romme et al. 2009, p. 97) describes:

What helped me was the support I got from the Hearing Voices Network. Feeling a part
of something and being accepted for who I was. I don't hear voices now, but I did till a
year ago. I heard voices for more than ten years without taking medication. Now I take
medication that suits me and at a low dose and I hardly hear voices at all now.

CRITICAL THINKING

The Hearing Voices Network is one of the largest mental health self-help groups
in the world. It was founded after discovering that at least one-third of people
who hear voices do so without any kind of assistance from mental health services
and largely cope well. Hearing Voices groups are generally run by people who hear
voices themselves, and people learn from each other how to manage and cope
with aspects of the experience that might cause problems. The Hearing Voices
Network stresses that voices are real, are a fundamental part of the person and
have meaning based on the person's life experience. Visit the website Intervoice
at <www.intervoiceonline.org> and read some of the personal testimony from
people who hear voices. From your reading, consider the following:

- What is it about hearing voices that may be distressing or pose a challenge to
  coping?
- Contrast the biomedical view of voice hearing as a symptom of mental illness
  with the view of members of the Hearing Voices Network. What are the areas
  of agreement and disagreement?

PSYCHOSIS: DISTINGUISHING BETWEEN THE 'REAL' AND 'UNREAL'

Cognitive and perceptual symptoms such as delusions and hallucinations are major features of 'psychosis'. You will often hear this term used in reference to mental health problems. Although there are varying definitions of psychosis, it may be understood as referring to a syndrome or cluster of symptoms found within a number of mental illnesses, including schizophrenia, bipolar disorder, schizo-affective disorder, substance-induced psychosis and puerperal or post-natal psychosis. Psychosis results in the person's loss of contact with reality due to the primary symptoms of thought disturbances such as delusions and/or perceptual disturbances such as hallucinations. Psychosis usually also includes the presence of disorganised thought processes ('loose associative thinking'), and sometimes the presence of bizarre or unusual behaviours (such as 'catatonic posturing').

The experience of psychosis can have significant meaning for service users, particularly in terms of the content and themes of hallucinations. For some, psychosis can be considered an existential crisis in which people question whether there is meaning in life or purpose to their existence. It is not unusual for service users to utilise religious and/or spiritual practices from which to draw strength. These can be of significant benefit as they can be a source of hope and help to prevent the person from acting on self-destructive impulses (Murphy 2000).

CASE STUDY

When Janet first became ill, she heard six different voices. One said it was going to kill her. Another told her to kill the mayor, and the rest said a variety of things. At the time she was attending college, where the voices helped her write papers. When she received failing grades she rewrote them without using the voices' suggestions. Occasionally, a voice said something positive like, 'I love you'. Janet said that, for her, the voices were real. From her religious background she knew about Satan and believed they came from him. Janet felt a lot of fear during this time; she thought she was lost to Satan. (Murphy 2000, p. 180)

Critical thinking

Reflect on what Janet has said about her experience of hearing voices. Imagine what it would be like to hear a voice continually telling you it would kill you.

- What feelings would you be likely to have?
- What behaviours might you develop?
- What beliefs about the voices might be contributing to distress, and how might these beliefs be modified or addressed?

One of the understandings of voices or hallucinations is that they are not 'real' or emenating from an external source; rather, they are self-generated. Discuss the issue of 'real' and 'unreal' voices:

- What attitudes come to mind when you think something is 'real'?
- Are these different to your attitudes towards things you consider 'not real'?
- Does it matter whether something a person experiences is 'real' or not?
- Are the emotions generated by an experience more important than the thought/experience itself (real or unreal)?

THE CONTESTED CONCEPT OF 'INSIGHT'

A symptom of mental illness that has been strongly critiqued in the field of mental health care is that of 'insight'. From a conventional psychiatric perspective, insight usually is understood to refer to the person's cognitive awareness of their mental illness and symptoms, as well as their related awareness of need for treatment, and hence their adherence (or not) to it.

In mental health settings, you may hear clinicians refer to a person's 'lack of insight', 'poor insight' or 'limited insight'. If a person is considered to have no insight or awareness into their illness, they are often referred to as being 'in denial'. It is, however, not surprising that people don't see their thoughts or the way they feel as necessarily symptoms of an illness or disease when in most cases people don't have a disease in the conventional sense. However, people always have insights into their situation, and the best way to account for insight is to ask people what their understanding is and to document this verbatim. It is unclear whether convincing people that they are ill is helpful in helping them to cope with their experiences or make sense of them.

SYMPTOMS RELATING TO MOOD

Another major group of symptoms relates to the person's experience of mood, or their internal feeling state. The terms 'mood' and 'affect' are often used interchangeably, but in mental health can be understood as referring to slightly separate features. While mood is a subjective or internal emotional state, affect can be seen externally in that it refers to the external manifestation of mood—that is, how the person appears to be feeling according to their non-verbal body and facial language. There are a number of mental health problems where altered mood states are a major feature (see Table 7.5 below for an overview).

Symptoms relating to mood are ones to which many of us can relate—we have all experienced sadness, happiness and joy. Some of us have felt depressed or very elated. A mood in the 'normal' range—that is, not being depressed or elevated—is sometimes called euthymic. Mood symptoms are those that, by their severity, duration and persistence, impact negatively on the person's ability to function in daily life. Symptoms of mood can range on a continuum of mild through to moderate or severe depth or intensity. These symptoms are often linked with cognitive symptoms such as 'flight of ideas' or 'poverty of thought', and behavioural symptoms such as 'psychomotor retardation' or 'agitation' and/or 'disinhibited' and/or 'self-destructive' behaviour, as discussed later in the chapter.

When people experience extremes of mood (as in mania or major depression), psychotic symptoms may emerge. Here, the person may have 'mood-congruent' delusions that, with a depressed mood for instance, may present with themes involving guilt or impending disaster and hallucinations involving derogatory voices. However, delusions and hallucinations may also be 'mood-incongruent', where the psychotic symptoms do not reflect the depressed mood.

Symptoms relating to depressed mood

Symptoms often associated with a depressed mood may be present over extended periods of time, such as weeks or months, and include:

- *Anhedonia*: A marked lack of pleasure in things normally experienced by the person as pleasurable—for example, the person no longer enjoys their favourite music.
- *Melancholia*: A severe despondency or feeling of depression in which the person has low enthusiasm or interest in activities.
- *Feelings of guilt or worthlessness*: Persistent and severe feelings of guilt over real or imagined wrongdoing, feeling unworthy of others' goodwill or attention or not feeling worthy enough to live.
- *Dysphoria*: A general term referring to an unpleasant feeling or mood, where the person feels, for example, uncomfortable, sad or irritable; this is the opposite of feeling euphoric and has been linked to a greater risk of suicide.
- *Changes in appetite*: Usually a loss of appetite and associated weight loss but sometimes weight gain associated with eating comfort food.
- *Reduced libido*: People often report a loss of libido or sexual drive.
- *Sleep problems*: Despite feeling tired, people often report poor sleep. Uncharacteristic early morning waking is considered an important indicator of some kinds of depression.
- *Suicidal thoughts or ideation*: The presence of thoughts ranging from more passive ones, where the person does not want to be alive, feels very down or depressed and wishes they were dead, through to more active thoughts and plans for taking their own life. Further detail on assessing for suicide risk is contained in Chapter 11.

Sometimes, a low or depressed mood may have a 'diurnal variation', in which the person's mood fluctuates during the day. People may feel worse in the earlier part of the day and better in the later part (for example, the afternoon). There may be myriad reasons why a person may experience depressive symptoms. There are at least four different broad clusters of symptoms with different causes: endogenous depression (sometimes called neurobiological); reactive or situational depression (induced by adverse life events—often losses); post-traumatic depression (often experienced after extremely traumatic events); and attachment- or abuse-induced depression (a consequence of poor attachment relationships in childhood) (Wehrenberg 2012).

CASE STUDY

Milo is a 35-year-old man who has been feeling increasingly down and sad over the past few weeks. He has stopped going out with his friends and is staying at home more and more, and not returning phone calls from his friends or family. He has lost interest in eating and cooking, which he usually enjoys, and has started to lose quite a lot of weight. He has been waking up early in the morning at around 3.00 a.m., and then finds it hard to get back to sleep. Recently, Milo was told by friends that his previous girlfriend had married.

At work, Milo feels very tired and is finding it increasingly difficult to concentrate. He has been unable to complete an important report that is due soon. He feels more and more guilty about this, and thinks he is not capable of doing the job and didn't deserve to get it in the first place. He thinks he has no future in the company and will never be any good at his job, and has started to think that everyone might be better off if he were no longer around. This is the first time Milo has experienced these symptoms, although his father has a history of similar symptoms.

Critical thinking

- Using the framework of cognitive/perceptual, mood and behavioural symptoms, identify the symptoms that Milo seems to have.
- How might Milo's symptoms be affecting his relationships with family, friends and work colleagues?
- What factors might be involved in the development of Milo's symptoms?
- Use the bio-psycho-social problem formulation grid (see Table 7.1) to create a formulation of Milo's problems.

A word on 'affect'

As discussed earlier, the terms 'mood' and 'affect' are often used interchangeably. However, 'affect' is distinct from mood in that it can be observed by others according to the person's facial/body language. There are a number of different forms of affect that can be considered unusual or that involve the presence or absence of usual expression of feelings, as well as affect that is considered to include a usual range of expression (see Table 7.4).

Table 7.4 Types of affect

Affect	Features
Blunted	A decrease in the intensity and range of emotional expression.
Flat	A total or near total absence of emotional expression. The person's face is immobile and their tone of voice is monotonous.
Reactive	Describes the person's ability to react and respond to situations with a range of facial expressions, voice tones and body movements. Considered a usual form of affect.
Restricted	An extensive decrease in the intensity and range of usual emotional expression.
Labile	Abrupt or rapid shifts in mood and affect.

Source: Adapted from Treatment Protocol Project (2000, p. 13).

Symptoms relating to elevated mood

An elevated mood refers to a 'high' or elated feeling. The person feels very excited or ecstatic, and experiences other symptoms including racing thoughts (flight of ideas), being very talkative (pressure of speech) and having a lack of inhibitions (disinhibited behaviour). Symptoms linked to an elevated mood, and which may be present for most of the day over an extended period of time, include:

- *Elevated or inflated self-esteem*: The person has an extremely high (but often fragile) opinion of themself and their abilities that does not seem related to actual achievement and/or abilities.
- *Grandiosity*: An exaggerated or inflated sense of the person's importance, power, knowledge and/or abilities. The person may be very boastful and consider themself superior to others.
- *Euphoria*: A feeling of extreme bliss or intense happiness.
- *A sense of energy*: Often people report not being able to sleep or not needing sleep. Indeed, sleep disturbance is often associated with the onset of an elated mood.
- *Disinhibition*: A reduction in observance of social boundaries. The person may be overly flirtatious, intrusive and engage in risk-taking behaviour.

The person may also experience 'labile' mood, where they alternate between extremes of mood: one minute they are euphoric and excited, then they shift to feeling very down or morose.

CASE STUDY

Over the past couple of weeks, her friends and family have noticed that Anastasia, a 27-year-old woman, has been increasingly loud and talkative, making lots of jokes, and laughing and talking on the phone constantly. She has been very excited about a whole lot of things. This morning she told her mother she was going to throw a huge party for her sister's birthday next month, and she would invite Elton John as she thought he would be 'really stoked' to come and it would be a 'piece of cake' to ring him and ask him to fly out from the United Kingdom.

Anastasia has also been out partying in nightclubs most nights for the past couple of weeks, and has been going home with a different man each night, which is unusual for her. She has been so busy she hasn't been eating much and has lost over 5 kilograms. Although she has been going to work, her supervisor has spoken to her and expressed concern at her lateness over the past week, as well as her lack of attention to and concentration on her work. She has warned Anastasia that she needs to improve this or she may be fired. Anastasia just laughs about it and tells her family that her supervisor is 'absolutely hopeless and she's just worried I'm going to take her job because I'm fantastic at it and she isn't'.

Critical thinking

- Identify the cognitive, mood and behavioural symptoms Anastasia appears to be experiencing.
- Discuss and debate the issue of Anastasia's apparent insights into her experiences, and the possible insights of her supervisor, family and friends. What meanings might they each find in Anastasia's symptoms?
- How might Anastasia feel after she has stopped experiencing these symptoms? What possible impacts might her behaviours have had on her self-perception and self-esteem?
- How might Anastasia's symptoms affect her work colleagues, family and friends?

SYMPTOMS RELATING TO ANXIETY

Most of us are familiar with the experience of anxiety. It is common to feel nervous and anxious when we are confronted with a situation in which we are required to perform in a particular way (such as being assessed on clinical skills), or in a situation that is unknown or unfamiliar (such as attending university for the first time). However, anxiety is not a one-dimensional state or symptom. 'Trait anxiety' can be understood as each person's predisposition or tendency (according to their temperament) to react to stressful situations, whereas 'state anxiety' is a temporary response induced by stressful environmental factors such as those described above (Lau, Eley & Stevenson 2006). Some people therefore have high trait anxiety, which may predispose them to respond in a heightened way to stressful situations.

From time to time, most of us will experience states of anxiety relating to our life circumstances, while 8–12 per cent of the population will experience a level of anxiety that affects their daily lives (Muir-Cochrane 2003). Peplau (1989) suggests that anxiety is an important theoretical construct for nurses to understand, and she has

Table 7.5 Mental health problems with mood symptoms as major features

Mental health problem	Features
Bipolar affective disorder	Includes episodes of mania (elevated mood) and major depression, sometimes weeks or months apart.
Cyclothymia	A chronic fluctuation in mood involving episodes of hypomania (below mania) and mild to moderate depression.
Major depression	One or more episodes of moderate to severe depression without a history of manic episodes. Symptoms include depressed mood, lack of interest in pleasure (anhedonia), significant weight loss or gain, insomnia or hypersomnia, fatigue, feelings of worthlessness or guilt, reduced concentration, recurrent thoughts of death and/or suicide.
Dysthymia	A less severe form of depression where the person has a chronically low or depressed mood.
Post-natal depression (PND)	A form of major depression that can emerge within the first few weeks after delivery and up to six months afterwards. PND can last for more than two years. Not to be confused with puerperal psychosis (PP), which is a rarer form of affective disorder that usually has features of mania and/or depression and psychosis. The onset of PP is sudden and occurs within two weeks of delivery.

written extensively about its characteristics. She suggests that anxiety is triggered when expectations of a given situation—with or without full awareness of the person—are not met. This gives rise to felt discomfort and what she terms relief behaviours. The experience of anxiety may be classified from mild to severe or panic. Mild anxiety can be adaptive, and be associated with improved performance, whereas, high levels of anxiety or panic involve impaired functioning and reflect a failure of relief behaviours to contain or reduce anxiety. There are a number of mental health problems where symptoms of anxiety are a major feature (see Table 7.6 for an overview). Note that all people may experience symptoms associated with anxiety disorders at some time, and some symptoms may be characteristic of particular personality types. A high degree of impairment and distress associated with symptoms marks the boundaries of illness or disorder.

Symptoms related to a state of anxiety can be grouped into cognitive, affective/mood, physical and behavioural (see Table 7.7). Often, symptoms of anxiety are experienced concurrently with symptoms of mood. Many service users who experience one group of these symptoms will also experience the other. The following account describes a service user's experience of having panic attacks. She had also experienced symptoms of obsessive-compulsive disorder and depression.

Table 7.6 Mental health problems with symptoms of anxiety as major features

Mental health problem	Features
Post-traumatic stress disorder	The person experiences long-term anxiety about memories of previous traumatic event/s. The person can have nightmares or flashbacks to the event/s, and will often avoid any cues that remind them of the event/s.
Generalised anxiety disorder	The person has marked and persistent worry about a number of aspects of their life, such as their job, family and friends, and finances.
Agoraphobia (with or without panic disorder)	The person has anxiety about being in situations from which escape would be embarrassing or problematic, or where help might not be easily accessible if they were to have a panic attack. This anxiety usually leads to them avoiding these situations—for example, being in crowded places like shopping centres or travelling on their own.
Social phobia	The person is anxious about being negatively evaluated or examined by others in case they do something that is humiliating, or they show obvious anxiety. This anxiety usually leads to avoidance of particular situations, such as eating, writing or speaking in public.
Simple phobia	The person has an irrational fear of specific objects or situations (e.g. spiders or flying in aeroplanes). They experience high levels of anxiety when exposed to the object of their fear, and go to great lengths to avoid it.
Obsessive-compulsive disorder (OCD)	The person experiences unpleasant and intrusive thoughts (obsessions), which are difficult to control. These can include concerns about dirt/germs/ contamination, or harming themselves or others. These obsessions often lead to compulsive rituals, which are difficult to control (e.g. urge to clean, wash, check or count objects).
Adjustment disorder (anxious type)	The person has a short-term period of feeling distressed and being emotionally disturbed following a significant life event or stressor (e.g. after illness or bereavement, including loss of partner, or loss of relationship or job).

Source: Adapted from Treatment Protocol Project (2000).

CASE STUDY

Jane described being an anxious child, but suggests that her problems really started when she was in her early teens. She said she felt different from her peers and conscious of being watched and judged. One day she was on a crowded, hot bus going to school and felt overwhelmed and fainted. When she regained consciousness, some classmates were laughing at her, with her clothes and possessions in disarray on the floor. She felt intensely ashamed, and began to avoid social situations. Things became progressively worse, however, and she would often find herself light-headed, have difficulty catching her breath and feel terrified of 'panic attacks' or losing control. She became afraid of going to school or even to shopping centres. She spent increasing amounts of time alone in her room.

Critical thinking

Jane's account provides a vivid description of the experience of symptoms of anxiety and panic.

- If you were the nurse listening to Jane's description, how might you respond to her?
- What effects did Jane's symptoms have on her life?
- How might her symptoms affect her relationships with family and friends, and her ability to hold a job and/or study?
- What might be the most useful way to conceptualise Jane's problem?

Table 7.7 Symptoms related to anxiety

Cognitive symptoms	Affective (mood) symptoms	Behavioural symptoms	Physical symptoms
Difficulty concentrating	Fear	Exaggerated startle reflex	Raised blood pressure
Feeling of disorientation	Terror	Irritability	Nausea
Persistent worry	Dread	Nail biting	Diarrhoea
Intrusive, unpleasant thoughts	Sense of impending doom	Motor tension (e.g. tapping foot, restlessness)	Choking sensation
Preoccupation	Apprehension	Withdrawal	Sweating
Thinking they are going 'insane'	Embarrassment	Avoidance of particular situations/objects	Hyperventilation Palpitations

Source: Adapted from Muir-Cochrane (2003, p. 214); Treatment Protocol Project (2000, pp. 236–7).

SYMPTOMS RELATING TO BEHAVIOUR

Many of the symptoms of mental health problems can be seen in the altered behaviour of the person. Behavioural symptoms refer to marked alterations from the person's usual behaviour, as well as behaviour considered to involve the presence of unexpected or unusual behaviour and/or the absence of expected or usual behaviour according to social and cultural norms. Some behaviours considered unusual in one culture or society may not be regarded as such in another, so we need to exercise caution in our interpretation of behaviours—particularly with service users from another cultural background to ours. It is important to check culturally relevant practices and norms so as to ensure that our response to their apparently altered behaviour is appropriate. Altered behaviours associated with mental distress occur for a range of reasons. Some behaviours (for example, echolalia) occur in conjunction with other symptoms to form the criteria for a particular mental health problem. Other behaviours (such as agitation) can be the response to or observable manifestation of other symptoms such as hallucinations, an adverse response to treatment (for instance, akathisia associated with neuroleptic use) or even be a reasonable or at least understandable response to the person's situation (for example, by being prevented from attaining goals).

For ease of understanding, Tables 7.8, 7.9 and 7.10 group common behavioural symptoms under three headings: those related to unusual or disturbed behaviour; those related to altered physical movements; and those related to altered social behaviours/skills. In psychosis, sometimes a distinction is made between what are called positive symptoms (those that represent an excess of usual functioning) and negative symptoms (those that reflect a diminishment of usual functioning). Positive symptoms such as hallucinations and delusions are generally thought to be more responsive to pharmacological treatments. Negative symptoms (see Table 7.11) tend to reflect a loss of drive and motivation, and difficulty engaging with the outside world; these can be disabling, and are sometimes exacerbated by pharmacological treatments.

Table 7.8 Symptoms related to unusual, disturbed or inappropriate personal behaviour

Symptom	Features
Sundown syndrome	Increased agitation, confusion and wandering that occurs in the late afternoon (as the sun goes down); occurs in some people who have dementia.
Disinhibited behaviour	Includes behaviours that are not usual for the person and/or not socially appropriate (e.g. stripping off clothes and being nude in public).
Self-destructive behaviour/s	Includes behaviours that are at risk of causing or do cause harm to the person, such as excessive gambling, spending, smoking, drinking and drug-taking; also self-harming behaviours such as cutting or burning the body or driving recklessly.
Echolalia	Involuntary imitation or echoing of another person's words. Can be in a sharp or mocking manner. Often accompanied by echopraxia. Can be a feature of schizophrenia.

Table 7.9 Symptoms related to unusual physical movements

Symptom	Features
Catatonic posturing (waxy flexibility)	Considered a disorder of muscle tone seen in people with catatonic schizophrenia, where the person's limbs can be maintained in awkward/unusual postures for lengthy periods of time without apparent distress. The person can look like a 'frozen' statue.
Psychomotor agitation or hyperactivity	Observable over-activity, restlessness, pacing and/or purposeless activity. Can be a feature in major depression (agitated type).
Psychomotor retardation	Observable under-activity, lack of movement and/or markedly slowed movements. Can be a feature of major depression and neurological diseases such as Parkinson's disease.
Stereotypical movements	Movements without pattern or purpose, which are performed repetitively in the same way. Can be a feature of schizophrenia and tardive dyskinesia.
Echopraxia	Involuntary repetition or imitation of another person's movements. Often accompanied by echolalia. Can be a feature of schizophrenia.

Table 7.10 Symptoms related to social behaviour/skills

Symptom	Features
Altered/reduced social skills	Includes use of appropriate verbal and non-verbal interactions and behaviours, as well as the ability to hold a conversation and be diplomatic with others. Social skills may be affected in autism, dementia and in schizophrenia.
'Acting out' behaviours	Refers to a range of behaviours considered to reflect the person's internal feelings or conflicts in ways that are disruptive to others and/or are socially undesirable. Includes sexual acting out/seductive behaviour, aggressive behaviour towards others, self-harming/suicidal gestures and disruptive/attention-seeking behaviours.
Hostility and/or aggression	Refers to verbal, non-verbal and physical forms of aggression, including threats and aggressive acts. These can be manifestations of a range of symptoms, including manic excitement, command hallucinations, paranoid delusions and the loss of cognitive inhibitions in substance intoxication, dementia and/or delirium. They can also be symptoms of the person's fear or distress.
Withdrawal	Refers to the person's physical and/or emotional withdrawal, where they retreat from contact with others. Can be a feature of depression and schizophrenia.
Negative symptoms	Refers to the absence of usual or expected behaviours. Often a feature of schizophrenia in the chronic or residual phase (see Table 7.2 for symptoms of schizophrenia).

Table 7.11 'Negative' symptoms

Domain	Term	Features
Altered communication	Alogia	Poverty of speech—for example, talks little, uses few words.
Altered affect	Blunted affect	Reduced range of emotions (perceptions, experience and expression)—for example, feels numb or empty, recalls few emotional experiences, good or bad.
Altered socialisation	Asociality	Reduced social drive and interaction—for example, little sexual interest, few friends, little interest in spending time with (or little time spent with) friends.
Altered capacity for pleasure	Anhedonia	Reduced ability to experience pleasure—for example, finds previous hobbies or interests no longer pleasurable.
Altered motivation	Avolition/amotivation	Reduced desire, motivation, persistence—for example, reduced ability to undertake and complete everyday tasks, may have poor personal hygiene.

Source: Adapted from Stahl & Buckley (2007, p. 6).

SYMPTOMS RELATING TO PERSONALITY

This final group of symptoms includes some of the most debated and contested in the area of mental health. Some mental health professionals even question whether these symptoms should be identified as belonging to mental disorders at all. This is due partly to the notion that many of the following symptoms related to alterations in personality can be attributed to the effects of trauma and problems with attachment at formative times in the person's development. As Horsfall (1999) identifies, we do not necessarily know how many people who receive mental health care have survived traumatic situations, including childhood sexual assault, violence in the home, war, natural disaster, torture, or the premature or violent death of a loved one, and therefore we may not know how these traumas have impacted on the person in the long term. There is evidence, though, that traumatic experiences such as child abuse are causally related to the development of a number of symptoms and mental disorders, including those related to personality, cognition and mood (Read et al. 2004).

The prevalence of mental health problems with personality features is reported as 10–50 per cent within the general community, and approximately 50 per cent for mental health service users. These symptoms often occur in adolescence, and peak in the early twenties. They can persist for some decades. Some symptoms do not resolve, but many do reduce over time (Svrakic et al. 2002). The symptoms begin with the personality traits that we all have, which manifest early in life and remain relatively stable throughout. They include personal traits or characteristics such as a tendency to be more or less optimistic, to be more or less extrovert (to enjoy the stimulation and energy from interacting with others), and to be more or less emotionally stable, including how quickly we respond to situations with emotions such as anger and anxiety.

According to Tredget (2001), the characteristics of clinical symptoms related to personality are those traits that have become extreme and persist over time, despite the difficulties they may create for the person and others.

Symptoms relating to personality may be grouped broadly according to:

- a lack of concern for the feelings of others
- marked self-centredness and/or lying
- blaming others for problems created by oneself
- expectations of being exploited or harmed.

These symptoms may then result in the person feeling insecure in personal relationships, demonstrating irresponsible behaviours and having a tendency to engage in reckless and thrill-seeking behaviours without consideration of the consequences (Melia, Moran & Wilkie 1999). There are a number of mental health problems where symptoms of personality are a major feature (see Table 7.12 for an overview).

For the person experiencing symptoms relating to personality, everyday life can be experienced as difficult, and they can feel judged and not accepted by others—including health professionals. One person describes it like this:

> It's awful. People think it's like an attitude problem, only an attitude problem that you should just pull yourself up and [your] life together. I had a psychiatrist [who] told me that I needed to grow up, get a job, and get a life . . . I mean, the criteria; I think it fits . . . anger, uncertainty about career choice, no friends, constant crises . . . stuff like that. It's always something. But to have the diagnosis means you are just screwed. Once you have that on a piece of paper in a medical file, it's over. It's just over. No one will touch me with a 10 foot pole. It's like you've got the plague. I don't even know what I'm supposed to be doing. Change, don't act like that. Okay. It's not that easy. I really don't know what I'm supposed to be doing . . . I know that there's not this little guy in my head pulling levers saying do this, do that, but it feels like it . . . (Nehls 1999, p. 287)

CRITICAL THINKING

Consider the above quote from a service user.

- What are your initial responses to it?
- How, if at all, has it affected your views on people with personality symptoms?
- If you put yourself in the position of this person, what might it be like to live on a daily basis with these symptoms and other people's responses to them?

Table 7.12 Mental health problems with personality symptoms as major features

Personality disorder	Features
Paranoid personality disorder	The person shows a pattern of mistrust and suspiciousness of others; believes that others have malicious reasons for every interaction.
Narcissistic personality disorder	The person shows a pattern of grandiosity and need for admiration, and a lack of empathy towards others.
Anti-social personality disorder	The person shows a pattern of disregard for, and violation of, others' rights.
Borderline personality disorder	The person shows a pattern of unstable interpersonal relationships, self-image and affects. They exhibit impulsive behaviours such as gambling, promiscuity and substance abuse.
Histrionic personality disorder	The person's behaviour is highly dramatic and emotional, and they may be perceived to be 'attention seeking'.
Avoidant personality disorder	The person shows a persistent pattern of social inhibition, feeling inadequate and being hypersensitive to criticism or negative evaluation from others.
Schizoid personality disorder	The person has a pattern of detachment from social relationships, shows emotional coldness or detachment, and a restricted range of expressed emotions.
Dependent personality disorder	The person shows an extreme need to be taken care of by others, leading to clinging and/or submissive behaviour and fear of separation.
Obsessive-compulsive personality disorder	The person has a preoccupation with orderliness and perfectionism. He or she tends to exert emotional and interpersonal control in relationships, which is at the expense of flexibility and openness.
Schizotypal personality disorder	The person shows a pattern of interpersonal and social deficits and an acute discomfort with, and reduced capacity for, close interpersonal relationships.

Source: Adapted from Marcus (2000, pp. 777–82).

CONCLUSION

This chapter has discussed the range of symptoms associated with major mental health issues. These have been grouped according to cognition, mood, personality, anxiety and behaviour. The aim has been to focus on the person and their experience of symptoms related to their mental health, rather than on the diagnosis or label that may be ascribed to a group of symptoms. This approach recognises the physical, mental, emotional and spiritual aspects of the individual in relation to the context within which their symptoms present, and to others in their environment.

REFERENCES

American Psychiatric Association (2006) Practice Guidelines, *Treatment of Patients with Delirium*, viewed 23 April 2013, <http://psycho.silverchair.com/pracGuide/pracGuideTopic_2.aspx>.

Arnone, D., Patel, A. & Tan, G.M-Y. (2006). The nosological significance of *folie à deux*: A review of the literature. *Annals of General Psychiatry*, 5. Viewed 20 February 2013, <www.annals-general-psychiatry.com/content/5/1/11>.

Beck-Sander, A., Birchwood, M. & Chadwick, P. (1997). Acting on command hallucinations: A cognitive approach. *British Journal of Clinical Psychology*, 36(1), 139–48.

Birchwood, M. & Chadwick, P. (1997). The omnipotence of voices: testing the validity of a cognitive model. *Psychological Medicine*, 27(6), 1345–53.

Crowe, M., Carlyle, D. & Farmar, R. (2008). Clinical formulation for mental health nursing practice. *Journal of Psychiatric and Mental Health Nursing*, 15(10), 800–8.

Davies, J. (2003). *A Manual of Mental Health Care in General Practice*. Canberra: Mental Health and Special Programs Branch, Commonwealth Department of Health and Ageing.

Garety, P., Freeman, D., Jolley, S., Ross, K., Waller, H. & Dunn, G. (2011). Jumping to conclusions: the psychology of delusional reasoning. *Advances in Psychiatric Treatment*, 17(5), 332–9.

Geekie, J. (2004). Listening to the voices we hear. In J. Read, L.R. Mosher & R.P. Bentall (eds), *Models of Madness: psychological, social and biological approaches to schizophrenia*. Hove: Brunner-Routledge, pp. 147–60.

Horsfall, J. (1999). Towards understanding some complex borderline behaviours. *Journal of Psychiatric and Mental Health Nursing*, 6(6), 425–32.

Insel, K.C. & Badger, T.A. (2002). Deciphering the 4 Ds: cognitive decline, delirium, depression and dementia—a review. *Journal of Advanced Nursing*, 38(4), 360–8.

Lau, J.Y.F., Eley, T.C. & Stevenson, J. (2006). Examining the state–trait anxiety relationship: a behavioural genetic approach. *Journal of Abnormal Child Psychology*, 34(1), 19–27.

Marcus, P.E. (2000). Behavioral disorders. In V.B. Carson (ed.), *Mental Health Nursing: the nurse–patient journey* (2nd edn). Philadelphia, PA: W.B. Saunders, pp. 773–98.

Melia, P., Moran, T. & Wilkie, I. (1999). Ashworth and after. *Mental Health Care*, 2, 205–7.

Muir-Cochrane, E. (2003). The person who experiences anxiety. In P. Barker (ed.), *Psychiatric and Mental Health Nursing*. London: Hodder, pp. 211–18.

Murphy, M.A. (2000). Coping with the spiritual meaning of psychosis. *Psychiatric Rehabilitation Journal*, 24(2), 179–83.

Nehls, N. (1999). Borderline personality disorder: the voice of patients. *Research in Nursing and Health*, 22(4), 285–93.

Nelson, H. (2005). *Cognitive Behavioural Therapy in Schizophrenia: a practice manual*. Cheltenham: Stanley Thornes.

Oliver, J.E., McLachlan, K., Jose, P.E. & Peters, E. (2012). Predicting changes in delusional ideation: the role of mindfulness and negative schemas. *Psychology and Psychotherapy: Theory, Research and Practice*, 85(3), 243–59.

Peplau, H.E. (1989). Theoretical constructs: anxiety, self, and hallucinations. In A.W. O'Toole and S.R. Welt (eds), *Interpersonal Theory in Nursing Practice*. New York: Springer, pp. 270–326.

Read, J., Goodman, L., Morrison, A.P., Ross, C.A. & Aderhold, V. (2004). Childhood trauma, loss and stress. In J. Read, L.R. Mosher & R.P. Bentall (eds), *Models of Madness: psychological, social and biological approaches to schizophrenia*. Hove: Brunner-Routledge, pp. 223–52.

Read, J., Os, J.V., Morrison, A.P. & Ross, C.A. (2005). Childhood trauma, psychosis and schizophrenia: a literature review with theoretical and clinical implications. *Acta Psychiatrica Scandinavica*, 112(5), 330–50.

Romme, M. & Escher, S. (2000). *Making Sense of Voices: A guide for mental health professionals working with voice-hearers*. London: Mind.

Romme, M., Escher, S., Dillon, J., Corstens, D. & Morris, M. (eds) (2009). *Living with Voices: 50 stories of recovery*. Ross-on-Wye: PCCS Books.

Shanley, E., & Jubb-Shanley, M. (2007). The recovery alliance theory of mental health nursing. *Journal of Psychiatric and Mental Health Nursing, 14*(8), 734–43.

Stahl, S.M. & Buckley, P.F. (2007). Negative symptoms of schizophrenia: a problem that will not go away. *Acta Psychiatrica Scandinavica*, 111(1), 4–11.

Stip, E. & Letourneau, G. (2009). Psychotic symptoms as a continuum between normality and pathology. *Canadian Journal of Psychiatry*, 54(3), 140–51.

Svrakic, D.M., Draganic, S., Hill, K., Bayon, C., Przybeck, T.R. & Cloninger, C.R. (2002). Temperament, character, and personality disorders: Etiologic, diagnostic, treatment issues. *Acta Psychiatrica Scandinavica*, 106(3), 189–95.

Treatment Protocol Project (2000). *Management of Mental Disorders* (3rd edn). Sydney: World Health Organization Collaborating Centre for Mental Health and Substance Abuse.

Tredget, J.E. (2001). The aetiology, presentation and treatment of personality disorders. *Journal of Psychiatric and Mental Health Nursing*, 8(4), 347–56.

Walker, M.T. (2006). The social construction of mental illness and its implications for the recovery model. *International Journal of Psychosocial Rehabilitation*, 10(1), 71–87.

Walsh, K. & Moss, C. (2007). Solution focused mental health nursing. In M. McAllister (ed.), *Solution-Focused Nursing: rethinking practice*. Hampshire: Palgrave, pp. 116–26.

Wehrenberg, M. (2012). Four faces of depression. *Psychotherapy in Australia*, 18(4), 14–19.

8

Sociological understandings of mental health and Indigenous social and emotional well-being

Main points

- Social determinants are factors that play an important role in mental health and families' and communities' well-being
- Social determinants can be positive factors that enhance well-being, where their opposite can have a negative impact on well-being (land rights vs alienation from land; social inclusion vs social marginalisation).
- The well-being of Aboriginal people and Torres Strait Islanders is impacted on by additional social determinants due to historical and contemporary social processes.
- There is a strong association between mental illness or disorder and issues such as child abuse, substance misuse and suicide.
- Primary, secondary and tertiary prevention strategies play an important role in reducing the incidence and impact of social determinants and/or addressing the harm that social determinants and issues may exert on the mental health and well-being of individuals, families and communities.

Definitions

Mental health: 'A state of well-being in which an individual realizes his or her own abilities, can cope with the normal stresses of life, can work productively and is able to make a contribution to his or her community.' (World Health Organization 2010)

Social constructivism: The way in which categories such as social class, gender, age, culture and ethnicity are created by human interaction within society's institutions.

Social determinants: The way in which society as a whole and someone's position within society influence life chances and so impact on health.

Social issues: Experiences or events in a person's or a group's social context that impact on health status.

Social and emotional well-being (SEWB): A broad concept developed by Indigenous leaders to register that the well-being of individuals is always related to their relationships to land, spirituality, culture, ancestors, community and family, and to broad societal issues.

INTRODUCTION

While we have focused on nursing issues relating to mental health so far in this book, we also recognise that a person's mental health issues do not occur in isolation, but rather are influenced by, and in turn influence, the broader social context. This chapter aims to increase nurses' compassion towards their clients by providing information on and insights into the complexity of factors that can bring a person to a point in their life where they will need your care. Health is inextricably related to historical issues from both the perspective of a person's own personal history and the perspective of the socio-political history of groups in society. This is something that Aboriginal people and Torres Strait Islanders[1] have long recognised, and their first national health policy, the National Aboriginal Health Strategy of 1989, spoke about health in terms of all aspects of their lives, not just in terms of a biomedical definition of health as an absence of disease (Eckermann et al. 2010, p. 168).

For these reasons, Indigenous leaders and policy-makers coined the term 'social and emotional well-being' as an explicit rejection of the term 'mental health', which implied that people's health or their distress arose from within individual minds. Rather, as Swann and Raphael (1995) clarify, the social and emotional distress experienced by Indigenous people is to do with reality factors—mostly arising from the ongoing experience of colonisation and subordination (see Cox 2007 for an historical overview).

It is this sociological understanding of issues of interest to mental health nurses, that is the focus of this chapter. Thus we explore 'social determinants' that may impact on the mental health and social and emotional well-being of the people you are nursing. We examine these issues for the population in general and also draw out specific issues impacting on Indigenous people. The second section of the chapter explores important *social issues* associated with mental health, and social and emotional well-being: child

---

1   We are aware that using terms such as 'Indigenous', 'Aboriginal 'and 'Torres Strait Islander' runs the risk of homogenising populations that are in fact extremely diverse. In everyday life, people refer to themselves using various identifiers such as geographical areas, language group, family names and so on. In this book, we use 'Indigenous' when discussing issues that may generally be relevant for all First Australians. We also use the terms 'Aborigines/Aboriginal' and 'Torres Strait Islander/s' when discussing issues specific to the mainland and to the Islands respectively.

abuse and substance misuse. As you will see, these are often related to the development of psychiatric disorders and to suicidal ideation, attempts and completions—the tragic outcomes of life circumstances that often exhibit a confluence of the social determinants and social issues that we discuss throughout the chapter.

However, it is also important that, as nurses, you gain some appreciation of the contributions you can make to ameliorate these factors. Therefore, before turning to a detailed exploration of social determinants, we briefly overview these now, picking up these threads in the case studies later in the chapter.

PROMOTION, PREVENTION AND RESILIENCE

As we have emphasised, mental health and illness can be understood as social constructions. They are categories or labels developed in society and taken for granted by mental health professionals and service systems as explaining particular symptoms and behaviours. The opportunity here is that since particular understandings of mental health/illness are constructed, they can be reconstructed or deconstructed to include other explanations and understandings. Thus strategies can be developed to support those disadvantaged in terms of their mental health.

Therefore, *primary prevention* (to prevent the onset of mental health problems), *secondary prevention* (to reduce the level of risk for those persons at risk of mental health problems and/or early detection of mental health problems) and *tertiary prevention* (to reduce negative effects of a mental health problem) strategies can be used in order to reduce and/or ameliorate the mental health problems that members of the population might face.

Resilience

It is also important to note that, while the focus in this chapter is on particular risks to a person's health, these can often be countered by the absence of these risks and by protective factors that can promote resilience. It is now recognised that resilience is not merely an 'inner' quality that individuals either have or are lacking. Rather, resilience is a social phenomenon, and aspects of people's social context enhance or diminish the likelihood that they can adequately deal with adverse life events (Lenette, Brough & Cox 2012).

So, rather than considering resilience as a trait, it is more helpful to see it as a process involving the interaction between personal and social factors that influences a person's capacity to cope with adverse life events. Personal factors that help people to cope include social competence and respect for others, self-worth and self-awareness, problem-solving skills, communication skills, autonomy and a sense of purpose about the future (Stewart & Sun 2004). Feeling connected and having a sense of belonging to family, community and society are other important aspects, while feeling supported and cared about are also protective attributes. Tedmanson and Guerin (2011) found that social relationships, community processes and social context are important factors in Indigenous mental health and well-being.

Research with Indigenous parents found a number of additional social factors that are believed to produce strong and resilient children who reveal values and priorities relevant to these social contexts. This research is reviewed in Heath and colleagues (2011), and themes that emerged included strong family support systems and role models, and a culturally inclusive position in the extended family that encourages children to prioritise and maintain their identity. This aspect is central to being able to cope with adversity. Good family communication and emotional support, guidance and protection, strong attachment bonds and following family traditions were all seen as important.

The availability of quality child care within and outside the family, knowing their child's health status, feeling connected to the child before and after birth, and opportunities for learning about culture and history were also important to Indigenous parents. Other factors included experiences of achievement and strength, socialisation within the Indigenous and the broader society, the instillation of a strong work ethic, a good education and study facilities at home. As for factors enabling resilience generally, being independent and learning from mistakes were also mentioned, and allowing high levels of risk-taking was thought to develop survival skills.

Research with Torres Strait Islander parents found that parental support, input from extended family, physical exercise, good nutrition, cultural identity, language, spiritual/ religious beliefs and financial security contributed to resilience (also see DOHA 2012, p. 8). Other resiliency practices included emphasis on self-reliance, large kinship systems and, in Torres Strait communities, the assignment of a mentor. Two factors were perceived to reduce resilience: poor self-esteem and a lack of discipline by parents.

In sum, parents, grandparents, aunts, uncles, cousins and siblings, family friends, peers, sport teams, neighbourhoods and the way in which society in general values young people and encourages their participation all contribute to feeling cared for and supported. As with health promotion activities, resilience is about building up the things that help us adapt to life's challenges, and reducing the environmental and social factors that create difficulty. Some of the issues identified as external stressors are rejection, harassment, bullying, loneliness and a lack of opportunities to be involved in community or social life.

From the above discussion, it is clear that addressing the role of society in fostering strong connections and real opportunities to be involved is crucial. Communities that genuinely encourage inclusivity, promote diversity, provide good services, have adequate opportunity and actively prevent bullying, racism and harassment are communities that foster resilience. Of course, nurses are part of the communities for which they work, so enhancing your knowledge of social determinants is in itself part of building compassion and creating a social ethos of care and understanding for one another. We turn to this discussion now.

SOCIAL DETERMINANTS

As noted at the start of the chapter, social determinants are important factors influencing a person's social and emotional well-being and mental health. By definition and due to the social character of these factors, they impact not merely on an individual but also on many others in the person's family, social networks and community. This is an important point as, due to the dominance of biomedical (psychiatric) understandings of health, mental health services in Australia tend to take an individualistic approach to mental illness and focus on the person's particular symptoms and concerns without necessarily attending to the broader historical and contemporary social context within which they occur. Such an approach clearly neglects important social aspects of a person's health (Cox 2009, 2010; Willis & Elmer 2011). Thus we need to recognise that the diagnostic systems of classifying mental health/illness are based on Western cultural values, which include the notion of an autonomous, stable, well-defined 'self'. This is a concept not necessarily shared by all cultural groups (Cox 2009, 2010), although it is commonly taken for granted by Western mental health clinicians.

The World Health Organization developed a list of social determinants of health (Wilkinson & Marmott 1998, cited in Eckermann et al. 2010, p. 168), applicable to any member of the population. The determinants include class, stress, early life, social exclusion, work/unemployment, social support, addiction, food and transport. Others have also listed additional social determinants of mental health, reflecting the socially constructed nature of health; these include factors such as age, gender and geographical location (Willis & Elmer 2011). In 2006, Wilkinson and Marmott expanded their list to include ethnic inequalities, ageing, neighbourhood features, housing and sexual behaviour. However, as a number of authors note, many of the social determinants listed are framed from a mainstream perspective, and so there are additional social determinants of health that impact on Indigenous people as depicted in Figure 8.1 below (Social Health Reference Group 2004, cited in Purdie, Dudgeon & Walker 2010, p. 76; Vickery et al. 2007; Henderson et al. 2007).

The remainder of this chapter overviews the Aboriginal and Torres Strait Islander populations and looks at specific factors impacting on their well-being. We then discuss examples of how social determinants impact on mental health in general, drawing out the cumulative effect on well-being experienced by Australia's First Peoples. This is followed by a discussion of a number of social issues and their impacts across the population. Table 8.1 provides an overview of social determinants, including those impacting on Indigenous Australians, Table 8.2 considers these for Aboriginal people and Torres Strait Islanders and Table 8.4 overviews relevant social issues.

ABORIGINAL PEOPLE AND TORRES STRAIT ISLANDERS

Prior to colonisation from 1788, the several hundred mainland Aboriginal language groups and two major language groups in the Torres Strait together constituted

100 per cent of the population of Australia and the Torres Straits and had done for upwards of 60 000 years (Cox & Taua 2013, p. 321). According to the National Mental Health Commission (NMHC 2012), in 2011 there were 669 700 Indigenous Australians—which represents 3 per cent of the population. Ninety per cent of the total Indigenous population identify as Aboriginal and 6 per cent identify as Torres Strait Islander (ABS 2011a, 2012). Almost one-third of the estimated Indigenous population (32 per cent) resided in major cities; 21 per cent lived in inner regional areas; 22 per cent in outer regional areas; 10 per cent in remote areas and 16 per cent in very remote areas. For the non-Indigenous population, a greater proportion lived in major cities (69 per cent) and less than 2 per cent in remote and very remote Australia (ABS 2006a). Another important aspect of Indigenous demographics is that in 2006, 38 per cent of the Indigenous population were aged fourteen or under which is double the proportion in this age bracket in the general population (ABS 2006a). The median age of Indigenous people is 21 compared with 37 for the non-Indigenous population (NMHC 2012).

The Torres Strait Islands are a group of approximately 200 islands situated between the tip of Australia's Cape York Peninsula and Papua New Guinea. Today, Torres Strait Islanders inhabit seventeen of these islands (Gab Titui Cultural Centre 2009). Approximately 38 per cent of Torres Strait Islanders identify as both Torres Strait Islander and Aboriginal, and the majority of Torres Strait Islanders reside in Queensland (61 per cent), while 15 per cent still reside in the Torres Straits (ABS 2010). Torres Strait Islanders are the only Australian Indigenous group to be named after the region where they originated (Arthur 2001). Torres Strait Islanders identify with the language group of their forebears. In 2008, 63 per cent of Torres Strait Islander adults (fifteen years and older) and about 48 per cent of Torres Strait Islander children (three to fourteen years) identified with a clan tribal or language group (ABS 2010). The two main language groups are Miriam Mir (Eastern Islands) and Kala Lagaw Ya (KLY) (Western and Central Islands); the latter consists of four dialects (DATSIP 2000).

One of the most significant factors contributing to the well-being of Indigenous Australians is strong connections to culture and country/place. Torres Strait Islanders of the Meriam language group use the traditional language term *ged*, meaning homeland (Aboriginal people use the term 'country'). However, one's *ged* or country is not limited to physical location, but rather refers to an intimate relationship between the land, the sea, the animals, the weather, the cosmos and the individual and their community (Scott & Mulrennan 1999). The Australian Health Ministers' Advisor Council reports that 'in 2002, 54 per cent of Aboriginal and Torres Strait Islander adults reported they identified with a clan or tribal group, 22 per cent currently lived in traditional lands, and 68 per cent had attended cultural events in the last twelve months' (AHMAC 2008, p. 12). In 2008, 70 per cent of Indigenous children had attended a cultural event in the past year, 47 per cent recognised their homelands and 42 per cent had spent time with an Elder (DOHA 2012, p. 6).

ABORIGINAL PEOPLE, TORRES STRAIT ISLANDERS AND SOCIAL DETERMINANTS

Everything is all interrelated. So if we look at health that is related to mental health, and employment, social inclusion. Aboriginal and Torres Strait Islander people still suffer racism in this country. We also have a history of colonisation that we have to deal with and reclaim our cultures. So that all compounds on the mental health of Aboriginal and Torres Strait Islander people. (Dudgeon, in NACCHO 2012)

Professor Dudgeon's comments reflect on the National Mental Health Commission's first report card, which stresses the importance of including Indigenous mental health in Close the Gap targets aimed at improving overall well-being (NACCHO 2012). Due to the ongoing impact of British invasion (colonisation) and genocide, and contemporary social experience, on the lives and well-being of Aboriginal people and Torres Strait Islanders, it can readily be appreciated that the brunt of the general list of social determinants, when considered with the unique social determinants impacting on well-being, will be amplified considerably (see Figure 8.1 and Table 8.1). Thus Aboriginal and Torres Strait Islander people experience a burden of disease and injury significantly greater than that of other Australians (Vos et al. 2007). Mental health was identified by Vos and colleagues (2007) as the second leading cause of disease burden (a range of cognitive, emotional and behavioural disorders) impacting on the lives and productivity of Indigenous people (AIHW 2009).

Specific social determinants for Indigenous Australians include complex unresolved grief and loss, which are partly to do with the earlier and excess morbidity of family and community members and the loss of family members to correctional facilities due to police harassment and over incarceration. However, behind these more obvious sources of loss and grief are a number of other unresolved issues, including removal from and loss of control over land and sea, and their resources, and their ceremonial and social significance. As indicated above, country and place are central to social identity and position in social networks, and the fact that those removed from country can no longer fulfil responsibilities to country is a little recognised and profound factor in ongoing social and emotional distress as new generations inherit these responsibilities. New generations create their own sense of belonging that reflects these sensibilities, even in urban areas that some might assume are far removed from such concerns (Bond 2007).

Thus land, sea and a sense of place are crucial to Indigenous peoples as determinants of mental health and well-being. Ironically, Malo, the god of the Meriam people in the Torres Strait, declared a law that people must keep their hands and feet off the land of others (Scott & Mulrennan 1999). In 1992, the High Court's *Mabo* decision ruled in favour of Eddie Mabo and the Meriam claimants, recognising the Meriam people's prior ownership of the land of their forefathers (Scott & Mulrennan 1999). This event led to the recognition of native title, but was preceded by the 1976 *Northern Territory*

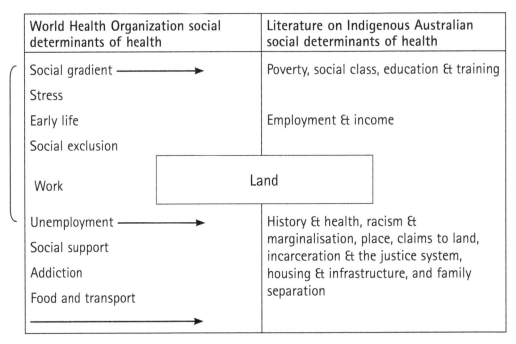

Figure 8.1 Social determinants of health identified by the WHO and their relationship to literature on Indigenous social determinants of health

Source: Vickery, J. et al. (2007, Table 1, p. 21). Used with permission of the authors.

Table 8.1 Social determinants in mental health and social and emotional well-being

Determinant	Social and emotional well-being
Colonisation and land	From an Indigenous perspective, a genocidal process involving alienation from land and the deliberate destruction of people and their social structures and institutions (e.g. lore/law; language, ceremony; family, kinship).
Genocide/family separation	Stolen generations/child removal statistics are a reflection of Australia's dominant racial perceptions and norms around Indigenous parenting and the dominance of Anglo parenting norms within Australia's child-protection system.
Racism	Many forms of racism are evident within Australia. According to Eckermann et al. (2010), these forms include personal, institutional and scientific racism.

Social exclusion, lack of safety	Limits to the ability to participate in society and benefit from its opportunities are barriers to jobs, wealth and services. Racism erodes trust and leads to social exclusion, and a lack of safety due to victimisation, discrimination and harassment. Results in social marginalisation, impacting on health.
Incarceration/police harassment	An exaggerated focus of law and order personnel on some members of the population, leading to highly inflated incarceration rates.
Being victim of crime	Murdered, sexually assaulted and assaulted.
Grief and loss	Intergenerational grief and trauma experienced by Aboriginal and Torres Strait Islander people associated with colonisation, separation from families and loss of land, sea, culture and identity, as well as historical and contemporary experiences of discrimination and human rights issues. Grief associated with the premature deaths of family and friends.
Age	Specific age groups—particularly the very young and the aged— are at higher risk of certain mental health problems, due to physical and/or social vulnerabilities
Gender	Gender refers to socially constructed categories of 'masculine' and 'feminine', and plays a significant role with respect to health status, the prevalence and diagnosis of particular mental health problems and responses to treatment and management.
Class/socio-economic status, poverty/wealth, social status, employment/unemployment; transport; food	Socio-economic factors are those affecting a person's ability to function independently, as well as interact with society. They include wealth and income, social status and power. In general, the lower a person's socio-economic status, the poorer their health.
Education	Education is strongly related to economic issues and health outcomes.
Housing; homelessness	Being homeless does not simply involve a lack of adequate housing, but also includes issues of social isolation, lack of adequate facilities and resources, and the experience of social marginalisation.
Rural, remote, regional location	Degree of 'remoteness' refers to the distance between a community and service centres. The more remote a community, the less access there is to jobs, education, transport and health care, compounding the impact of various social determinants. Lower income and natural disasters compound the existing impacts of remoteness itself. Poor dietary practices, as food and other necessities are all more expensive.

Sources: Purdie, Dudgeon & Walker (2010); Willis & Elmer (2011); AIHW (2009, 2011, 2012); Anderson (2004).

Lands Rights Act. (Readers are referred to the Human Rights and Equal Opportunity for material on land rights, native title and social justice, see <http://humanrights.gov.au/social_justice/index.html>.

Genocidal laws and policies such as Queensland's *Aboriginals Protection and Restriction of the Sale of Opium Act 1897* constituted a severe legislative apparatus that attempted to control every aspect of Indigenous people's lives (Cox 2007). Legislation outlawed the use of their own languages, and controlled where people could live and who they could marry, so the reproduction of Indigenous families, social structures and institutions was severely disrupted in many areas. Following the experience of profound social dislocation by removal from country, there was then the well-documented experience of removal of children (called the Stolen Generations), who then experienced abuse and neglect in reserves, missions, dormitories, orphanages and other institutions (Cox 2007). The Australian Institute of Health and Welfare (AIHW 2009) found that Aboriginal and Torres Strait Islander people who had been removed from their natural families experienced high levels of psychological distress.

Police harassment, violence and an extreme over-representation in the criminal justice system are other challenges to social and emotional well-being. Aboriginal and Torres Strait Islander people suffer higher levels of incarceration, making up 26 per cent of all prisoners in Australia (AIHW 2011). In 2008, 27 per cent of Torres Strait Islander people aged fifteen years and over reported being victims of physical or threatened violence in the last twelve months; 17 per cent had actually experienced physical violence in the previous year; 14 per cent had been arrested in the last five years; and 10 per cent had reported being incarcerated at some point in their lifetime (ABS 2010). These conditions increase the incidence of the children of sole parents being at high risk of experiencing lower socio-economic status, poor education and a lack of support. Indigenous children are twice as likely to live in one-parent families, with 47 per cent of Indigenous families with dependent children being one-parent families (AIHW 2011).

These issues both influence and are compounded by the marginalisation of Aboriginal people from the Australian workforce. Parker (2010, p. 5) reports that Indigenous people 'live in a situation of absolute poverty . . . where they have severe deprivation of basic human needs, including food, safe drinking water, sanitation facilities, health, shelter, education and information'. It is this level of racism, discrimination and social disadvantage that plays out in current social issues such as domestic violence, substance misuse, family breakdown and suicide.

These factors, among others, have gravely affected the mental health of many Aboriginal people and Torres Strait Islanders, and have led to widespread, devastating effects on their social structures and well-being. Combined, these factors have created one of the most disadvantaged populations within the Western world. While government efforts to close the statistical gap in health and social indicators between Indigenous and other Australians have seen some minor improvements, in overall terms things have stayed the same or grown worse (SCRGSP 2011). This disadvantage is clearly evident within the Australian Bureau of Statistics' health census data across a number of years of data collection, which show this minority population statistically has the worst health outcomes and mortality rates within Australia, with current life expectancy around 9.7 to 11.5 years less than other Australians (ABS 2012). It is important to note that changes to the current reduced life expectancy gap for Indigenous Australians have been worked out through reorganising mathematical statistical data arrangements, and many believe this to be an incorrect reflection as the data on which it originally was based have not changed (Purdie, Dudgeon & Walker 2010).

It is also important to note that these statistical depictions of poor Indigenous health and social disadvantage can in themselves become part of the problem in that they tend to create and solidify stereotypes of Indigenous Australians as all poor, all sick, all disadvantaged. Of course in the real world of everyday life Indigenous Australians are extremely socially and culturally diverse, live at all strata of society, and define health and well-being in myriad ways that are not captured in statistical collections which are always based on some non-Indigenous norm to which Indigenous people should presumably aspire. These issues concerning the creation and maintenance of stereotypes are of course part of the colonial relations of power that we've identified above as a social determinant of health, and to which we turn below in a discussion on the impact of racism and white privilege.

SOCIAL AND EMOTIONAL WELL-BEING, RACISM AND WHITENESS

It is well known that Australia, like many other colonial nations, has a long and strong 'legacy of racism' (Purdie, Dudgeon & Walker 2010, p. 35), which is still more than evident within today's society and its institutions, policies and practices. A national Australian survey reported that between half and three-quarters of respondees gave racist responses to key questions directly assessing racist attitudes, perceptions and beliefs (Purdie, Dudgeon & Walker 2010; Paradies & Cunningham 2009). With three-quarters of those surveyed currently holding racist views, it is no wonder that Indigenous Australians are subjected continually to an insidious and confronting level of racism that impacts on well-being. The current health and well-being of Indigenous Australians, then, is strongly related to policy and practice that are experienced as demeaning and non-beneficial, and also strongly related to 'whiteness' as a dominant paradigm against which all other ways of being are judged (see Cox & Taua 2013).

The Department of Health and Ageing (DOHA 2012, p. 8) sums up the impact of racism on Indigenous Australians:

> There are a number of pathways from racism to ill health, including: reduced access to societal resources such as education, employment and medical care; inequitable exposure to risk factors, stress and cortisol dysregulation affecting mental health,

immune, endocrine, cardiovascular and other physiological systems; and injury from racially motivated assault. Longitudinal and cross sectional studies both nationally and internationally have found a strong association between experiences of racism and ill health and psychological distress, mental health conditions, and risk behaviours such as substance use.

Racism is also evident in the extraordinary rates of removal of Aboriginal children from their families (see Table 8.2), which was often due not to neglect or abuse, as might be assumed, but to different parenting styles and a lack of understanding on the part of child protection workers of Indigenous Australians' social circumstances and cultural practices.

A glaring example of racism involved the dismantling of Australian's 1975 *Racial Discrimination Act*, allowing the Howard government to actively discriminate against Aboriginal people in implementing the Northern Territory Emergency Response (NTER). It continues to discriminate against Indigenous people in some areas, thereby worsening all the social determinates we have discussed here. The NTER was supported by successive governments, and is based on a fiction of widespread child sexual assault and neglect in communities when in fact there are very few substantiated cases in many communities (Cox & Taua 2013). One of the authors (Cox) has seen child protection workers inspecting Indigenous families' fridges for adequate food and deciding that an empty fridge is grounds for child removal. What the worker didn't know or think to find out is that the fridge was full yesterday and that 20 people have eaten from it since, and that it will be full again tomorrow.

Therefore, as nursing professionals, it is imperative that we are not only aware of racism but also actively practise cultural safety so as not to inflict greater harm on this population (see Chapter 14). In the practice of mental health nursing, our aim should be to reverse and address the effects of these devastating societal perceptions, beliefs and attitudes that contribute so strongly to the social determinants under discussion.

In the above discussion, we identified a number of social determinants that are common to the whole population, and social determinants that apply particularly to Indigenous Australians. We then demonstrated the extent to which some of these more general determinants impact on Indigenous Australians (economic status, housing and education), and detailed how the specific determinants compound and feed into the overall statistical picture of Indigenous well-being. Indigenous men have mental health admissions at 2.2 times the rate of others and Indigenous women at 1.5 times the rate of women generally (DOHA 2012, p. 54). We also cautioned against the tendency to create and solidify stereotypes from statistical pictures.

In the following, we use the social fact of suicide to show how several of the social determinants combine to culminate in this tragic act.

Table 8.2 Social determinants and Indigenous status

Social determinant	Indigenous status
Colonisation, land and sea rights/ native title	SEWB recognises the importance of connection to land and water, culture, spirituality, ancestry, family and community and how these affect the individual (AIHW 2009). Torres Strait Islanders residing in the Torres Strait reported higher levels of well-being then Torres Strait Islanders residing elsewhere (AIHW 2011).
Genocide, family separation/child removal	As of 2011, Indigenous children were removed from their families at seven times the rate of other children, an increase of 65% since 2007 (DOHA 2012, p. 97). Those removed from their natural families had high unemployment rates (41% compared with 26% of other Australians) (AIHW 2011).
Racism. Discrimination leads to high levels of psychological distress amongst Indigenous Australians (44% of Indigenous people compared with 26% of other Australians), fair/poor health (28% compared with 20%), binge drinking (42% compared with 35%) and illicit substance use (28% compared with 17%) (AIHW 2011).	AIHW (2009) found that 66% of Aboriginal and Torres Strait Islander people, who identified discrimination as a stressor, felt that the discrimination was against their Indigenous origin. Discrimination associated with Indigenous origin was reported by 27% of the Aboriginal and Torres Strait Islander population aged over fifteen years in 2008 (AIHW 2011). Indigenous Australians who experience discrimination were less likely to trust the police, their local school, their doctor and/or hospital and other people in general (AIHW 2011). AIHW (2009) found that Aboriginal and Torres Strait Islander adolescents were 1.6 times more likely to experience emotional and behavioural problems compared with their non-Indigenous counterparts.
Social exclusion/lack of safety	Some 7.6% of Indigenous Australians compared with 2.3% of other Australians experienced abuse or violent crime, and 9% of Indigenous Australians witnessed violence compared with 2.2% of others.
Incarceration/police harassment	Some 14.5% of Indigenous people had trouble with police compared with 2.6% of others and 12.8% of Indigenous people had a family member who had been in prison (DOHA 2012, p. 94).Variable data estimate that between one in ten and one in five Indigenous children (aged from birth to fourteen years) had a parent or other family member in prison. This results in a loss of parents for coming generations (SCRGSP 2011). Indigenous Australians are incarcerated at eleven times the rate of other Australians (Willis & Elmer 2011, p. 178).

continued

Social determinant	Indigenous status
Being a victim of crime	Variable across jurisdictions, however, in general 3 to 6 times more crime victimisation than non-Indigenous (SCRGSP, 2011).
Grief and loss	In a 2008 survey 39% of Aboriginal and Torres Strait Islander peoples had experienced the death of a family member or close friend (NMHC, 2012).
Class/socio-economic status, poverty/wealth, social status, employment/unemployment	There is a strong association between poverty, disadvantage, poor health and social marginalisation (Willis and Elmer 2011). In 2006 Indigenous people aged 18 years and over were almost four times more likely than non-Indigenous people to live in poverty (ABS 2010). Unemployment rates for Indigenous Australians are more than three times higher than the rate for others (5% in 2008). ABS reported a 69% employment rate of Torres Strait Islanders living in the Torres Straits, compared to 51% in the rest of Queensland and 54% elsewhere in Australia (ABS 2010). More Torres Strait Islander males then females reported participation in the labour workforce, 85% to 61% respectively (ABS 2010).
Education Past laws did not allow Indigenous Australians to complete schooling past year 3 or 6 depending on the geographical location (Eckermann et al. 2010, p. 25).This history impacts on today's participation rates and reflects the lack of attention to cross-cultural inclusion when educating children from differing cultures within an Anglo-Australian school-based system.	Indigenous students are less than half as likely to continue to year 12. 22% of Aboriginal and Torres Strait Islander people completed Year 12 in 2008. Torres Strait Islander residents of the Torres Strait region and Queenslanders report the highest rate, reporting a 38% and 35% year 12 completion rate respectively (ABS 2010). 40% of Aboriginal and 15% of Torres Strait Islander adults completed non-school qualifications in 2008 (ABS 2010). Torres Strait Islander women had more non-school qualifications then men, 57% and 41% respectively (ABS 2010). 3 to 7% of Indigenous people completed a bachelor degree vs. 25% of other Australians (ABS 2010; DOHA 2012).
Housing	Some 87% of Indigenous people in rural/remote Australia live in discrete communities that were once missions (AIHW 2011). 29% of Indigenous people own their own home vs. 69% of other Australians. 69% of Indigenous people's rent vs. 29% of other Australians rent (DOHA 2012, p. 73). 25% of Indigenous peoples live in overcrowded (often with structural problems) households vs. 4% of other Australians (DOHA 2012). Overcrowding is associated with communicable diseases, poor education and domestic violence (AIHW 2011).

Social determinant	Indigenous status
	Housing assistance needs for Indigenous people with a mental health problem is 5 times that for other Australians (NMHC 2012).
Rural, remote location	Mortality rates from various illnesses and suicide are higher in rural and remote locations. Housing, employment, education and health services are all less readily available (NMHC 2012). Although many Indigenous people live in urban areas, many more Indigenous people than other Australians live in very remote locations.

SUICIDE

The good news is that suicide deaths decreased between 1997 (2722) and 2006 (1799) (Harrison, Abou Elnour & Pointer 2009, p. 4)—a strong indication that suicide-prevention strategies can be successful. Nevertheless it is still a significant problem in Australia. As Willis and Elmer (2011) acknowledge, health and illness are social experiences; they occur within a social context. But not everyone's mental health or well-being is the same. As we have already established in this chapter, there are important differences between social groups, with some experiencing significantly poorer mental health than others. While not all people who commit suicide are diagnosed with a mental illness, it is fair to say that, in Australia, deaths relating to suicide are linked with particular social determinants such as gender, age, rural/remote location and Indigenous status.

We can see the influence of gender and location, in that males account for 78 per cent of all completed suicides and those who live in rural areas commit suicide at higher rates than urban men and than women, regardless of location (Willis & Elmer 2011, p. 122). We can see the influence of age in that, in 2006, the median age for suicide in males was about 45 years (Harrison, Abou Elnour & Pointer 2009). We can see the influence of the social determinants impacting on Indigenous people that we've reviewed in that the rate of suicide among Indigenous Australians is twice that among Australians generally, and is highest among those aged 15–29 years (DOHA 2012, pp. 54, 65).

Given that we've demonstrated how poverty impacts on mental health and well-being, we can safely assume that there is a greater risk for people from socio-economically disadvantaged backgrounds. We know that remote location is associated with lower income (AIHW 2011) and that 81 per cent of the Indigenous population counted in the Northern Territory lived in remote/very remote, and in Western Australia, 41 per cent of the Indigenous population lived in remote/very remote areas (ABS 2006c). We have also shown above that Indigenous people are much more likely to live in poverty—often in sub-standard housing, which is yet another social determinant. So we can see how these social determinants compound to produce high-risk social groups (such as young Indigenous males who live in remote areas, in poor housing and whose income level is below the nation's average).

Thus a new $30.2 million suicide-prevention program can be targeted at high-risk groups (DOHA 2012, p. 55). This program continues the efforts of national health policy and planning in an effort to prevent or intervene early with those at risk. The National Suicide Prevention Strategy in Australia commenced in 1999, and focuses on reducing risk across the lifespan through a range of prevention strategies involving the whole of government and the community. Strategies specifically target:

- people with substance-use problems
- people with mental health issues
- young men
- Aboriginal and Torres Strait Islander peoples
- people living in rural areas
- older people
- prisoners. (DOHA 2012)

Given that we have also outlined the over-representation of Indigenous people in correctional centres and in mental health admissions, the compounding effects of these social determinants on mental health and well-being should be abundantly clear. The high incidence of suicide means that a history of suicide attempts is another strong indicator of suicide. A major strategy developed as part of the National Suicide Prevention Strategy has been the Living is for Everyone (LIFE) framework. This is a resource that can be used by all segments of the community to develop suicide-prevention programs and strategies. See <www.livingisforeveryone.com.au/Home.html> for details of the framework.

CRITICAL THINKING
Using information from the LIFE framework, consider the risk factors noted above.

- How many of these factors can be changed or altered?
- If they can't be altered, how can their potential impact be reduced?
- What strategies (at an individual, family and community level) could be implemented to reduce the risk of suicide? Consider in your response the presence and impact of potential protective factors. These might include employment, strong family/social support, adaptive coping strategies, the ability to ask for and accept help, having a sense of humour and so on.

> • If you were to nurse a young male service user with symptoms of a mental health problem who lived in a remote area and was currently unemployed, how might you identify and address his potential risk for suicide?

The next section provides further consideration of social determinants in respect to mental health, and identifies the potential for preventative strategies that nurses can take to help reduce the incidence and/or impact of these factors.

A CLOSER LOOK AT GENDER AND MENTAL HEALTH

Gender is considered an important aspect of social difference in society, and there are specific links that can be made between a person's gender and their mental health. Women, for example, use psycho-active medications at a higher rate, and men (as already discussed) more often commit suicide (Willis & Elmer 2011). One of the controversies in the gendered diagnosis of some mental health problems is related to social attitudes towards so-called 'typical' gender roles, behaviours and stereotypes. These social constructions of gender relate to how we view 'masculine' and 'feminine' characteristics and qualities.

Some examples of 'masculine' stereotypes that may relate to mental health include that being masculine is to:

- not express emotions openly and not cry easily
- be uncomfortable talking about personal feelings with others
- be more aggressive
- take more risks.

Some examples of 'feminine' stereotypes that may relate to mental health include that being feminine is to:

- express emotions openly and cry easily
- be comfortable talking about personal feelings with others
- be more passive and acquiescent
- be more cautious.

CRITICAL THINKING

Consider the above examples of 'masculine' and 'feminine' social stereotypes.

- Do you agree/disagree with them? For what reason/s? Can you think of instances/people you know who have not conformed to these stereotypes?

- What role do you think cultural dominance plays in the development of such stereotypes?
- Think about the role of social and cultural context in how particular men and women might behave. Would an Aboriginal woman be more comfortable than an Aboriginal man talking about her feelings with non-Aboriginal others? Would it depend on that particular person?
- What implications might these and other stereotypes you can think of have for the diagnosis of particular mental health problems?
- How could concepts of 'masculine' and 'feminine' qualities/behaviours be constructed differently so that they are not fixed or polar opposites?

Table 8.3 Examples of mental health problems diagnosed more often in one gender than another

Mental health problem	Diagnosis of disorder
Alcohol misuse	Lifetime prevalence: 20% for men and 8% for women
Anti-social personality disorder	Lifetime prevalence: 5.8% for males and 1.2% for females
Major depression	Twice as common in women than men
Panic/anxiety disorders	Women predominate

Source: World Health Organization (WHO) (2013).

CRITICAL THINKING

Consider the mental health problems in Table 8.3 in terms of the previous examples of gender stereotypes.

- How much, if at all, do you think gender stereotypes might play a role in the diagnosis of these mental health problems?
- Research the known risk factors for these mental health problems.
- What other social determinants have been linked with these mental health problems?
- How many of the mental health problems in the table have been linked to social issues such as child abuse or substance misuse?
- What implications might these links have for the gender prevalence of the disorder?
- How could the risk of developing these mental health problems be reduced for a particular gender?

A CLOSER LOOK AT AGE AND MENTAL HEALTH

As identified in the discussion of suicide, age is another significant factor associated with mental health. For instance, many symptoms of mental health problems (such as psychosis, anxiety and mood symptoms) have been found to develop in mid- to late adolescence. This means that the focus of mental health promotion and prevention has increasingly been aimed at the childhood to adolescent/young person age group between twelve and 25 years, as this is a high-risk age group for the onset of mental health problems. Yet age—like gender—has a number of stereotypes and social constructions surrounding it. You may be able to think of some common social stereotypes about young people, for example. Yet the process of ageing does not have to be viewed from a narrow range of attitudes or expectations. While there are physical changes that occur with ageing, and being younger or older can be associated with physical and mental/emotional vulnerabilities, this is by no means inevitable. Nor is age the only factor in a person's mental health. However, it is important that the needs of particular age groups are recognised in terms of mental health.

Mental health problems in old age are different. It is not that older people are just adults grown older. In the same way that child and adolescent psychiatry is qualitatively different from adult mental health, for older people there are different conditions, different reactions to medication and different treatment strategies. There are strong arguments for having dedicated, discrete services for older people, as we do for children and adolescents, and specific mental health services for older people are now common in Australia.

In Australia in 2004–05, the prevalence of mental health problems was found to increase with age until 35–44 years, with 14 per cent of people in this age group reporting a mental or behavioural problem, declining to 10 per cent of people aged 75 years and over (ABS 2006b). There is also evidence that particular age groups have a higher prevalence of certain mental health problems. Over the past few decades, for example, there has been a significant increase in the incidence of mental health problems in children and young people aged between four and eighteen years. Yet only one in four young people with a mental health problem receives help for their problem (Select Committee on Mental Health 2006).

However, more recent evidence suggests that among older persons—those aged 65 years and over—mental health problems are prevalent; 24 per cent take medication for their mental health (Willis & Elmer 2011, p. 197). Dementia causes high levels of severe disability, and one in four people over 85 years has dementia. As the above shows, the needs of older persons are different in some respects to those of service users in younger age groups. In Australia, due to an ageing population of 'baby boomers' who were born in the period 1946–64, older persons constitute a social group whose mental health needs will continue to require particular attention.

IMMIGRATION AND MENTAL HEALTH AND WELL–BEING

Australia is a culturally diverse society. The Anglo-Australian population comprises the largest group, making up 36 per cent of the population. As of June 2011, 27 per cent of the Australian population was born overseas (ABS 2011b). The population is made up of people who identify with 160 different ancestral backgrounds and, in addition to Indigenous languages, over 200 languages other than English are used (ABS 2007).

For many groups in Australia, the process of immigration has exerted a significant impact on their emotional, social and physical well-being—particularly for those who are asylum seekers or from a refugee background. Psychiatry is a specific belief system based on Anglo-Saxon ideals of 'normal', so anyone not belonging to this dominant group is at risk of discrimination and racism. Of course, this is in addition to experiencing all the difficulties of settling into a new country, learning a new language and the attendant issues of finding housing, employment, a sense of belonging and adequate social support networks (Willis & Elmer 2011).

Some of these difficulties can be seen in the story of Cornelia Rau who, even though she was an Australian permanent resident and German citizen, was unlawfully detained on suspicion of being an illegal immigrant. Cornelia was held in a detention centre in 2004–05 when she experienced unrecognised and untreated symptoms of mental illness. Procter (2006) reminds us that Cornelia's experience resulted in the Palmer Inquiry, which concluded that reform was urgently needed to improve clinicians' attitudes towards, and skills in recognising, mental health problems in immigrants in detention centres.

CRITICAL THINKING

Research the story of Cornelia Rau online. Explore and identify any cultural and other factors (such as age, gender, socio-economic status) in her situation that seem to have played a role in her unlawful detention. (See, for example, <www.themonthly.com.au/often-she-cried-sometimes-she-screamed-she-begun-baxter-what-was-called-blue-compound-she-was-quickl>.

- How might your cultural background impact on your assessment of symptoms of mental health problems in someone you see as culturally different from yourself?
- What role does language play in the identification of mental health problems?
- How can nurses and other health professionals develop culturally safe practices with service users?

SOCIO-ECONOMIC STATUS, LOCATION, HOUSING AND MENTAL HEALTH

Socio-economic status includes wealth and level of income, level of education and degree of social influence. As demonstrated in the section on Indigenous social and emotional well-being, socio-economic status results in complex combinations of social determinants that have major impacts on health. Those in poverty tend to have higher morbidity and mortality rates, a fact reflected in mental health statistics showing that those with these conditions live ten to 32 years less than the general population (NMHC 2012). These outcomes are related to social and economic factors that impact on the ability to afford basics such as food, housing, education, health care and transport; to be a 'free agent'; to determine a path in life; to engage with and have influence upon society. For example, 13 per cent of those with a mental illness were homeless following discharge from a mental health facility and 42 per cent lived in unstable housing (NMHC 2012).

As also demonstrated above, rural and remote location has serious impacts on health and well-being, which were again compounded by Indigenous status and other social determinants such as gender, age, housing, education and employment. The National Mental Health Commission (2012) uses the example of health insurance to demonstrate that even if one has the best cover money can buy, it cannot be taken advantage of if one lives in some areas as the services simply do not exist there. In other words, there are losses associated with being at a socio-economic disadvantage that need to be recognised by health professionals as well as by the broader community.

We therefore urge nurses working in mental health to help service users and families understand that mental health problems are better viewed socially rather than as signs of individual failings. Problems occur in social contexts where issues such as history, social marginalisation, socio-economic status, geographical location and housing are extremely influential.

CASE STUDY

Serah is a 26-year-old single parent of two children; James, who is almost six, and Kate, who just turned eight. Due to the more affordable rents, the family lives in a small rural town and since the children's birth Serah has been a full-time mother and received the single parent's benefit. However, she has found it increasingly difficult to manage financially and emotionally since new Centrelink arrangements mean that when James is six she will be forced to return to part-time work and when he turns eight she will be moved off her parenting payment.

Serah didn't finish Year 10, and until Kate's birth she worked as a checkout operator in a supermarket. Serah is concerned about getting adequate child care, as there is a long waiting list at the nearest child-care centre, and in any case she does not have a car to get there and there is no public transport. Serah has no family living nearby who could help her.

Lately, she has been feeling increasingly down and disheartened about her situation, and has gone to her general practitioner, who has identified her as having symptoms of depression.

Critical thinking

- Research the Centrelink arrangements for mothers such as Serah.
- What social determinants may have influenced Serah's situation?
- How could nurses use preventative and health-promotion strategies in working with this family?
- What additional impacts might there be if Serah were from a refugee background?
- What additional impacts might there be if Serah lived in a very remote area?
- Research the statistics on and stories of homeless women and children.
- Given her situation, could Serah and her children be at risk of homelessness?
- Research the impacts of homelessness on mental health.
- What could mental health nurses do to reduce the risk of homelessness for people with mental health issues?

CRITICAL THINKING

Consider this quote from a young person about being homeless:

> That's the worst bits, the not having a stable anything, whether it be a place to stay, if you don't have a place to stay you don't have a place to keep your food. Everything's unstable. Not having a place of your own doesn't give you a stable anything whether it be just somewhere to relax or somewhere to keep your clothes, somewhere to keep your medication and take it, somewhere to feel safe, and that makes you stress out which makes everything harder. (Muir-Cochrane et al. 2006, p. 166)

- What images or thoughts come to mind when you think about homeless people?
- How did you feel when reading what it's like being homeless?
- If you were homeless, imagine how you would feel about yourself and others.
- Using the internet, research factors relating to homelessness in Australia. How do age, gender and Indigenous status interact with homelessness?
- What risk factors are there for being homeless?
- How do these risks relate to mental health?

SOCIAL EXPERIENCE AND ISSUES IN MENTAL HEALTH

In this section, the specific social issues of child abuse and substance misuse will be explored in relation to mental health.

Child abuse and mental health

In all states and territories of Australia, there are requirements and processes for mandatory reporting of suspected child abuse. As professionals who work closely with children and families, nurses play a major role in mandatory reporting. In most instances, nurses are specifically required to report any suspected child abuse to the relevant government department in their state/territory (AIFS 2012). There were 237273 reports of suspected child abuse and neglect in 2010–11 (AIFS 2012).

Table 8.4 Social experience and issues associated with mental health and well-being

Issue	Overview
Child abuse	Child abuse can be defined broadly as an act, or acts, performed by a parent or adult, older adolescent or caregiver endangering a child's/young person's physical or emotional health or development (AIFS 2012).
Substance misuse	Refers to the use of psychoactive substances, such as alcohol, cannabis, heroin, depressants and stimulants, at levels that may cause physical, social, cultural, emotional and psychological harm

Child maltreatment/abuse and neglect have five main sub-types:

- physical abuse
- emotional maltreatment
- neglect
- sexual abuse
- witnessing family violence (AIFS 2012).

One of the reasons why child abuse is an important social issue in terms of mental health is that there is evidence that victims of sexual abuse have increased risk of a lifetime diagnosis of multiple mental illnesses (Chen et al. 2010). These disorders—many of which are strongly associated with suicide—include post-traumatic stress disorder, panic attack, depression, dissociation, dissociative identity disorder, bipolar, schizophrenia, eating disorders and personality disorders (Adults Surviving Child Abuse 2008). Agar and Read (2002), for instance, found that 46 per cent of mental health service users in their study had histories of sexual or physical abuse. Apart from the need for mandatory notification of suspected child abuse by health professionals, it is also important to be aware that diagnosis formed on the basis of presenting symptoms such as hallucinations, sleep disturbance, hypervigilance and paranoia often overlook this underlying trauma.

CRITICAL THINKING

Primary prevention of child abuse is considered the most effective way to reduce the incidence of abuse.

- Brainstorm with your class some primary prevention strategies that nurses could use for child abuse. You may find it useful to group the strategies under headings such as Individual, Family and Societal.
- Do not restrict yourselves to hospital or community health settings. What other institutional and social settings might be relevant to such nursing work?

Although there can be significant health and other impacts from child abuse, as you may have seen by doing the above exercise, there is also opportunity to reduce its incidence and subsequent impacts if preventative strategies are implemented. While child sexual abuse has been linked with a number of mental health problems, this is by no means inevitable, and many survivors of abuse go on to lead fulfilling and successful lives—particularly if they receive adequate support and assistance from health professionals in managing the effects of the abuse.

CRITICAL THINKING

Consider and discuss the following quote.

> Abuse is not destiny. It is damaging, and that damage, if not always reparable, is open to amelioration and limitation. (Mullen & Fleming 1998, p. 12)

What might it suggest about the relationship between a potentially traumatic and damaging social issue, such as child abuse, and a person's ability to overcome adversity and trauma if they receive adequate support?

Substance misuse and/or dependence and mental health

The final social issue recognised for its considerable impact on mental health is the misuse of psychoactive substances, which exert specific effects on a person's central nervous system and alter thought processes, mood and/or behaviour. Table 8.5 provides an outline of some commonly used psychoactive substances in Australia and their legal status. Substance misuse or abuse refers to a person's substance use at levels that can be harmful to their physical and/or psychological health. Drug dependence or addiction involves the presence of increasing tolerance to the substance so that the person needs more and more of it to get the same effect and return to a state where they feel 'normal'. Addiction also involves the presence of withdrawal symptoms if the intake of the substance is abruptly stopped or markedly reduced.

Table 8.5 Commonly used/misused psychoactive substances

Legal/licit psychoactive substances		Illegal/illicit psychoactive substances	
Substance	Effect	Substance	Effect
Alcohol	Depressant	Heroin	Depressant
Tobacco	Stimulant	Gammahydroxybutyrate (GHB, liquid ecstasy)	Sedative/ hallucinogenic
Benzodiazepines (e.g. diazepam, clonazepam)	Sedative/hypnotic	Cocaine (including crack cocaine)	Stimulant
		Methamphetamine	Stimulant
		Cannabis/marijuana	Depressant
		Lysergic acid	Hallucinogenic
		Diethylamide (LSD) Solvents/volatile substances (e.g. glue, paint, nail varnish remover, liquid paper, cigarette lighter gas)	Depressant/ hallucinogenic depending on type of solvent
		Ecstasy	Hallucinogenic

The most commonly used illicit drug in Australia is cannabis, followed by ecstasy and hallucinogens, and 14.7 per cent of Australians aged over fourteen years had used illicit drugs in 2010 (AIHW 2011). In Australia, the most commonly misused legal substances are alcohol and tobacco. Although the rates of smoking have been declining over the past seventeen years, in 2010, 15.1 per cent of Australians over fourteen years smoked on a daily basis. One in five Australians drink alcohol on a daily basis and 28 per cent drink at least once a month at risky levels. As in our previous discussion of social determinants, research shows that those in remote areas, who are unemployed and with low levels of education, tend to use substances at riskier levels. Again, there are cumulative impacts where over 13 per cent of risky drinkers also have a dual diagnosis (comorbidity) of a mental illness (AIHW 2011).

There is a complex interrelationship between the development of comorbidity, and service provision is often fraught with difficulty. Many problems arise from the fact that in Australia alcohol and other drug services are separate from mental health services, so rather than being able to treat the person holistically, health professionals expend a lot of energy attempting to identify which issue developed first (the primary issue). The service structure also forces them to determine which issue requires the more urgent treatment so the client can be directed to that service. However, both the substance use disorder and the mental health issue must be addressed; if only one is treated and not the other, the person is much less likely to recover from either issue.

As the NMHC (2012, p. 131) point out—and as should now be clear from reading this chapter—substance abuse is just one of a complex mix of factors in mental ill-health and suicide that also include chronic unemployment, location, housing, grief and loss, financial stress, and disconnection from families and friends. The additional social determinants impacting on Indigenous Australians that we have discussed are other factors that also play into the issues of substance misuse in that population, along with a complex historical relationship to substances where they were used to pay Indigenous people (Cox 2007) and have since become a marker of equality with the dominant culture (Cox 2010).

CASE STUDY

There have been a number of devastating floods where Caroline is living on a farm with her husband, Graeme, and their four school-aged children. The family is under severe financial pressure and Graeme has symptoms of depression and is angry, drinking at least a six-pack of full-strength beer every night. His alcohol intake, combined with isolation, has contributed to his reducing ability to communicate or make appropriate decisions. He does not trust 'city experts', and will not ring anyone for help; nor will he go with Caroline to the nearby town to see anyone. Caroline does not go out because she is scared to leave him alone, and is also embarrassed by his drinking when they do go out, with Graeme tending to act the fool and pretend that all is well.

Critical thinking

- What social determinants can you identify in this case study? In particular, what impact might gender and location have in this situation?
- What role, if any, do discrimination or stigma about people with mental health problems/substance use issues play in this situation?
- How could Caroline and Graeme be assisted by mental health professionals?

In addition to alcohol, cannabis is a substance commonly associated with mental health issues. This is particularly the case for young people. There is considerable evidence that frequent use of cannabis is predictive of an increased risk of developing psychotic symptoms, and this is greater if there is also a family history of schizophrenia (Hall 2006). Regular (daily to weekly) cannabis use has also been closely linked with the development of mental health issues such as depression and bipolar disorder (van Laar et al. 2007).

CASE STUDY

Paul is seventeen, and has been smoking marijuana on a daily basis for the past three years. His parents are not aware he has been using drugs. Lately, Paul has been becoming more suspicious of others, and believes his friends are plotting against him and are going to tell his parents that he is smoking cannabis.

Critical thinking

As a nurse working in the local community mental health service, what secondary prevention strategies could you use to assist Paul and his family?

CONCLUSION

In this chapter, we have discussed a range of social determinants and their relationship to social experiences, including child abuse, substance misuse and suicide. Nurses have a significant role to play in helping to address these issues. Throughout the chapter, the social and historical context of mental health and social and emotional well-being has been emphasised, and the role of primary, secondary and tertiary prevention strategies to reduce the impact of these determinants and issues on mental health and well-being was discussed. Rather than seeing mental health issues, suicide or substance misuse as personal weaknesses and signs of moral failings, we have aimed in this chapter to give you information and insights as how difficulties develop and compound the impact of one another. The AIHW (2009) identified a correlation between positive well-being and better physical and mental health, less financial stress and improved labour force status. It is these social issues that lie at the heart of the distress of individuals, families and communities.

REFERENCES

Adults Surviving Child Abuse (ASCA) (2008). Abuse related conditions. Viewed 1 February 2013, <www.asca.org.au/displaycommon.cfm?an=1&subarticlenbr=45>.

Agar, K. & Read, J. (2002). What happens when people disclose sexual or physical abuse to staff at a community mental health centre? *International Journal of Mental Health Nursing*, 11(2), 70–9.

Anderson, I. (2004). Recent development in national Aboriginal and Torres Strait Islander health strategy. *Australia and New Zealand Health Policy*, vol. 1, no. 3, pp. 1–7.

Arthur, W.S. (2001). Autonomy and identity in Torres Strait: a borderline case? *Journal of Pacific History*, 36(2), pp. 215–44.

Australian Bureau of Statistics (2006a). *Population Characteristics, Aboriginal and Torres Strait Islander Australians*. Canberra: ABS. Viewed 23 January 2013, <www.abs.gov.au/ausstats/abs@.nsf/Lookup/6E6D19F5BB55AD66CA2578DB00283CB2?opendocument>.

—— (2006b). *Mental Health in Australia: a snapshot, 2004–05*. Canberra: ABS. Viewed 25 September 2007, <www.abs.gov.au/ausstats/abs@.nsf/productsbytitle/3AB354FFA0B0A31FCA256F2A007E5075?Open Document>.

—— (2006c). *Population Distribution, Aboriginal and Torres Strait Islander Australians*. Canberra: ABS. Viewed 31 January 2013, <www.abs.gov.au/AUSSTATS/abs@.nsf/Lookup/4705.0Main+Features12006?Open Document>.

—— (2007). *Year Book, Australia*. Canberra: ABS. Viewed 30 January 2013, <www.abs.gov.au/ausstats/abs@.nsf/0/2FD393B5CAC578E3CA257235007C111D?opendocument>.

—— (2010). *The Health and Welfare of Aboriginal and Torres Strait Islander Peoples*. Canberra: ABS. Viewed 26 October 2012, <www.abs.gov.au/AUSSTATS/abs@.nsf/lookup/4704.0Chapter880Oct+2010>.

—— (2011a). *Census Population and Housing- Counts of Aboriginal and Torres Strait Islander Australians*. Canberra: ABS. Viewed 13 October 2012, <www.abs.gov.au/websitedbs/c311215.nsf/web/Aboriginal+and+Torres+Strait+Islander+Peoples+-+Population>.

—— (2011b). *Australia's Population by Country of Birth*. ABS: Canberra. Viewed 23 November 2012, <www.abs.gov.au/ausstats/abs@.nsf/Products/84074889D69E738CCA257A5A00120A69?opendocument>.

—— (2012). *Topics at a Glance: Aboriginal and Torres Strait Islander peoples' health*. Canberra: ABS. Viewed 13October2012,<www.abs.gov.au/websitedbs/c311215.nsf/web/Aboriginal+and+Torres+Strait+Islander+Peoples+-+Health>.

Australian Health Ministers' Advisory Council (AHMAC) (2008). Aboriginal and Torres Strait Islander Health Performance Framework: Report 2008 Summary. Canberra: DOHA. Viewed 1 February 2013, <http://www.health.gov.au/internet/main/publishing.nsf/Content/health-oatsih-pubs-framereport-summary>.

Australian Institute of Family Studies (AIFS) Child Family Community Australia (2012). What is child abuse and neglect? Viewed 1 February 2013, <www.aifs.gov.au/cfca/pubs/factsheets/a142091/index.html>.

Australian Institute of Health and Welfare (AIHW) (2009). *Measuring the Social and Emotional Well-being of Aboriginal and Torres Strait Islander Peoples*. Canberra: AIHW.

—— (2011). *National Drug Strategy Household Survey Report*. Drug Statistics Series No. 25. Canberra: AIHW. Viewed 1 February 2013, <www.aihw.gov.au/publication-detail/?id=32212254712>.

—— (2012). *Australia's Health 2012*. Australia's Health Series no. 13. Canberra: AIHW. Viewed 31 January 2013, <www.aihw.gov.au/publication-detail/?id=10737422172>.

Bond, C. (2007). 'When you're black, they look at you harder': narrating Aboriginality within public health. PhD thesis. Brisbane: University of Queensland.

Chen, L.P., Hassan Murad, M., Paras, M.L., Colbenson, K.M., Sattler, A.L., Goranson, E.N. et al. (2010). Sexual abuse and lifetime diagnosis of psychiatric disorders: systematic review and meta-analysis. *Mayo Clinic Proceedings*, 85(7), 618–29.

Cox, L. (2007). Fear, trust and Aborigines: the historical experience of state institutions and current encounters in the health system, *Health and History* 9 (2) pp. 70–92.

—— (2009). Queensland Aborigines, multiple realities and the social sources of suffering: psychiatry and moral regions of being, part 1. *Oceania*, 79(2), 97–120.

—— (2010). Queensland Aborigines, multiple realities and the social sources of suffering: psychiatry and moral regions of being, part 2. *Oceania*, 80(3), 241–62.

Cox, L. & Taua, C. (2013). Socio-cultural considerations and nursing practice. In J. Crisp, C. Taylor, C. Douglas & G. Rebeiro (eds), *Fundamentals of Nursing* (4th edn). Sydney: Elsevier, pp. 320–40.

Department of Health and Ageing (DOHA) (2006). *Suicide Prevention*. Canberra: Commonwealth Government. Viewed 14 August 2007, <www.healthconnect.gov.au/internet/wcms/publishing.nsf/Content/mental-suicide-overview>.

—— (2012). *Aboriginal and Torres Strait Islander Health Performance Framework: 2012 report*. Canberra: Commonwealth Government. Viewed 30 January 2013, <http://www.health.gov.au/internet/main/Publishing.nsf/Content/E1C132BA79E38973CA2578CB001C217D/$File/hpf-2012.pdf>.

Eckermann, A.K., Dowd, T., Chong, E., Nixon, L., Gray, R. & Johnson, S. (2010). *Binang Goonj: bridging cultures in Aboriginal health*, Sydney: Elsevier.

Gab Titui Cultural Centre (2009). *The Torres Strait*. Viewed 2 February 2013, <www.gabtitui.com.au/index.php?option=com_content&view=article&id=6&Itemid=12>.

Hall, W.D. (2006). Cannabis use and the mental health of young people. *Australian and New Zealand Journal of Psychiatry*, 40, 105–13.

Harrison, J., Abou Elnour, A. & Pointer, S. (2009). *A Review of Suicide Statistics in Australia*. Canberra: AIHW. Viewed 31 January 2013, <www.aihw.gov.au/publication-detail/?id=6442468269>.

Heath, F., Bor, W., Thompson, J. & Cox, L. (2011). Diversity, disruption, continuity: parenting and social and emotional well-being amongst Aboriginal peoples and Torres Strait Islanders. *Australian and New Zealand Journal of Family Therapy*, 32(4), 300–13.

Henderson, G., Robson, C., Cox, L., Dukes, C., Tsey, K. & Haswell, M. (2007). Social and emotional well-being of Aboriginal and Torres Strait Islander People within the broader context of the social determinants of health. In I. Anderson, F. Baum & M. Bentley (eds), *Beyond Bandaids: Exploring the underlying social determinants of Aboriginal health*, papers from the Social Determinants of Aboriginal Health Workshop, Adelaide, July 2004. Darwin: Cooperative Research Centre for Aboriginal Health, pp. 136–64.

Lenette, C., Brough, M. and Cox, L. (2012). Everyday resilience: narratives of single refugee women with children. *Qualitative Social Work*, 11(5), 1–17.

Muir-Cochrane, E., Fereday, J., Jureidini, J., Drummond, A. & Darbyshire, P. (2006). Self-management of medication for mental health problems by homeless young people. *International Journal of Mental Health Nursing*, 16(3), 163–70.

Mullen, P.E. & Fleming, J. (1998). *Long-term Effects of Child Sexual Abuse*. Issues Paper no. 9. Canberra: National Child Protection Clearinghouse.

National Aboriginal Community Controlled Health Organisation (NACCHO) (2012). Make Aboriginal mental health a national priority. *Aboriginal Health News Alerts*. Viewed 1 February 2013, <http://nacchocommunique.com/2012/12/05/make-aboriginal-mental-health-a-national-priority-commission>.

National Mental Health Commission (NMHC) (2012). *A Contributing Life: the 2012 national report card on mental health and suicide prevention*. Sydney: NMHC. Viewed 1 February 2013, <www.mentalhealth-commission.gov.au/our-report-card.aspx>.

Paradies, Y. & Cunningham, J. (2009). Experiences of racism among urban Indigenous Australians: findings from the DRUID study. *Ethnic and Racial Studies*, 32(3), 548–73.

Parker, R. (2010). Australian Aboriginal and Torres Strait Islander mental health: an overview. In N. Purdie, P. Dudgeon & R. Walker (eds), *Working Together: Aboriginal and Torres Strait Islander mental health and well-being principles and practice*. Canberra: AGPS, pp. 3–12.

Procter, N. (2006). 'They first killed his heart (then) he took his own life': reaching out, connecting and responding as key enablers for mental health service provision to multicultural Australia. *Australian e-Journal for the Advancement of Mental Health*, 5(2). Viewed 7 May 2007, <www.ausienet.com/journal/vol5iss2/ proctoereditorial.pdf>.

Purdie, N., Dudgeon, P. & Walker, R. (eds) (2010). *Working Together: Aboriginal and Torres Strait Islander mental health and well-being principles and practice.* Canberra: AGPS.

Queensland Department of Aboriginal and Torres Strait Islander Policy and Development (DATSIP) (2000). *Mina mir lo ailan mun: proper communication with Torres Strait Islander people* (rev. ed). Thursday Island: Department of Aboriginal and Torres Strait Islander Policy and Development. Viewed 29 January 2013, <http://trove.nla.gov.au/work/23415664>.

Scott, C. & Mulrennan, M. (1999). Land and Sea Tenure at Erub, Torres Strait: Property, sovereignty and the adjudication of cultural continuity, *Oceania*, vol. 70, no. 2, pp. 146–76.

Steering Committee for the Review of Government Service Provision (SCRGSP) (2011). *Overcoming Indigenous Disadvantage: Key Indicators 2011.* Canberra: Productivity Commission. Viewed 23 January 2012, <www.pc.gov.au/__data/assets/pdf_file/0018/111609/key-indicators-2011-report.pdf>.

Stewart, D. & Sun, J. (2004). How can we build resilience in primary school aged children? The importance of social supports from adults and peers in family, school and community settings. *Asia Pacific Journal of Public Health*, 16, (supplement), s37–41.

Swan, P. and Raphael, B. (1995). *Ways Forward: National Consultancy Report on Aboriginal and Torres Strait Islander Mental Health*, Part 1 and 2. Canberra: Commonwealth of Australia.

Tedmanson, D. & Guerin, T. (2011). Enterprising social well-being: social entrepreneurial and strength based approaches to mental health and well-being in a 'remote' Indigenous community contexts. *Australis Psychiatry*, 19, Suppl. 1, S30–3.

Vickery, J., Faulkhead, S., Adams, K. & Clarke, A. (2007). Indigenous Insights into oral history, social determinants and decolonisation. In I. Anderson, F. Baum & M. Bentley (eds), *Beyond Bandaids: Exploring the underlying social determinants of Aboriginal health*, papers from the Social Determinants of Aboriginal Health Workshop, Adelaide, July 2004. Darwin: Cooperative Research Centre for Aboriginal Health, pp. 19–36.

Vos, T., Barker, B., Stanley, L. & Lopez, A. (2007). *The Burden of Disease and Injury in Aboriginal and Torres Strait Islander Peoples.* Brisbane: University of Queensland. Viewed 23 January 2013, <www.pc.gov.au/__data/assets/pdf_file/0018/111609/key-indicators-2011-report.pdf>.

Wilkinson, R. & Marmott, M. (eds) (2006). *Social Determinants of Health* (2nd ed.). Oxford: Oxford University Press.

Willis, K. and Elmer, S. (2011). *Society, Culture and Health: an introduction to sociology for nurses.* Melbourne: Oxford University Press.

World Health Organization (WHO) (2010). Mental health: strengthening our response. Factsheet N220. Viewed 21 January 2013, <www.who.int/mediacentre/factsheets/fs220/en>.

—— (2013). Gender disparity in mental health. Viewed 1 February 2013, <www.who.int/mental_health/prevention/genderwomen/en>.

PART III

TREATING MENTAL ILLNESS

9

Physical treatments in mental health care

Main points
- Modern psycho-pharmacology has seen the development of many medications, such as the anti-psychotics, anti-depressants, anti-anxiety drugs and mood stabilisers.
- Psychotropic medication (medication that has an effect on the mind) is a prevailing treatment for people with mental illness.
- Although medications can help improve the symptoms of an illness, they do not cure the underlying condition that causes the symptoms.
- Electro-convulsive therapy (ECT) is a treatment that involves using an electric shock to the brain for specific conditions; its use remains controversial.
- Trans-cranial magnetic stimulation (TMS) is a treatment that delivers an electric current through a coil held close to the head for specific conditions; it has fewer cognitive side-effects than ECT.

Definitions
Akathisia: Excessive and repetitive movements such as pacing, foot tapping and rocking that are generally not controllable.

Anti-psychotics: A drug group used most frequently for treatment of psychosis. This group includes more than one family of drugs.

Dystonia: Muscle spasm that can occur as a side-effect of anti-psychotic medications. The muscle spasm is prolonged, can be very painful and may affect various parts of the body, such as the jaw, tongue, neck and hands, or the whole body. The acute tonic muscle spasms, while sudden and often severe in onset, will respond readily to medication treatments.

Extra-pyramidal side-effects: (EPSE) include the physical symptoms of tremor, slurred speech, akathisia, anxiety, dystonia and distress associated with incorrect, excessive or uncommon reactions to anti-psychotic medications.

Neuroleptics: Another term for anti-psychotic medications. Neuroleptics (anti-psychotics) are a major tranquillising group of drugs that work as antagonists to neurotransmitter receptor sites called dopamine and serotonin receptors.

Non-adherence: An individual's personal decision not to continue with a recommended plan of treatment and/or therapy.

Psychotropic drugs: The word 'psychotropic' is based on Greek words meaning 'mind' and 'turning', and refers to any drugs that may have effects on the psychological functioning of a person.

Polypharmacy: The use of many drugs by a person that may be excessively prescribed.

INTRODUCTION

In this chapter, the physical treatments available to service users will be examined. The first section will focus on psycho-pharmacology and the second will discuss electro-convulsive therapy (ECT) and trans-cranial magnetic stimulation (TMS). The following information, readings and activities focus on mental health nurses' roles and responsibilities in an ever-changing environment.

PSYCHO-PHARMACOLOGY

> [T]hey were drinking a drug which takes away grief and passion and brings forgetfulness of all ills (Homer, The *Odyssey*, Book IV, line 221, ninth century BC).

Psycho-pharmacology (drugs specifically designed and used to treat mental conditions) represents another branch of interventions in mental health care. While psycho-pharmacological agents are prescribed by the mental health nurse, the use of psycho-pharmacology requires knowledge and expertise for mental health nurses to fulfil their legal and ethical responsibilities in administering medications to people diagnosed with psychiatric conditions. The decisions about choice, amount and frequency of a drug treatment are the domain of the prescribers (mostly the treating psychiatrist) in consultation with the service user and significant others.

Mental health nurses are central members of the health-care team, who work in consultation with service users concerning their medication. Part of the nurse's professional role and responsibility is to help service users and carers deal with medication issues, including education and information, assessment, observation and documentation. Because nurses work within the treatment team, they need to advocate on behalf of the service user and carer while still maintaining a therapeutic relationship with them.

During the past 50 years, expansion in the use of psycho-pharmacology has led to psychotropic drugs taking a leading role among treatments for many mental illnesses such as mania, depression and schizophrenia. Sedatives and tranquillisers appeared on the scene in the late 1800s, followed by barbiturates and amphetamines in the early 1900s. But it was anti-psychotic drugs (for example, chlorpromazine), which were introduced in the Western world in the 1950s, that dramatically changed the public's perception about mental illness (Gardner & Teehan 2011): 'For Psychiatry, the 1950s might now be seen as . . . one Golden Age, for the 1950s saw the explosive birth of psychopharmacology.' (Cunningham Owens 1999, p. 1)

In the same manner as any other medication, psychotherapeutic medications do not have the same effect on everyone. Some people may respond better to one type of medication than to another. Other people may need larger dosages, and some will experience aggravating side-effects, while others will not experience any problems. Factors that can influence the effect of a medication include age, sex, body size, body chemistry, physical illnesses, other treatments, diet and lifestyle habits such as smoking and exercise. Genetic factors have now also been recognised as playing a large role in determining risks of side-effects, adverse reactions and drug responses for the service user. When undertaking a medication profile, and to examine responses to pharmaco-therapy, the interactions of genetics, environment and cultural aspects need to be taken into consideration (Wong & Pi 2012).

The medications used to treat mental health conditions are classified according to the effects they have on the central nervous system. These include the anti-depressants, the mood stabilisers (anti-manic), the anxiolytics (anti-anxiety), the anti-psychotics (also called neuroleptics) and the anti-cholinergics (anti-Parkinsonian drugs). The following sections will outline these groups of medications and look at some of their most important side-effects. An exploration of issues surrounding psycho-pharmacology education, the issue of adherence and non-adherence, interventions for increasing adherence, nursing interventions and dual diagnosis will all be discussed.

PSYCHO-PHARMACOLOGY EDUCATION

Before any form of therapy is administered, information explaining the treatment should be shared with service users (and include family and carers), such as risks involved and whether there are any side-effects or adverse effects. Informed understanding of treatment is needed in order to give consent and participate in treatment. Details such as how to take the medication, when to stop and any interactions with other medications, diet and daily activities should be discussed. An understanding of the medications will allow the service user to be involved as a knowledgeable and active partner in managing their mental health.

For some individuals, there may be times when medication will be prescribed without the consent of the service user. In these circumstances, it is important that the service user is fully informed about the medication, beneficial outcomes and any possible side-effects. Equally, the reasons for prescribing should be discussed, and everyone concerned should be given the opportunity to ask questions. Ongoing medications education for the service user and their carers should include verbal as well as written instructions, and should form the basis of relapse prevention planning (AMH 2013; Treatment Protocol Project 2004).

THE PROBLEM OF NON-ADHERENCE TO DRUG TREATMENTS

An issue for all mental health nurses, irrespective of their workplace, is the fact that up to 50 per cent of service users do not adhere to pharmacological treatments as prescribed (Gray et al. 2010). Non-adherence to drug treatments has enormous ramifications for our health-care resources, as well as being a leading cause of morbidity and mortality for people diagnosed with psychiatric conditions (specifically those diagnosed with schizophrenia). There are two broad questions that flow on from the issue of non-adherence:

- What factors influence non-adherence?
- What nursing interventions can target the issue of non-adherence?

CRITICAL THINKING

Think about the last time you were prescribed medication (e.g. an antibiotic).

- Did you take the course right to the end, as recommended, or did you stop when you started feeling better?
- Do you hang on to your medication without checking the use-by date?

Non-adherence has been linked with increases in hospitalisations, relapse and increases in symptomatology and decreased quality of life. Most research on the topic of non-adherence concentrates on measuring the number of readmissions a patient may have within a year, and therefore compares groups of service users who adhere to treatment with groups of those who do not. Readmission rates have been found to decrease if medication adherence occurs (Gray et al. 2010). Therefore, medication adherence is a very important issue for the mental health nurse.

Non-adherence may not be as simple as not taking any medication after discharge. It might also include self-medicating, sporadically taking recommended dosages and even taking excessive dosages. Two issues arise here: the careful history-taking of self-medication; and establishing knowledge and understanding of medication. The advent and use of dosage boxes can assist with prevention of varying dosages and times of dosage to a point, but ultimately it remains the choice of the service user as to whether they take the prescribed medication.

CASE STUDY

David, aged 23, was diagnosed with schizophrenia nearly five years ago, and has had several readmissions in the last two years. David has been taking Risperidone for two years and is continually worried that the medication is altering his 'special gifts' of mind control and thought broadcasting. Hearing voices is generally not problematic for David; however, on occasion—and much more commonly lately—the voices say some terrible things such as 'Kill them . . . they are evil' or 'You are not worth it, why don't you jump?' David tells you he does not want to change his medication, and that experimenting with tablets or any new medication is not good for his health and well-being.

A plan is made by David's case manager to spend 30 minutes per week for the next two months assessing medication adherence.

Critical thinking

- What physical issues do you think might affect David's medication adherence?
- What psycho-social issues might also affect David's medication adherence?
- How can the case manager's plan assist in the issue of non-adherence?

You may hear the term 'compliance' or 'persistence' used in place of 'adherence' (Chong, Aslani & Chen 2011). The notion of compliance suggests that the service user is passive in relation to the treatment plan. The doctor makes the orders, the nurse administers and the service user takes what is given. This language does not promote a sense of partnership; it is working at, not with, the service user. Because of its passive inferences, Gray and colleagues (2010) recommend replacing the notion of compliance with the idea of concordance, which the authors feel captures the notion of working together to promote recovery and well-being. Concordance with or adherence to recommended medication means that the service user has the right to make decisions on their medication treatment based on up-to-date psycho-pharmacology education as well as any changes to lifestyle.

If people accept that they are experiencing problems that have a negative impact on the life they wish to lead, they may more readily adhere to treatment that offers relief (Gray et al. 2010). Similarly, when people do not perceive their mental state as a problem that needs fixing, they are less likely to take medication as prescribed. Some of the symptoms of mental illness, such as paranoia, grandiosity and delusions, can influence service users' attitudes to treatment.

MEDICATION ADHERENCE EXERCISES

There are five possible exercises that a mental health nurse might utilise in adherence therapy:

- *Structured medication problem solving:* sorting and solving practical issues such as side-effects and good regimes for taking medications.
- *Review previous experiences:* using reflection for positive and negative events in medication taking.
- *Assessing and discussing ambivalence:* exploring what are the 'good and the not so good' aspects of medication and considering a variety of ways of changing this.
- *Exploring and explaining beliefs about medications:* looking at where these ideas and concerns have come from and how they might be undermining medication education and use.
- *Explaining the role of medication in future events:* how will medication help to achieve life goals?

(Adapted from Gray et al. 2010)

Akathisia (motor restlessness) and other extra-pyramidal side-effects (EPSE) are possible causes for non-adherence (although this is changing rapidly, due to the use of second-generation anti-psychotics). If EPSE are interfering with a service user's quality of life, this may affect adherence. For example, experiencing involuntary muscle movement or being constantly restless may influence adherence. 'Weight gain, sedation, EPS (extra-pyramidal syndrome), excessive sleep, diminished sociability, sexual anhedonia and metabolic syndrome' are the items on the current list of possibilities for non-adherence, according to research by Fischel et al. (2012). What does appear to have some impact on adherence is the notion that taking medication can help keep the service user out of hospital, and can assist psycho-social areas of life such as meeting and maintaining friendships. For example:

> I take my medication as a kind of insurance policy. Because I don't want to go back to hospital ever again, and because I don't want my child to live through my absence, or to be around me if I should go mad again—it's just not worth it, but I'm lucky, because I don't have bad side effects from the drugs I take. (Service user, pers. comm.)

Interventions for increasing adherence: what works and what doesn't?

The following three areas are most cited by authors as categories to consider when planning your interventions:

- education
- behavioural interventions
- cognitive-behavioural interventions.

CASE STUDY

The weather was getting warm, and summer was coming. Julie had come to dread the summer more than anything else in her life. The warm weather meant fewer clothes and less cover on the body, and that's where Julie's seasonal-based embarrassment began. After taking medication for her mental health condition, Julie had developed unfortunate but not uncommon skin discolourations and irritations that had become more or less permanent while she stayed on the medication. In order to protect her skin, her self-esteem and whatever remained of her vanity, Julie tried to constantly cover up her arms with long-sleeved coats, jackets and shirts, and always wore long pants. Summer meant that this would become a constant source of unhappiness for Julie as she suffered through the heat. Maybe this year Julie would give up the medication, just for a while. It would be so good to not have this burden.

Critical thinking

- How might Julie be assisted with her particular difficulties?
- What other problems similar to this one might be of concern to people taking medication for mental health conditions, but be something they don't want to discuss openly?

Education involves the provision of information on the nature and outcomes of the mental illness as well as information regarding treatments and medications. In considering this form of intervention, it is important to clarify whether education is to occur on an individual basis, as part of a group or as a combination of both. It is also important to consider the family and carers as an integral part of the education process.

The delivery of education may be written (such as pamphlets, booklets and documents), verbal (such as groups led by nurses and other mental health carers), individually based (one to one at home or as an in-patient) or, preferably, a combination of them all. Online learning might involve the use of YouTube as well as a variety of reliable and well-resourced websites and podcasts managed by state-based groups or national groups such as the following:

- GROW (<www.grow.net.au>) is a national organisation that provides a peer supported program for growth and personal development to people with a mental illness and those people experiencing difficulty in coping with life's challenges.
- The Black Dog Institute (<www.blackdoginstitute.org.au>) is a world leader in the diagnosis, treatment and prevention of mood disorders such as depression and bipolar disorder.
- The Mental Illness Fellowship of Australia (<www.mifa.org.au>) is a national network of service providers, with members in every state and territory working alongside individuals and families affected by serious mental illness.

The timing of education is also an important factor: it should begin as soon as the first treatment is prescribed. However, it is important to note that education is an ongoing process, is individually tailored to the service user's needs and is an essential part of treatment—whether inside the hospital unit or based in the community.

Behavioural interventions include assisting the service user to adapt the medication regime to their lifestyle and daily routine. Taking medication is also attached to daily activities such as mealtimes, before leaving the house or first thing when getting out of bed. Calendars, dosage boxes and labels are useful behavioural interventions aimed at encouraging adherence.

The reasons why service users do not adhere to their medication treatment may not be addressed by behavioural interventions alone. Motivational interviewing may be used to encourage service users to consider the positive and negative consequences of taking medication. By engaging in conversation about the advantages and disadvantages of medications, the service user is more able to make an informed decision, and there is opportunity to correct false beliefs about medication and suggest strategies for minimising the impact of side-effects.

Gray, Wykes and Gournay (2002, p. 283) suggest these important points to follow when developing interventions to promote adherence:

- a collaborative approach to working with service users
- providing service users with information about the illness and its treatment
- tailoring medication regimes to suit the service user
- the use of motivational interviewing techniques such as exploring ambivalence and testing beliefs about medication.

CRITICAL THINKING

Imagine that you have been given a diagnosis that will require you to adhere to a medication treatment plan.

- What critical questions would you ask?
- Who would be involved?

- How would you cope?
- How would this affect your daily activities?
- Would adherence be an issue? Why?

THE USE OF PRN MEDICATION AS A NURSING INTERVENTION

Most often the use of PRN (*pro re nata*, or 'as needed/required') nurse-initiated medication falls into the domain of nursing staff decisions. Therefore, one could say that the decision processes, assessment, intervention and outcomes of PRN medicating are, as Usher, Lindsay and Sellen (2001, p. 383) describe it, 'largely an autonomous nursing role', and are 'influenced by safety, knowledge of the patient and patient distress' (Usher, Baker & Holmes 2010, p. 558).

It is estimated that between 70 and 90 per cent of people in any form of mental health care will be offered or receive PRN medication during their stay, and that the most likely drugs are anti-psychotics and benzodiazepines that have been initiated and provided by the mental health nurse (Molloy et al. 2012). Therefore, all mental health nurses need to have sufficient knowledge, expertise and education to administer PRN medication appropriately and safely

What medication to give

Once the situation has been assessed and discussed with the service user and other nursing staff, the choice of what medication to give may be as simple as what is prescribed by the licensed medical officer. However, there may be a choice of 'as needed' medications that will depend on what circumstances have arisen—for example, an anxiolytic for unresolved anxiety or an anti-psychotic for excessive delusional ideation. There is also often a choice of which route to give the PRN medication—for example, in tablet form, in liquid form or in an injectable form. The decision of which route to provide the PRN should depend on collaboration and negotiation with the service user and fellow staff, as well as how quickly the desired effects are required.

When to give it

Broadly, while the perceived need to issue PRN medication may occur at any time of the day, a number of authors claim that night-time and evenings are most common. Specifically, PRN medication is most useful in relieving service user distress as it begins to escalate and when other alternatives or interventions have failed to assist.

CASE STUDY

Robert had been in the acute care unit now for six days, getting treatment for his second episode of psychosis. He had come to know many of the nursing staff, but tonight there were staff rostered on who he had not seen before. As his headache got worse, Robert became more anxious. What if they deliberately gave him the wrong drug, he kept thinking—what if they did not believe him . . .

All he wanted was a couple of headache tablets, but it might be difficult to explain—especially as he had taken an overdose of Panadol a year or so ago when he was trying to take his own life. All this worry made his headache worse . . .

Critical thinking

- What considerations are most important for the nurse in dispensing medication to Robert?
- What issues relating to the use of PRN medication should the nurse address here?
- What therapeutic communication skills are required in these circumstances?

Under what circumstances should it be given?

The most commonly cited reason for the nurse to issue PRN medication is when the service user requests it to alleviate agitation and as an aid for sleeping (Cleary et al. 2012). However, PRN medication is also utilised to de-escalate aggressive and violent situations. Other common reasons may include inability to sleep, restlessness, unresolved anxiety, over-activity, withdrawal symptoms and distress from auditory hallucinations and delusions.

Documentation

It is a legal requirement that all medication dispensed in a hospital be signed for by a registered nurse (and, in some cases, enrolled nurses with appropriate qualifications and endorsements), and the same applies to PRN medication. Research has shown that nurses do not always document the decision-making rationale for PRN medication or the outcomes of this treatment (Usher et al. 2010). The lack of consistent and appropriate documentation makes it difficult for fellow nurses to judge the ongoing effects of PRN medication on an individual, the pattern of illness/health outcomes for the patient and any external environmental effects that might be compounding the usage of PRN medication.

PSYCHO–PHARMACOLOGY AND DUAL DIAGNOSES

Although a number of texts describe dual diagnosis as a term used to denote two illnesses, a more accurate definition might be the coexistence of a condition and a psychiatric condition within the same person. If you expand the definition of dual diagnosis, it will also cover those persons diagnosed with a medical condition and a mental illness and those with mental retardation (developmental disability) and mental illness (Lunsky & Balogh 2010).

WORLD HEALTH ORGANIZATION DEFINITION OF DUAL DIAGNOSIS

A general term referring to comorbidity or the co-occurrence in the same individual of a psychoactive substance use disorder and another psychiatric disorder. Such an individual is sometimes known as a mentally ill chemical abuser [*sic*] (MICA). Less commonly, the term refers to the co-occurrence of two psychiatric disorders not involving psychoactive substance use. The term has also been applied to the co-occurrence of two diagnosable substance use disorders (*see* multiple drug use). Use of this term carries no implications of the nature of the association between the two conditions or of any etiological relationship between them. *Synonym:* comorbidity.

Source: <www.who.int/substance_abuse/terminology/who_lexicon/en>.

Given the prevalence of both substance abuse and mental illness (dual diagnoses), there is a great challenge for the nurse to assess for substance misuse and/or usage in their service users before administering prescribed medications to avoid adverse side-effects and drug interactions. People diagnosed with schizophrenia are considered four times more likely to have problematic substance use than the general population, and the rate is higher still for people with mood disorders.

The following paragraphs provide you with an outline of the uses, precautions, adverse drug reactions/side-effects, professional responsibilities and issues of the more common medications used in the treatment of mental illness. The first group will be the anti-depressants, followed by the mood stabilisers, then the neuroleptics, then the anticholinergics and concluding with the anxiolytics.

Before starting any medication, a thorough assessment needs to be undertaken. Assess:

- service user knowledge base
- barriers to communication, such as language
- attitudes to their health and medication
- for any other treatable causes (for example, alcohol/illicit drug misuse)

- psychiatric examination, including past history, treatment responses
- physical examination, including baseline testing (for example, blood counts, electro-cardiogram)
- signs and symptoms for later assessment of treatment
- current medications for assessment of interaction potential
- any previous responses to anti-depressant therapy, including allergies
- the side-effects or adverse reactions of the drug
- the individual's response to a particular drug
- the safety of the drug (for example, in case of overdose). (AMH 2013; Boyd 2012)

Anti-depressants
Uses
Anti-depressants are used to provide relief from psychological and some physical symptoms of depression. Depression is a state of intense and profound sadness, and can be a response to a life event, or can come about without any apparent cause. More specifically, non-clinical depression is sadness, which is a normal reaction to what goes on around us any day of the week and will dissipate in time. Clinical depression, however, is a disorder where no exact trigger can be found, but a physical change is occurring within the brain, causing (or caused by) a chemical imbalance of neurotransmitters. This type of depression will not generally resolve without medical intervention (usually medication). Anti-depressant drugs can enhance the functional capacity of the service user, and also reduce the likelihood of self-harm or suicide. The anti-depressant drugs which will be focused upon in the following pages are tricyclic anti-depressants (TCAs), mono-amine oxidase inhibitors (MAOIs) and selective serotonin reuptake inhibitors (SSRIs) (see Table 9.1). More than 60 per cent of patients with major depression respond to anti-depressant treatment (compared with 30 per cent response to placebo), and relapse is relatively common.

Anti-depressant drugs are generally equal in their efficacy, although individual patient response will vary markedly. Similarly, although the anti-depressant classes have different adverse effects, no class is superior in terms of tolerability (AMH 2013).

Side-effects
Side-effects of TCAs include anti-cholinergic effects (for example, dry mouth, blurred vision, constipation, urinary hesitancy or retention, orthostatic hypotension), sedation, weight gain and sweating. Other less common side-effects include reduced GI (gastro-intestinal) motility, delirium, impotence, loss of libido, other sexual adverse effects, tremor, dizziness, agitation and insomnia. Other important considerations with TCAs include the need:

- to check BP (supine and standing) before and after starting treatment and after each dose change

Table 9.1 Anti-depressants: drug groups, generic and trade names

Drug group	Generic name	Trade name
Selective serotonin reuptake inhibitors (SSRIs)	Citalopram	Cipramil
	Fluoxetine	Prozac
	Sertraline	Zoloft
	Paroxetine	Aropax
	Escitalopram	Esitalo
	Fluvoxamine	Luvox
Serotonin and noradrenaline reuptake inhibitors (SNRIs)	Desvenlafaxine	Pristiq
	Duloxetine	Cymbalta
	Venlafaxine	Efexor
Tricyclic anti-depressants (TCAs)	Amitriptyline	Tryptanol
	Clomipramine	Anafranil
	Dothiepin	Dothep
	Doxepin	Sinequan
	Imipramine	Tofranil
	Nortriptyline	Norpress
	Trimipramine	Surmontil
Mono-amine oxidase inhibitors (MAOIs)	Phenelzine	Nardil
	Tranylcypromine	Parnate
	Moclobemide	Aurorix
Other anti-depressants:	Agomelatine	Valdoxan
(Tetracyclic Anti-depressant (TeCA),	Mianserin	Tolvon
Noradrenergic and Specific Serotonergic Anti-depressant	Mirtazapine	Avanza
(NaSSA), Methanesulfonate Salt	Reboxetine	Edronax

- to be aware that, although adverse effects may appear early, therapeutic response is usually delayed by two weeks
- to be conscious that increased suicidal thoughts and behaviour are possible soon after starting anti-depressants
- to be aware that the use of high-strength TCA tablets and capsules is in maintenance treatment only, as overdose with high-strength products is associated with increased mortality compared with low strengths
- to understand that the use is as a single dose at night to aid adherence; if insomnia develops or daytime anxiolytic effect is desirable, it can be given in two or three divided doses
- to alter the dose in increments every two to three days as needed
- to withdraw TCAs slowly to avoid withdrawal symptoms. (Adapted from AMH 2013)

Side-effects of MAOIs include anti-cholinergic effects (for example, dry mouth, blurred vision, constipation, urinary hesitancy or retention, hypotension), insomnia, sedation, weight gain, postural hypotension, reduced GI motility, delirium, impotence, loss of libido, other sexual adverse effects, tremor, dizziness, sweating and agitation. MAOIs:

- are used for atypical depression and psychotic depression; and in some circumstances for post-traumatic stress disorder
- may increase suicidal behaviour and thoughts soon after commencing medication
- have a number of potentials for drug interactions and this may persist for two to three weeks after cessation
- may cause an initial hypotensive state; however, this is usually temporary (cease if it persists). (Adapted from AMH 2013)

Side-effects of SSRIs include nausea, agitation, insomnia, drowsiness, tremor, dry mouth, diarrhoea, dizziness, headache, sweating, asthenia, anxiety, weight gain or loss, sexual dysfunction, rhinitis, myalgia and rash. When using SSRIs:

- be aware that they are less likely to affect driving or manual machinery operations than other anti-depressants
- understand that the dosage increase may not provide further improvement, except where some psychiatric comorbidities exist
- realise that the dosage for managing OCD or eating disorders is often higher than needed for depression
- begin with only half the normal dose for anxiety compared with that of depression
- understand that, when stopped, the dosage needs to have been tapered down over several weeks first to avoid withdrawal symptoms; reduce the daily dose by half no faster than weekly
- be aware that the drugs can increase suicidal thoughts and behaviour soon after commencement
- be aware that they can cause sexual dysfunction, and that this may affect adherence. (Adapted from AMH 2013)

Revision points
- The synaptic hypothesis of depression proposes that depletion in the synaptic levels of noradrenaline and serotonin underlies the condition. Anti-depressant drugs work by raising the levels of one or both of these neurotransmitters (Bullock & Manias 2010).

CRITICAL THINKING

- As significant therapeutic benefits of anti-depressant therapy are not apparent for some weeks, adherence may be an issue. Outline some approaches that you think could promote adherence to drug therapy.
- Record the recommended daily dose for each of the medications listed in Table 9.1.

Mood stabilisers

Uses

Lithium is the most commonly prescribed drug for treatment of bipolar or mood conditions, and rumours of its healing qualities have been talked of for more than two centuries (Schioldann 2009). Lithium is used to reduce the frequency and severity of manic states, and may also reduce the frequency and severity of depression in bipolar conditions. It is not known how lithium works to stabilise a person's mood. Most recently, researchers have claimed that 'despite six decades of intensive research and an accumulating number of known cellular targets, lithium's mechanism of action still needs to be unravelled' (Toker, Belmaker & Agam 2012, p. 93). Lithium is a naturally occurring element, and its anti-manic properties were discovered in 1949 by Australian psychiatrist John Cade and published in the *Medical Journal of Australia* that year (Cole & Parker 2012).

Side-effects

Common side-effects include nausea, diarrhoea, a metallic taste in the mouth, weight gain, and increased thirst and fluid intake. Less common side-effects include acne, tremor, hypothyroidism and increased urine output.

Lithium toxicity is an issue of major concern. This occurs when the blood level of lithium is elevated, and at very high levels toxicity can cause convulsions, acute renal failure, coma and death. With prevention, this occurs rarely; however, assessment for toxicity should become an ongoing priority. Dehydration is a cause of toxicity; therefore, early warning signs of toxicity need to be acted upon. These include nausea, vomiting, diarrhoea, unsteadiness and mild confusion. Some important points in managing lithium include:

- Acute mania will probably require hospitalisation.
- Therapeutic levels of lithium may take six to ten days, so it may be useful to provide the service user with a benzodiazepine or anti-psychotic in severe mania.

- Titrate the lithium dose to achieve concentration for prophylaxis; treat for six to twelve months.
- Check renal and thyroid function as well as serum calcium concentration at baseline, then check every three to six months (at least annually).
- Conduct an ECG at baseline for patients with significant cardiac disease.
- Anti-depressants may be used with lithium during the depressive phase of bipolar illness.
- Do not stop lithium treatment abruptly; withdraw gradually to avoid relapse. (Adapted from AMH 2013).

Sodium valproate and carbamazepine are increasingly being used as alternative mood stabilisers when lithium is considered too dangerous or is poorly tolerated by the service user. They are sometimes used with each other or with lithium.

Revision points

- Lithium carbonate is a mood stabiliser that acts to deplete synaptic noradrenaline levels. Close monitoring is required, as lithium has a low therapeutic index.
- Some anti-seizure drugs are also used to stabilise mood. They act to stabilise erratic firing patterns in pathways that control mood (Bullock & Manias 2010)

Anti-psychotics (also known as neuroleptics and major tranquillisers)
Uses

The treatment of psychosis was transformed by the discovery of anti-psychotics in the 1950s. They are thought to act by blocking dopamine receptors in the brain, particularly in the limbic system. Benefits for patients who respond to treatment include reducing or eliminating hallucinations, delusions and agitation, which are considered 'positive symptoms' of schizophrenia. There are also sedative and tranquillising effects in very disturbed or aggressive patients. The patient may feel more relaxed and in control. Anti-psychotics also reduce relapse rates after an acute episode. The conventional or typical anti-psychotics are listed in Table 9.2.

The atypical anti-psychotics (particularly clozapine) appear to be more effective in reducing the 'negative symptoms' of schizophrenia, such as lack of motivation, inactivity, restricted affect and speech. They also are more effective for service users for whom treatment has not been successful, and can decrease relapse rates. Some examples are listed in Table 9.3.

If adherence is an issue, long-acting depot injections (intramuscular injections) of conventional anti-psychotics are used for maintenance treatment.

Side-effects

Not all service users will respond uniformly to every medication. There are many side-effects that can occur with anti-psychotic medication. Atypical agents are less likely to

Table 9.2 Conventional (typical) anti-psychotics: drug groups, generic and trade names

Drug group	Generic name	Trade name
Phenothiazines	Chlorpromazine	Largactil
	Thioridazine	Melleril
	Trifluperazine	Stelazine
	Fluphenazine	Modecate
	Pericyazine	Neulactil
Butyrophenones	Haloperidol	Serence
	Droperidol	Droleptan
Diphenylbutylpiperidines	Pimozide	Orap
Thioxanthines	Thiothixene	Navane
	Zuclopenthixol	Clopixol
	Flupentixol	Depixol

Table 9.3 Atypical anti-psychotics: drug groups, generic and trade names

Drug group	Generic name	Trade name
Dibenzapines	Amisulpride	Solian
	Clozapine	Clozaril
	Olanzapine	Zyprexa
	Quetiapine	Seroquel
	Risperidone	Risperdal
	Paliperidone	Invega
Dopamine antagonist	Sertindole	Serlect
Phenylindole derivative	Ziprasidone	Geodon
Additional anti-depressant or anti-manic properties	Aripiprazole	Abilify
	Asenapine	Saphris

cause acute and chronic extra-pyramidal side-effects (EPSE), which are listed in more detail below. Hyperglycaemia, weight gain and Type 2 diabetes mellitus are more likely with atypical agents.

The atypical drug clozapine has some serious side-effects, including agranulocytosis (a marked decrease in white blood cells), which can occur in less than 1 per cent of the population. The monitoring of white blood cells is essential, and agranulocytosis can occur up to a year after treatment; however, the majority of cases occur six months after commencement of treatment.

The points below list some of the considerations for dispensing and managing and educating on the use of typical and atypical anti-psychotic medications.

- Preference is for the lowest effective dose, especially if continuous treatment will be required.
- Long-acting injections are not for commencement of treatment; rather, they may be suitable once dose titration is achieved.
- Avoid using anti-psychotics routinely for short-term management of anxiety, agitation or disturbed behaviour in non-psychotic disorders, and consider that benzodiazepines may be more appropriate.
- Monitor carefully for clinical improvement, and document possible reasons for non-response.
- Check weight, blood glucose and BP when first commenced and regularly thereafter.
- Routine full blood counts and liver function tests are advisable.
- Use of a benzodiazepine may allow anti-psychotic dose reduction in acute psychotic states exhibiting acute agitation.
- Avoid use of more than one anti-psychotic, except in periods of 'cross-over' from one drug to another.
- Supervise and carefully monitor when switching from one anti-psychotic drug to another.
- Individualise treatment duration: prophylaxis is usually continued for one to two years after remission of a first psychotic episode in order to prevent relapse (which may occur several weeks after stopping treatment), and for longer after more than two episodes.
- Total daily oral dose may be given at night once stabilised (due to the long half-life of most anti-psychotics).
- Slowly withdraw any anti-psychotics, monitoring for tachycardia, sweating and insomnia (due to prominent anti-cholinergic effects). (Adapted from AMH 2013)

Neuroleptic malignant syndrome (NMS) is a rare, serious and potentially fatal condition occurring as a result of anti-psychotics. Trollor and colleagues (2012) found in their recent study of NMS cases in Australia over the past 20 years that both the typical and atypical anti-psychotic drugs were possible causes of the syndrome; however, the atypical sufferers (second-generation anti-psychotic medications) were younger, more likely to be diagnosed with a psychotic disorder and less likely to present with extra-pyramidal symptoms, and mortality was lower than for sufferers from the typical (first-generation) anti-psychotic drugs.

Major signs of NMS can include increased body temperature and rigidity. It is similar to severe Parkinsonism with hyperthermia, and treatment is urgent. It can also occur as a result of anti-depressant use, but this is even less common (Bullock & Manias 2010).

Extra-pyramidal side effects

Some people who commence anti-psychotic medications may have a reaction to this group of drugs where the extra-pyramidal (motor) system is affected due to the effects of blocking dopamine. These effects are commonly seen in people suffering from Parkinson's Disease and Huntington's Disease. Parkinsonism is characterised by a mask-like facial expression, muscle rigidity, 'pillrolling' tremor, shuffling gait, festination (involuntary acceleration in rate of walking), retropulsion (involuntary backward walking or running) and diminished arm swing.

An acute episode of dystonia is characterised by involuntary sustained spasm of the muscles, especially those of the head and neck—for example, facial grimacing, protrusion of the tongue, opisthotonos (tetanic spasm in muscles of the back, causing the head and lower limbs to bend backward and arching of the body so that it rests on the heels and the head), oculogyric crisis (involuntary contraction of the eye muscles, resulting in a gaze that is usually in an upward direction). In the longer term, dystonia is demonstrated by sustained involuntary spasm of skeletal muscles, resulting in abnormal posture.

(Tardive) akathisia is represented by the subjective feeling of 'inner restlessness' with a drive to move, frequent changes of posture, inability to sit still and constant walking.

Tardive ayskinesia is indicated by abnormal involuntary movements of the face, tongue and lips, with chewing movements, tongue movement, puckering of lips and grimacing. It may be associated with slow writhing, involuntary or irregular movements of the extremities (AMH 2013).

CRITICAL THINKING

- Geraldine has been ordered to take Risperidone. What education would be of benefit to her?
- Record the recommended daily dose for each of the medications listed in Tables 9.2 and 9.3.

Revision points

- Anti-psychotics are used in the treatment of psychoses in conditions such as schizophrenia, dementia and severe agitation.
- All anti-psychotics affect dopamine and serotonin receptors, and antagonise dopaminergic activity in the central nervous system.
- There are two principal groups: typical and atypical.

- Typical anti-psychotics act on D2 receptors and cause EPSEs.
- Atypical anti-psychotics act principally on D4 receptors and tend not to cause EPSEs.
- Anti-psychotics have a diverse and potentially debilitating adverse effect profile. (adapted from Bullock & Manias 2010)

The use of Anti-Parkinsonian/anti-cholinergic medications

Anti-Parkinsonians affect and reduce acetylcholine, thereby reducing EPSE caused by traditional anti-psychotics—especially drug-induced Parkinsonism, dystonias and akinesia.

Tremor and akathisia respond less well to anti-Parkinsonians, and there can be a worsening of tardive dyskinesia. Common anti-Parkinsonians are shown in Table 9.4. The tertiary amines 'act centrally and peripherally and have the full range of adverse effects, including anti-nicotinic action at higher doses. Quaternary amines are less active orally and tend to have fewer CNS effects'. (AMS 2013)

Table 9.4 Anti-Parkinsonian drugs: generic and trade names

Tertiary amines	Quaternary amines
Benzhexol	Glycopyrrolate
Benztropine	Hyoscine butylbromide
Biperiden	Propantheline
Darifenacin	
Hyoscine hydrobromide	
Orphenadrine	
Oxybutynin	
Solifenacin	
Tolterodine	

Side-effects

Side-effects—which are usually dose-related—include dryness of the mouth, dilation of the pupils, nausea, blurred vision, gastric upset and urinary hesitancy. Less common side-effects include dizziness, hallucinations, delirium and tachycardia. It is important to not suddenly stop taking the anti-Parkinsonian/anti-cholinergic medications, as an acute exacerbation of the side-effects may reappear (AMS 2013). Misuse of anti-cholinergics, whereby excessive doses are taken, can cause hallucinations and highly toxic effects. This can lead to fatalities and must be treated as a medical emergency.

Other drugs to treat EPSEs include anti-histamine and benzodiazepines.

Benzodiazepines

The World Health Organization (<www.who.org>) claims that Benzodiazepines are some of the most widely used and misused drugs in the world today, despite their use for treatment of anxiety and as hypnotics. The issue of dependence and misuse must be considered alongside their many therapeutic values.

Uses

The drugs in this group are most commonly used as muscle relaxants and anti-convulsants, to alleviate stress and anxiety, and to promote sleep. Benzodiazepines increase the strength of the outcome of gamma-aminobutyric acid (GABA) throughout the central nervous system, resulting in anxiolytic, sedative, hypnotic, muscle-relaxant and anti-epileptic effects.

Table 9.5 Minor tranquillising drugs: generic and trade names

Generic name (examples)	Trade name (examples)
Alprazolam	Xanax
Bromaepam	Lexotan
Chlordiazepoxide	Librium
Clobazam	Frisium
Diazepam	Valium
Flunitrazepam	Rohypnol
Lorazepam	Ativan
Nitrazepam	Mogadon
Oxazepam	Serepax
Temazepam	Normison
Triazolam	Halcion
Zopiclone	Imovane
Buspirone	Buspar
Zolpidem	Stilnox

Side-effects

Common side-effects include drowsiness, over-sedation, light-headedness, memory loss, ataxia and slurred speech.

Infrequent side-effects include headache, vertigo, hypotension, disorientation, confusion, paradoxical excitation, euphoria, aggression and hostility, anxiety, decreased libido, anterograde amnesia, pain and thrombophlebitis with IV injection, and respiratory arrest with IV use.

Rare side-effects include blood conditions (including leucopenia and leucocytosis), jaundice, transient elevated liver function tests and allergic reactions (including rash and anaphylaxis).

Tolerance of and dependence on benzodiazepines may occur, so withdrawal symptoms may develop when the medication is stopped suddenly. These withdrawal symptoms include anxiety, dysphoria, irritability, insomnia, nightmares, sweating, memory impairment, hallucinations, hypertension, tachycardia, psychosis, tremors and seizures. Withdrawal symptoms may not occur until several days after stopping, and can last for several weeks or longer after prolonged use. To prevent or alleviate withdrawal symptoms, gradual dose reduction is required (AMH 2013; Treatment Protocol Project 2004).

CRITICAL THINKING
Record the recommended daily dose for each of the medications listed in Tables 9.4 and 9.5.

Revision points

- There are divergent groups of hypnotics and sedatives; benzodiazepines are the most common group.
- Benzodiazepines act on the GABA receptor complex.
- Benzodiazepines can be addictive and have undesirable adverse effects.
- With most anxiolytics, the anti-anxiety effect is related to their sedative effect. (Galbraith et al. 2004)

ELECTRO-CONVULSIVE THERAPY

Electro-convulsive therapy (ECT) is an intervention utilised primarily in the treatment of depression, and to some extent for the affective or mood disturbances of schizophrenia. ECT has always been regarded as a highly controversial intervention, and this remains true in the twenty-first century (Andre 2009). The very actions of ECT remain unclear, and may provoke strong reactions in mental health practitioners and service users alike.

This section discusses information on the history, indications for treatment and nursing interventions concerning ECT. An overview is also provided of trans-cranial magnetic stimulation (TMS), a newer form of treatment that is perhaps seen as an alternative to ECT.

CRITICAL THINKING

Listen to the song 'Mother's Little Helper' by the Rolling Stones, the lyrics of which can be downloaded from <www.youtube.com/watch?v=7ETX7i_adnw>.

- Is this song as relevant today as it was in the 1960s and 1970s? Why/why not?
- Are the lyrics sympathetic to motherhood? If so, in what way?

What is ECT?

An electric current is passed through the temples (either unilaterally or bilaterally) of an anaesthetised patient in order to induce a grand mal seizure (Stuart & Laraia 2005). The amount of voltage used is based on the minimum possible to achieve the grand mal seizure, and will depend on the history and severity of the patient's condition. The number of treatments given will again depend on the case history of the patient, but will generally fall into a pattern of six to twelve treatments, administered two or three times a week. Currently, ECT is also provided as an out-patient treatment.

History of ECT

ECT has been accepted as an (albeit controversial) treatment, primarily for depression, over the past 60 years. It is currently regarded as being a safe, efficient and effective form of treatment (Kelly & Zisselman 2000; Nuttall et al. 2004)—perhaps more effective than psycho-pharmacology treatment (Pagnin et al. 2004; UK ECT Review Group 2003), and valuable when a rapid response is needed or when other types of therapy have failed (Mitchell 2004). This has not always been the case, and the use of ECT remains controversial among some service users and the public (Andre 2009). *The Journal of ECT* (which also covers related therapies) is published regularly, and covers scientific, medical, sociological, ethical and legal issues relating to this therapy, It is available at <http://journals.lww.com/ectjournal/pages/default.aspx>.

Epileptic seizures have been known throughout the centuries to produce improvement in some psychiatric symptoms for a variety of psychiatric complaints. Different substances were used to induce seizures, but most were too difficult to control, or the effects were fatal. ECT was formally introduced in the late 1930s in Europe (Boyd 2012).

It remains unclear how ECT helps to alleviate the symptoms of depression; however, there are many theories. A number of these are suggested by Kneisl and Trigoboff (2012) and listed below:

- ECT may act as a 'brain defibrillator'.
- It may act as an anti-convulsant.

- It may restore equilibrium between brain hemispheres.
- It may have a placebo effect—that is, it works because people expect it to work.

Contemporary and past depictions of electro-convulsive therapy (ECT) have usually implied that it is a cruel punishment for people who do not conform in society, or that it is used to 'clear a patient's head so that he or she no longer feels depressed' (Walter 2004). Most of the information that service users and the general public have concerning ECT has been acquired from movies, newspaper reports or novels. For example, movies such as *One Flew Over the Cuckoo's Nest* (1975) and *Frances* (1982) are responsible for negative images and ideas of ECT (Walter 2004; Walter et al. 2002). Anti-ECT lobby groups, such as the Scientology movement, and anti-psychiatry groups have also played a part in portraying ECT negatively.

There continues to be a debate in the community regarding the safety of ECT. Authors such as Andre (2009) claim that important questions about the use of ECT remain unanswered, and this is simply not good enough when considering evidence-based practices. For example, does ECT permanently damage the brain, and does it cause ongoing amnesia and cognitive damage?

Indications for the use of ECT

The most common indicators for the use of ECT are aptly described by the Treatment Protocol Project (2004). These include:

- depressive conditions (including those with psychotic features, those of unipolar affective conditions and those that have not responded to anti-depressant drug therapy)
- mania (severe unremitting mania that has not responded to psycho-pharmacological treatments and as an alternative to neuroleptics)
- schizophrenia (specifically, catatonic states, comorbid affective states, those that have not responded to psycho-pharmacological treatments and underlying anti-social behaviours)
- neuro-psychiatric conditions (severe catatonic states and neurologically malignant states)
- older people (where psycho-pharmacology is contra-indicated with other pharmacological treatments)
- pregnancy (where rapid resolution is paramount, psycho-pharmacology is contra-indicated and previous treatment indicates good recovery with ECT)
- people experiencing physical illness (where no contra-indications are present).

The law and ECT

ECT is commonly used as a treatment for severe depression. It may only be given to a person with the status of 'voluntary patient', and requires the service user's informed and signed consent. The Mental Health Review Tribunal must approve all plans to administer ECT to involuntary patients (see Chapter 5 for more information).

Nursing interventions

The service user's and their family's questions need to be addressed in depth, and available treatment options, risks involved and consequences of ECT must be discussed fully. Nursing involvement before the procedure may include reviewing consent, service user education, fasting before the procedure, laboratory tests and baseline vital signs. After the procedure, the service user needs to be monitored, as does any post-anaesthetic patient. The mental health nurse should specifically monitor vital signs, observe for any confusion and, if the service user is going home, remind family members to observe how the service user manages at home throughout this therapy. Follow-up appointments need to be organised, and mental health and depression must be monitored carefully (Boyd 2012).

Side-effects

The immediate side-effects of which service users may complain include amnesia, headaches, nausea and confusion. Research undertaken by various health professionals states that no long-term effects on memory or intelligence are evident, but long-term memory loss is a frequent subjective complaint of ECT patients. Also unanswered is the matter of whether ECT saves lives in the case of acute risk of suicide. O'Reilly, Bell and Chen (2010) suggest that more research needs to be undertaken in collaboration with both health-care professionals and service users.

Lawrence's (1996) study endeavoured to detect areas of concern among service users who had undergone ECT and 'to give previously unheard voices a chance to speak out' (for more information see <www.ect.org/resources/voices.html>). Questions continue to arise regarding service users' subjective experiences, and the issue of whether memory problems stem from the underlying depression remains unresolved and is at times highly controversial (Andre 2009).

In summary, ECT has a long and often controversial history, and may require significant understanding from the mental health nurse in order to provide support and strong current evidence-based psycho-education to service users and their families. Regularly updating current knowledge on policies, procedures, side-effects and research on this topic will help provide the basis for evidence-based mental health nursing practice.

TRANS-CRANIAL MAGNETIC STIMULATION (TMS)

TMS involves the use of magnetic fields to stimulate the brain with indirect electric current, which disrupts neuronal firing (Kneisl & Trigoboff 2012). Electro-magnetism is produced by magnetic fields moving electrical charges. These changing magnetic fields can then produce electric currents. When working in succession, this triggers the occurrence of trans-cranial magnetic stimulation. Further information can be found at <http://sulcus.berkeley.edu/mcb/165_001/papers/manuscripts/_905.html>.

CRITICAL THINKING

After reading a number of the articles pertaining to ECT in the references section, list the advantages and disadvantages of ECT and, if possible, discuss your responses in small groups. Also consider/discuss how a nurse might provide support for the service user and their family if the service user is a conscientious objector to this form of therapy.

- Outline the common and most significant side-effects of ECT.
- How can informed consent be obtained?
- What is the nurse's role in ECT psycho-education?
- What alternatives to ECT might be discussed with the service user?
- What preparations should the nurse provide prior to ECT?
- List any adverse effects that a nurse should monitor for post-ECT.
- How might the nurse provide emotional support to the service user and their family?

TMS is delivered through a coil, which is held close to the head. TMS seems to be a safe, promising tool for the treatment of depression. It is considered painless, does not require anaesthesia, does not induce seizure and appears to have fewer cognitive side-effects and risks than electro-convulsive therapy. TMS can be restricted to a small area within the skull in a highly specific manner. It appears to work by causing disruption in order to change patterns of thinking (Kneisl & Trigoboff 2012). TMS is being examined as an alternative to ECT, and is being implemented in such countries as Australia, the United Kingdom and Canada. Research is continuing worldwide in the field of neuro-stimulation techniques, which are being seen as useful options for severely depressed patients who have found medication and psychotherapy unhelpful. ECT has been seen as the proven technique, but there are newer stimulation techniques under development (Carpenter 2006).

CONCLUSION

Throughout this chapter, the physical treatments currently available for mental health conditions have been discussed and explored. As you would have come to realise by this point, many of these treatments are of a pharmacological nature, and therefore include inherent issues relating to a reliance on medication as a potential cure-all. Nurses need to have an understanding of the process and procedure of medication as a form of treatment, and how this affects the service user and carer. The future of physical treatments in mental health care may depend on our understanding of causation, neurobiology and even genetics. The next chapter explores other non-pharmacological therapies.

REFERENCES

Andre, L. (2009). *Doctors of Deception: what they don't want you to know about shock treatment*. New Brunswick, NJ: Rutgers University Press.

Australian Medicines Handbook (AMH) (2013). Viewed 20 February 2013, <www.amh.net.au>.

Boyd, M.A. (2012). *Psychiatric Nursing Contemporary Practice* (5th edn). Philadelphia, PA: Wolters Kluwer/ Lippincott Williams & Wilkins.

Bullock, S. & Manias, E. (2010). *Fundamentals of Pharmacology* (6th edn) Sydney: Pearson Education.

Carpenter, L.L. (2006). Neurostimulation in resistant depression. *Journal of Psychopharmacology*, 20, 35.

Chong, W.W., Aslani, P. & Chen, T.F. (2011). Effectiveness of interventions to improve anti-depressant medication adherence: a systematic review. *International Journal of Clinical Practice*, 65(9), 954–75.

Cleary, M., Horsfall, J., Jackson, D., O'Hara-Aarons, M. & Hunt, G.E. (2012). Patients' views and experiences of *pro re nata* medication in acute mental health settings. *International Journal of Mental Health Nursing*, 21(6): 533–9.

Cole, N. & Parker, G. (2012). Cade's identification of lithium for manic-depressive illness: The prospector who found a gold nugget. *The Journal of Nervous and Mental Disease*, 200(12), 1101–4.

Cunningham Owens, D.G. (1999). *A Guide to the Extra-pyramidal Side Effects of Anti-psychotic Drugs*. Cambridge: Cambridge University Press.

Fischel, T., Krivoy, A., Kotlarov, M., Zemishlany, Z., Loebstein O, Jacoby, H. et al. (2012, in press). The interaction of subjective experience and attitudes towards specific anti-psychotic-related adverse effects in schizophrenia patients. *European Psychiatry*. Viewed 20 February 2013, <http://dx.doi.org/10.1016/j.bbr.2011.03.031>.

Galbraith, A., Bullock, S. & Manias, E. (2004). *Fundamentals of Pharmacology*. Sydney: Pearson Education.

Gardner, D. M. & Teehan, M.D. (eds) (2011). *Anti-psychotics and Their Side Effects*. Cambridge: Cambridge University Press.

Gray, R., White, J., Schulz, M. & Abderhalden, C. (2010). Enhancing medication adherence in people with schizophrenia: an international programme of research. *International Journal of Mental Health Nursing*, 19, 36–44.

Gray, R., Wykes, T. & Gournay, K. (2002). From compliance to concordance: a review of the literature on interventions to enhance compliance with anti-psychotic medication. *Journal of Psychiatric and Mental Health Nursing*, 9, 277–84.

Kelly, K. & Zisselman, M. (2000). Update on electroconvulsive therapy (ECT) in older adults. *Journal of the American Geriatrics Society*, 48(5), 560–6.

Kneisl, C.A. & Trigoboff, E. (2012). *Contemporary Psychiatric–Mental Health Nursing* (3rd ed.). Upper Saddle River, NJ: Pearson Education.

Lawrence, J. (1996). Voices from within: a study of ECT and patient perceptions 1986–1996. Viewed 13 December 2012, <www.ect.org/resources/voices.html>.

Lunsky, Y. & Balogh, R. (2010). Dual diagnosis: a national study of psychiatric hospitalization patterns of people with developmental disability. *Canadian Journal of Psychiatry*, 55(11), 721–8.

Mitchell, P.B. (2004). Australian and New Zealand clinical practice guidelines for the treatment of bipolar disorder. *Australian and New Zealand Journal of Psychiatry*, 38(5), 280–305.

Molloy, L., Field, J., Beckett, P. & Holmes, D. (2012). PRN psychotropic medication and acute mental health nursing: reviewing the evidence. *Journal of Psychosocial Nursing & Mental Health Services*, 50(8),12–15.

Nuttall, G.A., Bowersox, M.R., Douglass, S.B., McDonald, J., Rasmussen, L.J., Decker, P.A. (2004). Morbidity and mortality in the use of electro-convulsive therapy. *The Journal of ECT*, 20(4), 237–41.

O'Reilly, C.L., Bell, J.S. & Chen, T.F. (2010). Pharmacists' beliefs about treatments and outcomes of mental disorders: a mental health literacy survey. *Australian and New Zealand Journal of Psychiatry*, 44(12), 1089–96.

Pagnin, D., de Queiroz, V., Pini, S. & Cassano, G.B. (2004). Efficacy of ECT in depression: a meta-analytic review. *The Journal of ECT*, 20(1), 13–20.

Schioldann, J.S. (2009). *History of the Introduction of Lithium into Medicine and Psychiatry: birth of modern psychopharmacology*. Adelaide: Academic Press.

Stuart, G.W. & Laraia, M.T. (2005). *Principles and Practice of Psychiatric Nursing* (8th edn). St Louis, MO: Mosby.

Toker, L. Belmaker, R.H. & Agam, G. (2012). Gene-expression studies in understanding the mechanism of action of lithium. *Expert Review of Neurotherapeutics*, 12(1), 93–7.

Treatment Protocol Project (2004). *Acute Inpatient Psychiatric Care: a source book* (2nd edn). World Health Organization and the Centre for Mental Health and Substance Abuse. Sydney: Brown Prior & Anderson.

Trollor, J.N., Chen, X., Chitty, K. & Sachdev, P.S. (2012). Comparison of neuroleptic malignant syndrome induced by first- and second-generation anti-psychotics. *British Journal of Psychiatry*, 201(1), 52–6.

UK ECT Review Group (2003). Efficacy and safety of electroconvulsive therapy in depressive disorders: a systematic review and meta-analysis. *The Lancet*, 361.9360, 799.

Usher, K., Baker, J.A. & Holmes, C.A. (2010). Understanding clinical decision making for PRN medication in mental health inpatient facilities. *Journal of Psychiatric and Mental Health Nursing*, 17(6), 558–64.

Usher, K., Lindsay, D. & Sellen, J. (2001). Mental health nurses' PRN psychotropic medication administration practices. *Journal of Psychiatric and Mental Health Nursing*, 8, 383–90.

Walter, G. (2004). 'About to have ECT? Fine, but don't watch it in the movies': the sorry portrayal of ECT in film. *Psychiatric Times*, 21(6), 65–7.

Walter, G., McDonald, A., Rey, J.M. & Rosen, A. (2002). Medical student knowledge and attitudes regarding ECT prior to and after viewing ECT scenes from movies. *The Journal of ECT*, 18(1), 43–6.

Wong, F.K. & Pi, E.H. (2012). Ethnopsychopharmacology considerations for Asians and Asian Americans. *Asian Journal of Psychiatry*, 5, 18–23.

10

Treatments in mental health: complementary and other therapies

---

Main points

- A range of natural or complementary therapies are used for mental-health problems—particularly anxiety and depression.
- Naturopaths are trained in Australia as primary care practitioners in natural and complementary medicines, including diet and lifestyle modifications and herbal medicine.
- Mental health nurses can play an important role in the use of complementary and alternative therapies.
- Two important issues in natural and complementary therapies are safety and the efficacy of products and procedures.
- Service users, nurses and other health practitioners need to be aware of potential interactions that may arise with concurrent use of conventional medications, dietary supplements (drug–nutrient interactions) and herbal medicines (drug–herb interactions).

Definitions

Complementary and alternative medicines or therapies (CAM): A group of diverse medical and health-care systems, practices and products that are not generally considered part of conventional medicine.

INTRODUCTION

Mental health problems are very common in the general population. Even phenomena such as hearing voices are thought to be experienced by most people at some time in their lives (Beavan, Read & Cartwright, 2011). Most people deal with mental health problems without the assistance of a specialist mental health professional, or even medicine. Many people, when feeling stressed or experiencing mood problems, difficulty with sleeping or feeling out of balance, make changes to their lifestyle, draw on a supportive relationship, or slow down and reflect on what needs to be done to restore equilibrium. For many problems, these are just the kinds of things that need to be done. They are what a competent health professional would recommend. The majority of Australians also routinely use what might be called 'complementary and alternative medicine' (CAM) (Xue et al. 2007).

What counts as a complementary or alternative medicine can sometimes be a little blurry. Complementary and alternative medicines or therapies comprise a diverse range of practices, products and approaches to health that are generally not considered part of conventional or orthodox medicine, nursing and allied health. Some practices, such as acupuncture for pain relief or massage for stress relief, when used with conventional medicine may be referred to as 'complementary medicine'. Other practices—for example, the use of St John's wort—may replace conventional anti-depressant medicines and might be considered an 'alternative' medicine.

People with chronic health problems, and particularly mental health conditions, are more likely to use CAM (Spinks & Hollingsworth 2012). Interventions such as diets, nutritional supplements or approaches to health used by celebrities are widely promoted and described favourably in popular magazines (Dunn & Phillips 2010). CAM therapies may be classified in terms of practices (see Table 10.1), and include the use of natural products, mind and body medicine, manipulative and body-based practices, movement therapies, and practices based on energy fields. Specific CAM practices may have little empirical support but they are very popular (e.g. homœopathy), while others confer general benefits rather than disease-specific ones.

Practitioners of CAM vary in their training and expertise. For example, osteopaths in Australia are a regulated profession and undertake a higher degree in order to gain an expert knowledge of the workings of all body systems. Naturopaths (while presently unregulated) may also obtain higher degree-level qualifications to gain expert knowledge in nutrition, lifestyle and herbal medicine. Practices such as Traditional Chinese Medicine (TCM) or Ayurvedic medicine are actually whole medical systems, and can't easily be reduced to a set of practices. Like contemporary Western medicine, they encompass assumptions about health, illness, methods of diagnosing problems and particular therapeutic techniques. Some practices, such as acupuncture, have become assimilated into Western medicine. Table 10.2 outlines some common CAM practices that people use to address mental health problems.

Many CAM practices are safe when used judiciously or as recommended by appropriately trained practitioners. They are likely to confer considerable health advantages, and attempts often are made to integrate them into routine professional practice. For example, various kinds of meditative practices such as yoga are likely to be helpful for

Table 10.1 Types of complementary and alternative therapies and examples

Natural products
- Herbal medicines (botanicals)
- Vitamins and minerals
- Probiotics and other dietary supplements

Mind and body medicine
- Meditation
- Yoga
- Acupuncture
- Hypnotherapy
- Relaxation exercises
- Qui Gong and Tai Chi
- Traditional Chinese Medicine

Manipulative and body-based practices
- Spinal manipulation
- Massage therapy

Movement therapies
- Alexander technique
- Pilates

Energy field
- Light therapy
- Magnet therapy
- Healing touch

Whole medical systems
- Ayurvedic medicine
- Traditional Chinese Medicine
- Homœopathy
- Naturopathy

Source: NCCAM (2012).

people in reducing anxiety, blood pressure and improving quality of life (Panesar & Valachova 2011; Smith et al. 2007). In recent years, 'mindfulness'—a set of practices derived from meditation and Eastern philosophy—has been incorporated into a range of mainstream therapies. Mindfulness in these contexts encourages people to pay attention to their thoughts and emotions in the present moment without judgement, evaluation or attempting to change them. The evidence for the effectiveness of the practice of mindfulness is beginning to accumulate. It is incorporated in cognitive behavioural therapy (Chiesa & Serretti 2011), in general stress reduction in health care (Smith et al. 2005) and in therapies such as dialectic behavioural therapy (DBT) and acceptance and commitment therapy (Baer 2003). Thus practices that might once have been considered alternative are gradually being assimilated, tested and evaluated in mainstream mental health care.

Table 10.2 Some complementary and alternative therapies used for mental health issues

Uses related to therapy	Description	Uses related to mental health
Homœopathy	Diluted medicinal remedies, where the original substance is no longer present but the diluent is presumed to be highly energised. Treats the whole person by including their mental, emotional and physical symptoms, and matches remedy to individual or specific symptoms. Not to be confused with herbal medicines or Bach flower remedies. Developed over two centuries ago by German physician Samuel Hahnemann. These ought to be administered by a trained homœopath.	Depression (mild to moderate) Insomnia
Bach flower remedies	Flower remedies or essences that are thought to work as energy patterning using water as a means of delivery. Blossoms are infused in water and then removed. Treats the person through energetic patterns of the remedy resonating with emotional patterns of the person. Influences the person's life-force and promotes emotional equilibrium. Developed in the early twentieth century by British doctor and homœopath Edward Bach. May be self-administered by choosing the remedy from a table of current emotional symptoms.	Irritability, stress and tension Despondency and despair Fear and uncertainty Loneliness Lack of interest in everyday life Over-care for others' welfare
Acupuncture	Involves the stimulation of defined points on the skin by inserting needles, and/or by manual pressure (acupressure) and/or electrical or laser stimulation. The concept involved is that the flow of chi (a term referring to vital force or energy) has been disrupted, which has caused the issue/disorder. Treatment aims to stimulate relevant points on the body's surface to unblock or enhance the flow of chi and so treat the disorder. Together with herbal medicines and other treatments, acupuncture is part of Traditional Chinese Medicine, and has been used for over 5000 years. Can also be used as a single therapy. Acupuncture is a regulated therapeutic activity in Australia, and must be conducted by a qualified and experienced practitioner.	Alcohol and other drug abuse and dependence Smoking cessation Tension headaches Anxiety and depression Insomnia
Healing or therapeutic touch	A holistic method that aims to heal or help by using the hands to redirect and rebalance the body's energy field through focusing on the body's energy meridians. Assumes people have the potential to heal naturally, and that energy fields are the basic unit of living beings.	Anxiety Grief Fatigue Relaxation

Uses related to therapy	Description	Uses related to mental health
	Developed in the 1970s by nurse Dolores Kreiger and psychic Dora Kunz. Derived from the 'laying on of hands'.	
Qigong and Tai Chi	*Qi* means 'life-force' and *gong* means 'practice', so Qigong refers to the practice of working with *qi* to improve health through a combination of physical movements, abdominal breathing exercises and meditation or concentration. Tai Chi was derived from Qigong, and was originally used as a martial art, but has therapeutic uses. Can be done either sitting or standing, and many styles are used. Both considered part of Traditional Chinese Medicine, along with herbal medicines and acupuncture, and have been used for several thousand years.	Stress reduction
Relaxation therapy	Various techniques used to counteract the effects of stress on the body and mind, such as hypertension, anxiety and over-active thinking. Techniques include diaphragmatic breathing (using the abdomen for deep breathing), guided imagery (visualisation of pleasant scenes, etc. using pictures, aromas, music, sounds of nature or verbal suggestions) and meditation (gaining peace through non-resistant and calm dwelling or focusing on a word, sound or object and/or a feeling; usually includes attention to breathing). To be helpful, these techniques need to be practised regularly.	Relaxation Stress reduction Anxiety Insomnia Depression Grief and bereavement Low self-esteem
Reflexology	A treatment where varying degrees of pressure are applied to different parts of the body, usually the feet or hands, in order to promote health and well-being. Zones or reflexes are considered to run through the body and terminate in the hands and feet, and all body systems and organs are considered to be reflected on the surface of the skin. Treats the person through gentle pressure being applied to these areas in order to effect change in other parts of the body. Has been in existence for over 5000 years. More recent developments attributed to Dr William Fitzgerald at the end of the nineteenth century.	Relaxation Stimulating various parts of the body
Herbal medicines	The use of whole plant materials to promote recovery from disease and to enable healing through mobilising the vital force or life energy of the person. Methods include infusions (herbal teas), capsules, external applications (creams, lotions), tinctures (concentrated herbal extract in water and alcohol) and juices.	Relaxation Stress reduction

Uses related to therapy	Description	Uses related to mental health
	Common herbal medicines include ginseng, liquorice, St John's wort, foxglove (digitalis), meadowsweet and willow (aspirin). Use is evident from the first century BC in ancient Greek, Egyptian and Chinese cultures. Therapeutic doses should only be prescribed by a qualified herbalist or naturopath.	
Humour and laughter therapy	Humour therapy refers to a humorous intervention used by the service user or health professional to produce a beneficial response in the service user. Laughter therapy is an intervention used by the service user or health professional to produce laughter in the service user. Humour can occur without laughter, and laughter without humour. Physical and emotional responses to humour and laughter can have positive effects on all organ systems. Interventions include watching funny films, telling/hearing jokes, telling/hearing funny stories. Used therapeutically from the thirteenth century.	Anxiety Fear Agitation and anger Tension and stress Facilitate communication and develop therapeutic rapport
Music therapy and music-as-therapy	A systematic process where the therapist helps the service user to achieve health using musical experiences, and the relationships that can develop through this process, in order to effect change. Usually performed by a qualified music therapist. Music-as-therapy is the use of music to accomplish therapeutic aims such as restoring, maintaining and improving mental health. Can be used informally by nurses and service users. Includes the use of music as background listening, or more formally in group sessions, live concerts or creating/playing music. Used as therapy since the eighteenth century.	Relaxation Stress reduction Fear and anxiety Anger and agitation
Aromatherapy	The therapeutic use of essential oils from plants. Often mixed with carrier oils for use on the body. Primarily uses the sense of smell and absorption of the oil through the skin as healing aids. Can be used via a number of applications (e.g. massage, inhalations, compresses, baths and vaporisers). Common oils include lavender, clary sage, peppermint, orange, eucalyptus, tea tree, rose, bergamot, ylang ylang, geranium. Modern-day use developed in the early twentieth century, and the practice was named by French chemist Rene-Maurice Gattefosse.	Relaxation Anxiety and agitation Insomnia Stress reduction Enhance mood Headaches

Sources: Benor (2001); Biley (2001); Busby (2001); Griffiths (2001); Lennihan (2004); Linde et al. (2001b); Lovas (2001); Mallett (2001); Meyer (2001); Wren & Norred (2003).

As healers and educators, nurses are well placed to provide care that is holistic and acknowledges service users' use of CAM (Grimaldi 2004). The increasing attention given worldwide to CAM since the late 1980s has seen an emergence of interest in these therapies in nursing, as the notions of healing, spirituality and energy can be seen to resonate with nursing's interest in the many facets of caring (Watson 1999). As service users of CAM in the general community, nursing students are likely to have some knowledge of complementary and alternative therapies, as they may have used them in their personal lives. Generally, however, nursing students' knowledge and understanding of CAM has been found to be limited (Uzun & Tan 2004). Given the common use of CAM by the general public, gaining knowledge about these medicines and therapies in your nursing education may assist you to respond more effectively to service users' questions, and enhance your capacity to provide comprehensive nursing care in mental health and other health settings. One area in which it is essential for nurses to have some understanding of CAM is in the area of promoting positive mental health.

CRITICAL THINKING

Consider a version of the solution focused 'miracle question' outlined in Chapter 13:

Suppose you were to wake up tomorrow morning to find that a miracle had occurred and you had learned how to be mentally healthy. Make a list of the things you would do, how you might behave and how you might experience the world. From this list, what 'lifestyle' recommendations could you make that might be useful to promoting mental health?

LIFESTYLE INTERVENTIONS

Many CAM practitioners are concerned about promoting healthy lifestyles, and are able to offer coaching in areas of lifestyle that health professionals are often poorly equipped to address. Promoting mental health has been so far outside the traditional sphere of interest of mental health services as to be verging on the alternative, although this is changing rapidly. The greatest threats to quality of life, and the main causes of mortality and morbidity in the developed world are the so-called lifestyle diseases, such as cardiovascular disease, obesity, diabetes and cancer. These are strongly determined by lifestyle, and in particular a bad diet, lack of exercise, alcohol intake and smoking. People diagnosed with and treated for mental illness have been found to have rates of such disease many times higher than the rest of the community, and consequently they have a life expectancy that is between ten and 32 years less than the general population

(National Mental Health Commission 2012). Psychiatric treatments themselves often contribute to heightened risk. Walsh (2011) suggests that mental health professionals have greatly under-estimated the importance of lifestyle factors in the aetiology of multiple psycho-pathologies, both for fostering individual and social well-being and preserving cognitive functioning.

Making positive lifestyle change

The components of positive mental health are much like the elements of good health generally. It also seems that what is helpful for the general mental health of people is at least as helpful for people with diagnosed mental health problems. A team of people in Western Australia developed a social marketing campaign to promote positive mental health for individuals and groups called Act-Belong-Commit (see <www.actbelongcommit.org.au>). They suggest that people can become more mentally healthy by following the A-B-C guidelines outlined in Figure 10.1.

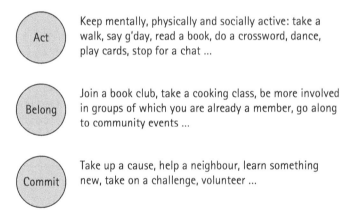

Figure 10.1 The A-B-C guidelines for positive mental health provide a simple approach that we can adopt to become more mentally healthy

Source: <www.actbelongcommit.org.au>.

Making therapeutic lifestyle changes can help prevent the development of mental health problems, and may be as effective as psychotherapy or pharmacotherapy for some problems (Walsh 2011). Lifestyle changes can offer many health advantages—particularly those involving exercise, improved diet, better relationships, recreation and relaxation, spending time in nature, religious or spiritual involvement and providing service to others (Walsh 2011).

CRITICAL THINKING

There is little doubt that engaging in regular physical exercise contributes to improved mood and general well-being. Indeed, exercise is often found to be as effective as anti-depressants in improving mood (Conn 2010; Freeman et al. 2010). What remains to be clarified is what kind of exercise intensity and frequency might best suit an individual. Studies are conflicting on this issue and at the present time it may be best to tailor an exercise regime to the individual which includes a mixture of low intensity, resistance and stretching exercises with aerobic exercise added if tolerated. Group exercise may confer motivational and social advantages. Practitioners such as exercise physiologists have expertise in tailoring exercise regimes for individuals.

Diet

Like exercise, diet has a profound effect on mood. Deficiencies in essential nutrients such as folic acid, vitamin B12 and zinc are strongly associated with psychiatric problems, and where deficiencies are likely, then supplementation is recommended (Abou-Saleh & Coppen 1986; Lai et al. 2012). Similarly, deficiencies have been examined in bipolar disorder and some promising results have been found with omega-3 fatty acids and chromium supplementation. People diagnosed with schizophrenia who have a diet high in sugar and saturated fat have worse long-term outcomes (Peet 2004). Furthermore, surveys of people diagnosed with schizophrenia have found that they often adhere to a diet that contributes to poor mental health and metabolic syndrome (Dipasquale et al. 2012). It appears that adherence to a healthy diet is a lifestyle change that might have profound positive effects on people's overall health.

There has been considerable interest in what is known as the Mediterranean diet and its mental health-enhancing properties (SánchezVillegas et al. 2006). This dietary pattern is characterised by a relatively high level of consumption of fruits, nuts, vegetables, legumes, cereals, olive oil and fish, moderate alcohol intake and low meat and dairy consumption. The Mediterranean diet is particularly rich in folic acid, the B vitamins and anti-oxidants, and these nutrients play a protective role in cardiovascular disease, Alzheimer's disease and depressive disorders. While their mechanisms of action in chronic disease are not completely known, vitamin B6 and B12 are involved in converting homocysteine into substances that are involved in the synthesis of important neurotransmitters. Thus a decreased intake of B vitamins leads to an accumulation of homocysteine and a decreased synthesis of monoamines in the brain, which are likely to contribute to psychiatric symptoms in the long term (SánchezVillegas et al. 2006).

A controversial CAM approach to nutrition is called 'orthomolecular medicine'. This involves determining and evaluating the concentrations of substances normally present in the human body and the prescription of supplements to address this deficiency (Robinson & Pauling 1974). Orthomolecular medicine proponents often advocate the administration of large doses of vitamins and minerals. Large doses of vitamin C, nicotinic acid and other minerals were once given to people diagnosed with schizophrenia, but randomised clinical trials have failed to support the efficacy of such treatments, which have been found to carry risks (Petrie & Ban 1985). It appears that moderation and supplementation when there is a clear deficiency (as in thiamine or vitamin B1 deficiency in alcoholism) is the safest option for people. There is also no diet that suits everyone; like exercise, diet ought to be tailored to the individual, ensuring that it includes essential vitamins, minerals and fatty acids.

Sleep

Sleep disturbances affect between 50 and 80 per cent of all people diagnosed with mental health problems, and it is well known that the quality and amount of sleep people experience have profound impacts on their mental well-being (Kallestad et al. 2012). The regulation of sleep and wake cycles is an area of intense research, and treating sleep disturbances can involve the use of CAM (see Wickboldt et al. 2012 for a review of assessment and treatment). As with most problems, the causes of sleep disturbances should be sought and addressed, and physiological problems such as sleep routines or the iatrogenic effect of medical treatments ought to be ruled out. Common factors associated with insomnia include stress, intrusive thoughts, poor sleep routines, poor diet or activity scheduling, excessive use of stimulants such as caffeine and uncomfortable sleep environments.

Pharmacological approaches to addressing sleep disturbances are limited because people rapidly habituate to common sedative/hypnotics. Alternative approaches tend to be safer and confer other advantages. Many herbal preparations, including valerian, hops, passionflower, kava-kava and peppermint, are thought to aid sleep quality although most have received very little research attention (Antoniades et al. 2012). Acupuncture, relaxation training and guided imagery, aromatherapy and music therapy all may be of use in promoting sleep (Cuellar, Rogers & Hisghman 2007). Diet and exercise are probably also related to sleep, and moderate amounts of exercise obtained through a variety of means can be sufficient to improve sleep quality (Buman & King 2010).

Relationships and belonging

The A-B-C health promotion campaign urges people to extend and strengthen their social networks, join a group or make a commitment to helping others. This is exceptionally good advice, even for people with the most severe mental health problems. Our sense of connection to other people and affiliation with groups is fundamental to our identity. The quality and types of relationships we enjoy have a strong bearing on our mental health, and when relationships break down this can contribute to depression and despair. Social networks can provide a buffer against stress and provide sources of support (Kawachi & Berkman 2001).

A considerable body of evidence has accumulated regarding the benefits associated with belonging to self-help organisations such as Alcoholics Anonymous or GROW. What seems pivotal to the success of self-help groups is the opportunity for people to assist others as well as the sense of belonging that such involvement entails (Lakeman, Watts & Howell 2010). Research of the effect on volunteering on the physical and mental health of older people supports this proposition. Volunteering has been found to slow decline in self-reported health and functioning and improve well-being (Lum & Lightfoot 2005).

Some of the most important relationships experienced by adults are intimate and sexual. Most research and commentary on sexuality in the mainstream mental health field relates to the adverse impacts of sexual abuse and trauma, sexual risk-taking or sexual dysfunction associated with medical treatments. Very little research addresses the undoubted health benefits of a good sex life. Achievement of orgasm causes a massive flood of prolactin and other 'feel-good' chemicals—particularly when achieved through sexual engagement with another person (Brody 2009). In large representative surveys, people's sense of well-being, as well as their satisfaction with their intimate relationships, has been found to be directly related to the frequency of sexual intercourse. The mechanisms by which positive sexual functioning relates to well-being and impacts on relationships are complex and poorly understood, but nevertheless sexual functioning is bound inextricably to both physical and mental health (Diamond & Huebner 2012). Professionals such as sex therapists, who are trained in and at ease with discussing sexual problems as well as promoting positive sexual behaviour, are likely to make a positive contribution to people's well-being.

EVALUATING AND RECOMMENDING COMPLEMENTARY AND ALTERNATIVE MEDICINE

The widespread use of complementary and alternative medicines and therapies is a global phenomenon. For example, up to 80 per cent of the populations in developing countries rely on traditional medicines due to their cultural traditions or a lack of alternatives. In developed countries such as Australia, people often seek out natural remedies with the assumption that they are safe (WHO 2004). Indeed, in Australia the complementary and alternative medicine industry is booming and the public is increasingly aware of the various forms of these treatments through media advertising and information (MacLennan, Wilson & Taylor 2002). For example a representative population survey in Australia estimated that 52.1 per cent of the population used at least one complementary or alternative medicine. A profile of users indicated that they were most likely to be female and commonly used alternative medicines such as herbal medicines, Chinese medicines and aromatherapy. Nearly a quarter of the respondents had consulted alternative therapists such as reflexologists, acupuncturists, aromatherapists and herbal therapists (MacLennan, Wilson & Taylor 2002).

Professional organisations such as the Royal College of Nursing Australia (RCN) (1997) and the New South Wales Nurses' Association (2006) have policies on the use of complementary therapies in nursing practice. These argue that many traditional nursing interventions might be considered complementary and the nursing profession has a right to interpret complementary therapies within the context of nursing theory and practice, with the caveat that the profession has a responsibility to provide evidence for the efficacy of complementary therapies employed as nursing interventions. The New South Wales Nurses' Association goes further by stating that the practice of complementary therapies ought to be supported by written policies; practices and outcomes need to be documented; informed consent should be provided; the treating medical practitioner should be informed (where appropriate); and nurses ought to have an appropriate qualification in any therapy they practise (NSW Nurses' Association 2006). Nurses must be extremely cautious in recommending any therapy, and in particular making claims about the therapeutic efficacy of products.

In general, CAM has been considered under-researched, with a resulting lack of evidence as to their efficacy (Linde et al. 2001a, 2001b). Some therapies have been exhaustively examined and found to be ineffective. For example, homœopathy—which is a popular system of medicine (particularly in Europe)—has frequently been found to yield clinical effects no better than control treatments or placebo (Ernst 2002). The positive subjective effects of homœopathy and similar treatments such as Bach flower remedies is probably due to the placebo effect, which is increasingly being recognised as a substantial part of the efficacy of all manner of healing rituals within and outside of medicine (Kaptchuk 2002). It ought to be noted that many contemporary mental health treatments such as anti-depressants have been found to be only marginally more effective than placebo (Pigott et al. 2010). However, the finding of no efficacy creates a conundrum for health professionals, who cannot ethically recommend a treatment that has no efficacy for a specific problem—although they may propose that it might make a person feel better. A risk with approaches such as homœopathy stems from people delaying or not receiving appropriate treatment if they erroneously believe that it might address a specific disease, such as an infection. Unlike medicines and herbal remedies, they are unlikely to cause any side-effects or adverse effects.

In Australia, any product for which therapeutic claims are made is regulated by the Therapeutic Goods Administration (TGA), and must be listed, registered or included in the Australian Register of Therapeutic Goods (ARTG). Some herbal remedies are listed on the ARTG, but many other preparations are marketed with no therapeutic claims or as foods. Many CAM therapies make no claims about treating specific diseases, but rather are purported to play a supportive role in promoting health.

Arguably, many (but not all) CAM approaches are orientated towards promoting health rather than treating illness. Some non-conventional systems of health care might even be considered holistic (addressing the whole person), whereas much of medicine is technocratic or concerned with a technical or scientific response to highly circum-scribed problems (Davis-Floyd 2001). Many human processes such as childbirth, death and dying, or living a fulfilling and healthy life require a different response to that provided within the technocratic medical paradigm. This poses a dilemma for those working within mental health systems in that the cultures of mental health services often emphasise framing problems as symptoms of an illness in need of an evidence-based treatment (Lakeman 2012). Rarely are CAMs framed as treatments in this way by CAM practitioners, and nor are there the large financial incentives available to research what may help promote mental health, as there are for researching and extending the market for psychiatric drugs. Thus many CAM approaches cannot be evaluated in the same way as medical treatments. For example, Ayurvedic medicine has been used to treat mental health problems for over 3000 years, and involves massage, diet, the regulation of life-style and complex mixtures of herbs. A few scientific trials have shown promise in the treatment of schizophrenia compared to psychiatric drugs (Agarwal et al. 2007), but it is difficult to compare a whole system of care or range of interventions prescribed for an individual to the provision of a single drug.

Some CAM treatments have been examined and found to be effective for specific mental health problems, and there is at least some empirical support for commonly used treatments for anxiety and depression (Kessler et al. 2001), such as the herb St John's wort (*Hypericum perforatum*). This wildflower has anecdotally been used widely for centuries to treat various forms of depression, including major depression and dysthy-mia, as well as anxiety, obsessive compulsive symptoms, anorexia, insomnia, seasonal affective disorder and fatigue. Hypericin, the active ingredient in St John's wort, has been found to work on a number of neuro-receptor sites and inhibits the uptake of serotonin, dopamine and norephinephrine in the brain (Wren & Norred 2003). There is evidence that St John's wort is as effective for mild to moderate depression, and that it causes fewer side-effects than traditional anti-depressants (Linde, Berner & Kriston 2008). One randomised controlled study, for example, examined the effectiveness of St John's wort for major depression in comparison to Sertraline, a conventional anti-depressant. The results found no significant difference between Sertraline and St John's wort compared with a placebo, and therefore did not support the efficacy of St John's wort for moderate to severe depression (Hypericum Depression Trial Study Group 2002). Note that the study also found that Sertraline was no more effective than the placebo, so in this case neither the conventional nor the alternative medicine was more effective than no active treatment.

A review of CAM treatments in major depression (Freeman et al. 2010) found suffi-cient evidence for the use of St John's wort, S-adenosyl-L-methionine supplementation and light therapy to recommend these as mono-therapy (or sole treatments). They also suggested that there was sufficient evidence for the usefulness of exercise and omega-3 fatty acid supplementation as adjunctive treatments in depression (Freeman et al. 2010).

Other treatments, such as mindfulness-based cognitive behavioural therapy (CBT) or problem-solving therapy are low risk and might be helpful, but there is not a strong enough research base to make recommendations specific to depression.

The World Health Organization (2004) recommends that service users ask themselves the following questions when considering the use of CAM (although these are good questions to ask about any treatment). You may find this list useful when discussing CAM with service users:

- Is the therapy or medicine suitable for the service user's disease or condition?
- Does the therapy or medicine have the potential to prevent, improve and/or cure symptoms or in other ways contribute to the service user's improved health and well-being?
- Does a qualified traditional medicine/CAM practitioner with adequate training and experience, skills and knowledge (preferably one who is registered and certified) provide the therapy or medicine?
- Are any herbal medicines of assured quality? What are the contra-indications and precautions related to the medicines?
- Are the therapies or medicines available at a competitive price?

GUIDELINES FOR NURSES WHEN USING CAM IN MENTAL HEALTH

- Information about any CAM the service user is currently using needs to be included in the initial assessment in a mental health service and, if possible, service users should be supported to continue their use of CAM unless they pose a risk to their health (or that of others) and/or interact with prescribed medications (especially psychotropics).
- Be aware of potential interactions between the service user's current medications and any herbal or CAM they may be considering using. If unsure, consult the prescribing medical officer and check with the Therapeutic Goods Administration if necessary.
- Document the details of any CAM administered/used during treatment, and cease their use immediately and report to the medical officer if any adverse effects occur.
- Regularly review service users' satisfaction with, and desired and/or adverse effects of, their use of CAM.

CRITICAL THINKING

Identify any of the CAM described in Table 9.2 with which you are unfamiliar. Choose one and investigate it further, using reliable information such as credible journal articles.

- How could this particular CAM be used effectively in the field of mental health?
- What benefits might it offer?
- How could nurses incorporate this CAM into their work with mental health service users?
- What would nurses need to know and do in order to use this CAM effectively?
- What problems or difficulties might occur with using this CAM? How could these be overcome?
- Who might have the most training and experience in the proper use of the CAM?

CONCLUSIONS

Complementary and alternative medicines typically are viewed favourably by service users, who often choose to use CAM to support their health. In general then, CAM can provide a number of benefits compared with the use of traditional medicines and therapies. These include the following:

- Service users can feel that using CAM provides a nurturing, supportive and non-judgemental management of their mental health-related issue.
- Like over-the-counter pharmaceutical products, many CAM approaches do not require a prescription or visit to a health practitioner, so may be considered by service users to be more time- and cost-effective in managing symptoms.
- Using CAM can enhance service users' feelings of self-efficacy and sense of empowerment.

Nurses can support people's choice to engage in practices that support their health. While nurses need to be cautious in recommending specific therapies for specific problems, there is sufficient evidence to support recommending supportive therapies and to support people accessing CAM practitioners. There is a pressing need for nurses to collaborate with service users and other health professionals in promoting positive lifestyle changes to enhance mental health and well-being.

This chapter has outlined the use of complementary and alternative therapies in mental health. These therapies increasingly are being recognised as effective for a number of mental health issues or problems, and can offer service users a further range of therapeutic approaches from which to select. Nurses working in mental health need to be aware of and understand the relative benefits of and limitations to each of these broad therapeutic approaches. Nurses need to be particularly alert to potential drug–nutrient and drug–herb interactions. With further education and training, nurses can provide some of these approaches themselves, and so enhance their provision of comprehensive nursing care for service users experiencing a wide range of mental health issues; however, they also need to recognise their scope of practice, and refer people or work collaboratively with other qualified practitioners.

SOME USEFUL AUSTRALIAN WEBSITES ON CAM

Australian Acupuncture & Chinese Medicine Association (AACMA): <www.acupuncture.org.au>.

Australia's Therapeutic Good Administration site on Complementary Medicines: <www.tga.gov.au/cm/cm.htm>

National Herbalists Association of Australia: <www.nhaa.org.au>.

Australian Traditional Medicine Society: <www.atms.com.au>.

The US National Centre for Complementary and Alternative Medicine: <http://nccam.nih.gov>.

Australian Society of Sex Educators Researchers and Therapists: <www.assertnsw.org.au>.

Information on drug–nutrient interactions: <http://edis.ifas.ufl.edu/he776>.

Information on drug–herb interactions: <www.consumerreports.org/cro/2012/05/beware-of-risky-herb-drug-combos/index.htm>.

REFERENCES

Abou-Saleh, M.T. & Coppen, A. (1986). Psychiatric progress: The biology of folate in depression—implications for nutritional hypotheses of the psychoses. *Journal of Psychiatric Research*, 20(2), 91–101.

Agarwal, V., Abhijnhan, A. & Raviraj, P. (2007). Ayurvedic medicine for schizophrenia. *Cochrane Database of Systematic Reviews*, 4, Art. CD006867.

Antoniades, J., Jones, K., Hassed, C. & Piterman, L. (2012). Sleep . . . naturally: a review of the efficacy of herbal remedies for managing insomnia. *Alternative and Complementary Therapies*, 18(3), 136–40.

Baer, R.A. (2003). Mindfulness training as a clinical intervention: a conceptual and empirical review. *Clinical Psychology: Science and Practice*, 10(2), 125–43.

Beavan, V., Read, J. & Cartwright, C. (2011). The prevalence of voice-hearers in the general population: a literature review. *Journal of Mental Health*, 20(3), 281–92.

Benor, R. (2001). Bach flower remedies. In D. Rankin-Box (ed.), *The Nurse's Handbook of Complementary Therapies* (2nd edn). Edinburgh: Bailliere Tindall.

Biley, F.C. (2001). Music as therapy. In D. Rankin-Box (ed.), *The Nurse's Handbook of Complementary Therapies* (2nd edn). Edinburgh: Bailliere Tindall, pp. 223–8.

Brody, S. (2009). Satisfaction (sexual, life, relationship, and mental health) is associated directly with penile–vaginal intercourse, but inversely with other sexual behavior frequencies. *Journal of Sexual Medicine*, 6, 1947–54.

Buman, M.P. & King, A.C. (2010). Exercise as a treatment to enhance sleep. *American Journal of Lifestyle Medicine*, 4(6), 500–14.

Busby, H. (2001). Herbal medicine. In D. Rankin-Box (ed.), *The Nurse's Handbook of Complementary Therapies* (2nd edn). Edinburgh: Bailliere Tindall, pp. 179–84.

Chiesa, A., & Serretti, A. (2011). Mindfulness based cognitive therapy for psychiatric disorders: a systematic review and meta-analysis. *Psychiatry Research*, 187(3), 441–53.

Conn, V. (2010). Depressive symptom outcomes of physical activity interventions: meta-analysis findings. *Annals of Behavioral Medicine*, 39(2), 128–38.

Cuellar, N.G., Rogers, A.E. & Hisghman, V. (2007). Evidenced based research of complementary and alternative medicine (CAM) for sleep in the community dwelling older adult. *Geriatric Nursing*, 28(1), 46–52.

Davis-Floyd, R. (2001). The technocratic, humanistic, and holistic paradigms of childbirth. *International Journal of Gynaecology & Obstetrics*, 75, S5–S23.

Diamond, L.M. & Huebner, D.M. (2012). Is good sex good for you? Rethinking sexuality and health. *Social and Personality Psychology Compass*, 6(1), 54–69.

Dipasquale, S., Pariante, C.M., Dazzan, P., Aguglia, E., McGuire, P. & Mondelli, V. (2012). The dietary pattern of patients with schizophrenia: a systematic review. *Journal of Psychiatric Research*, 47(2), 197–207.

Dunn, A. & Phillips, C. (2010). Complementary and alternative medicine: representation in popular magazines. *Australian Family Physician*, 39(9), 671–4.

Ernst, E. (2002). A systematic review of systematic reviews of homeopathy. *British Journal of Clinical Pharmacology*, 54(6), 577–82.

Freeman, M.P., Fava, M., Lake, J., Trivedi, M.H., Wisner, K.L. & Mischoulon, D. (2010). Complementary and alternative medicine in major depressive disorder: the American Psychiatric Association Taskforce report. *Journal of Clinical Psychiatry*, 71(6), 669–81.

Griffiths, P. (2001). Reflexology. In D. Rankin-Box (ed.), *The Nurse's Handbook of Complementary Therapies* (2nd edn). Edinburgh: Bailliere Tindall, pp. 241–50.

Grimaldi, D. (2004). Complementary and alternative mental health treatments. *Journal of Psychosocial Nursing and Mental Health Services*, 42(7), 6–7.

Hypericum Depression Trial Study Group (2002). Effect of Hypericum perforatum (St John's wort) in major depressive disorder. *Journal of the American Medical Association*, 287(14), 1807–14.

Kallestad, H., Hansen, B., Langsrud, K., Ruud, T., Morken, G., Stiles, T.C. & Grawe, R.W. (2012). Impact of sleep disturbance on patients in treatment for mental disorders. *BMC Psychiatry*, 12, 179.

Kaptchuk, T.J. (2002). The placebo effect in alternative medicine: can the performance of a healing ritual have clinical significance? *Annals of Internal Medicine*, 136(11), 817–25.

Kawachi, I. & Berkman, L. (2001). Social ties and mental health. *Journal of Urban Health*, 78(3), 458–67.

Kessler, R.C., Soukup, J., Davis, R.B., Foster, D.F., Wilkey, S.A., Van Rompay, M.I. & Eisenberg, D.M. (2001). The use of complementary and alternative therapies to treat anxiety and depression in the United States. *American Journal of Psychiatry*, 158(2), 289–94.

Lai, J., Moxey, A., Nowak, G., Vashum, K., Bailey, K., & McEvoy, M. (2012). The efficacy of zinc supplementation in depression: Systematic review of randomised controlled trials. *Journal of Affective Disorders*, 136(1–2), e31–9.

Lakeman, R. (2012). Talking science and wishing for miracles: understanding cultures of mental health practice. *International Journal of Mental Health Nursing*, 322(2), 106–15.

Lakeman, R., Watts, M. & Howell, M. (2010). Growing leaders in mental health recovery. *British Journal of Wellbeing*, 1(9), 7–9.

Lennihan, B. (2004). Homeopathy: natural mind–body healing. *Journal of Psychosocial Nursing and Mental Health Services*, 42(7), 30–40.

Linde, K., ter Riet, G., Hondras, M., Vickers, A., Saller, R. & Melchart, D. (2001a). Systematic reviews of complementary therapies—an annotated bibliography. Part 2: Herbal medicine. *BMC Complementary and Alternative Medicine*, 1(5).

Linde, K., Vickers, A., Hondras, M., ter Riet, G., Thormahlen, J. & Melchart, D. (2001b). Systematic reviews of complementary therapies—an annotated bibliography. Part 1: Acupuncture. *BMC Complementary and Alternative Medicine*, 1(3).

Linde, K., Berner, M.M. & Kriston, L. (2008). St John's wort for major depression. *Cochrane Database of Systemic Reviews*, 4, CD000448.

Lovas, J. (2001). Relaxation—the learned response. In P. McCabe (ed.), *Complementary Therapies in Nursing and Midwifery: from vision to practice*. Melbourne: Ausmed, pp. 162–74.

Lum, T.Y. & Lightfoot, E. (2005). The effects of volunteering on the physical and mental health of older people. *Research on Aging*, 27(1), 31–55.

MacLennan, A.H., Wilson, D.H. & Taylor, A.W. (2002). The escalating cost and prevalence of alternative medicine. *Preventive Medicine*, 35(2), 166–73.

Mallett, J. (2001). Humour and laughter therapy. In D. Rankin-Box (ed.), *The Nurse's Handbook of Complementary Therapies* (2nd edn). Edinburgh: Bailliere Tindall, pp. 195–208.

Meyer, M. (2001). Aromatherapy. In P. McCabe (ed.), *Complementary Therapies in Nursing and Midwifery: from vision to practice*. Melbourne: Ausmed, pp. 131–45.

National Centre for Complementary and Alternative Medicine (NCCAM) (2012). What is complementary and alternative medicine? Viewed 20 March 2013, <http://nccam.nih.gov/health/whatiscam>.

National Mental Health Commission (2012). *A Contributing Life: the 2012 National Report Card on Mental Health and Suicide Prevention*. Sydney: NMHC.

NSW Nurses' Association (2006). *Policy on Complementary Therapies in Nursing and Midwifery Practice*. Viewed 14 December 2012, <www.nswnma.asn.au/infopages/2948.html>.

Panesar, N. & Valachova, I. (2011). Yoga and Mental Health. *Australasian Psychiatry*, 19(6), 538–9.

Peet, M. (2004). Nutrition and schizophrenia: beyond omega-3 fatty acids. *Prostaglandins, Leukotrienes and Essential Fatty Acids*, 70(4), 417–22.

Petrie, W.M. & Ban, T.A. (1985). Vitamins in Psychiatry: do they have a role? *Drugs*, 30(1), 58–65.

Pigott, H.E., Leventhal, A.M., Alter, G.S. & Boren, J.J. (2010). Efficacy and effectiveness of antidepressants: current status of research. *Psychotherapy and Psychosomatics*, 79(5), 267–79.

Robinson, A.B. & Pauling, L. (1974). Techniques of orthomolecular diagnosis. *Clinical Chemistry*, 20(8), 961–5.

SánchezVillegas, A., Henríquez, P., BesRastrollo, M. & Doreste, J. (2006). Mediterranean diet and depression. *Public Health Nutrition*, 9(8A), 1104–9.

Smith, C., Hancock, H., Blake-Mortimer, J. & Eckert, K. (2007). A randomised comparative trial of yoga and relaxation to reduce stress and anxiety. *Complementary Therapies in Medicine*, 15(2), 77–83.

Smith, J.E., Richardson, J., Hoffman, C. & Pilkington, K. (2005). Mindfulness-based stress reduction as supportive therapy in cancer care: systematic review. *Journal of Advanced Nursing*, 52(3), 315–27.

Spinks, J. & Hollingsworth, B. (2012). Policy implications of complementary and alternative medicine use in Australia: data from the National Health Survey. *Journal of Alternative and Complementary Medicine*, 18(4), 371–8.

Uzun, O. & Tan, M. (2004). Nursing students' opinions and knowledge about complementary and alternative medicine therapies. *Complementary Therapies in Nursing & Midwifery*, 10, 239–44.

Walsh, R. (2011). Lifestyle and mental health. *American Psychologist*, 66(7), 579.

Watson, J. (1999). *Postmodern Nursing and Beyond*. Edinburgh: Churchill Livingstone.

Wickboldt, A.T., Bowen, A.F., Kaye, A.J., Kaye, A.M., Rivera Bueno, F. & Kaye, A.D. (2012). Sleep physiology, abnormal states, and therapeutic interventions. *The Ochsner Journal*, 12(2), 122–34.

World Health Organization (WHO) (2004). New WHO guidelines to promote proper use of alternative medicines. Viewed 25 June 2013, <www.who.int/mediacentre/news/releases/2004/pr44/en/print. html>.

Wren, K. & Norred, C.L. (2003). *Complementary and Alternative Therapies*. Philadelphia, PA: Saunders.

Xue, C.C., Zhang, A.L., Lin, V., Da Costa, C. & Story, D.F. (2007). Complementary and alternative medicine use in Australia: a national population-based survey. *Journal of Alternative and Complementary Medicine*, 13(6), 643–50.

PART IV

MENTAL HEALTH NURSING ROLES AND PRACTICE

11

Mental health and illness assessment

Main points

- The context and content of the mental health assessment are important initial parts of gaining an overall understanding of the service user.
- The purpose of the mental health assessment is to methodically gather information about a person's mental and general health status.
- Tools for mental health assessment include history, mental state examination, psychosocial and current life events, physical, neurological and psychological examination.
- The skills required for mental health assessment include interviewing and communication techniques.
- Throughout the assessment process, the aims are to continually build on service user strengths and to meet immediate needs.
- Contemporary mental health assessment should include risk assessment for self-harm, suicide, drug and alcohol, aggression and violence.

Definitions

Mental health assessment: An overall picture of a person's mental, general and physical state.

Marginalisation: The movement and demotion of a group of people to a lower or outer edge from the main group.

Iatrogenic: Illness arising from or caused by health care.

Risk: Potentially negative event arising from a characteristic or behaviour.

INTRODUCTION

In a very broad sense, nursing assessment is a systematic process of gathering, checking, confirming, reporting and sharing information about service users. A skilful ongoing assessment process is a fundamental competency of the mental health nurse in any setting. The general aims of nursing assessment include collecting, creating and updating documentation of a service user's state of health, including past, present and future health status and goals.

Mental health assessment is generally the starting point for diagnosis and the development of a treatment and care plan. A mental health assessment will most likely take place alongside a physical assessment, and although the assessment process is continuous and ongoing, medical professionals such as nurses and/or doctors usually undertake the initial assessment.

Mental health nursing assessment incorporates the assessment criteria utilised by medical staff, but the focus is on linking assessment to nursing interventions and nursing outcomes. This chapter will discuss the key components of a mental health nursing assessment, such as mental status, psycho-social assessment, assessment of substance use, medical and physical assessment and finally risk assessment. Throughout this chapter, we continue to focus on building on strengths and aim to view the assessment process from the service user and carer's perspective.

Before we begin to discuss the topic of mental status and map out the principles involved in a mental state examination, there are important prerequisites to consider overall. First, the assessment process should not be a passive one for the service user (Barker 2004). This means that throughout all assessments, the aims should be to incorporate collaboration and shared information where possible. For example, assessment should not be something that is done 'to you'; rather, it should be something that is done 'with you'.

Many parts of the mental health assessment are also inherently subjective. This means that in order for us to gather data that can be used objectively within a mental status assessment, we have already subjectively determined categories of what falls within and outside of an expected response. Therefore, in any evaluation or assessment there is a tendency to make judgements based firstly on our own values and biases. To counteract the tendency towards a potential inherent bias, we need to make a conscious decision to recognise our own biases and then deliberately set them aside before making any assessments. This is a crucial step in the assessment process. Because assessment is an ongoing process, this will mean that we need to be constantly aware of our own values in the assessment role.

As you read through this chapter, hold in mind any tensions you can see between nursing purposes where you need to 'describe' the service user—even 'monitor' them—and nursing purposes where you need to develop and maintain a warm, positive and non-judgemental relationship with that person. Think about how you could find out and facilitate what is important to the service user as you read through the following assessment frameworks.

CONTEXT OF MENTAL HEALTH ASSESSMENT

The circumstances or background in which a mental health assessment is undertaken will vary substantially from person to person, as will the environment in which the assessment occurs. It may be the first or only mental health assessment, or it may be one of many. Perhaps the assessment is in relation to a court order, individual request or sought by family and carers. Different contexts will mean potentially different outcomes for the assessment, so it is worth keeping in mind at the outset what the context of the assessment is, why it is being undertaken and how this might influence the assessment.

SERVICE USER, FAMILY, SIGNIFICANT OTHERS AND THE ENVIRONMENT

You may have come to understand assessment as a linear process within the overall nursing process of assessment, diagnosis, interventions and evaluations (Frisch & Frisch 2011). Although it is important to be mindful of these categories, it is also important to remember that each category will be dependent on the context of the assessment, the setting and the service user's specific needs and concerns. From a service user's perspective, receiving information about mental health care, shared decision-making (more on this concept in Chapter 3) and about the service user's rights are issues of most concern during an admission to mental health services (Matthias et al. 2012; Thapinta et al. 2004).

In the acute setting, you may find that the admission procedures and policy will often dictate the assessment process in the clinical field. Irrespective of the service user's needs, the assessment process will be time-bound (Hamilton et al. 2004). This means that within a set period of time (usually 24 hours), an assessment by a psychiatrist and the nursing staff will need to be conducted in order to determine eligibility for compulsory assessment or treatment. This timeframe, while varying from one state or territory of Australia to another, forms a part of the requirements of the principle of providing the least restrictive environment, as contained in mental health legislation.

There is an ongoing inherent danger of recasting or reorganising assessment information into a nursing or medical framework to suit the mental health professional and the health service environment. By doing this, we risk reconstructing the service user's concerns and immediate needs, thereby disempowering and marginalising the service user (Hamilton et al. 2004). All is not lost, though, as we can learn from our past and aim now to work towards a shared assessment experience with the service user, particularly by including family and significant others in the process. It is important to remain true to the service user's story while also ensuring that the clinical decision-making process is transparent and enhancing our communication with all other health-care professionals. Within the context of the mental health assessment, you can ask yourself what the assessment means for the service user. For example, why have the concerns of the service user been interpreted in this way, and can they be restated with the service user to gain a shared perspective?

CASE STUDY

The police had found Johnno sitting on the kerb of a very busy highway late last night, and had brought him in to the mental health unit for an assessment. Since his arrival, Johnno had watched the nurses hurry past him to get back to the nurses' station. They barely made eye contact with him, and no one stopped to assist him or even acknowledge him—for hours, or so it seemed. Johnno knew he smelt bad and looked unkempt—even dirty—but he just could not find it in himself to care anymore. What did any of it matter when all he wanted to do was to die?

Critical thinking

- How would you begin to engage Johnno in an assessment process?
- What priorities might you consider in the assessment partnership process for Johnno?

CONTENT OF MENTAL HEALTH ASSESSMENT

Purpose

The purpose of a mental health assessment is to systematically collect information about a person so that decisions can be made about his or her health status (Keltner, Bostrom & McGuinness 2011) and about the best way to provide care for the person. A comprehensive assessment enables the mental health professional to make sound clinical judgements and plan appropriate interventions (Varcarolis & Halter 2010). People are entitled to a comprehensive, timely and accurate assessment, in which all data is reviewed regularly, and the person should not be a passive recipient within the assessment process (Barker 2004).

CONSTRUCTION OF MENTAL HEALTH ASSESSMENT

The elements of a mental health assessment involve mental status, communication, initiation of therapeutic relationships and meeting immediate needs. Information is shared between the mental health professional and the service user. The first aspect is mental status; while this is important, it is no more important than other aspects. First, though, we will discuss mental status and examine a few different methods for assessing it.

When we talk about mental status, we mean the mental functioning of a person and whether there are areas of strengths, problems or deficits. Broadly speaking, mental status encompasses a number of categories and characteristics. A systematic inventory, checklist, assessment criteria form—even an examination—are some of the various methods we may use to categorise the different aspects of mental status.

Elements of assessment

The Council of Australian Governments' National Action Plan on Mental Health (2006–11, <www.coag.gov.au>) required that mental health professionals provide 'effective assessment and triage within all parts of the system to ensure care needs are identified accurately and early, and that people with mental illness are referred to the services from which they will benefit most'. The elements of the mental health assessment will depend on issues such as the phase of a mental illness, whether a person is at risk of an acute episode and how assessment and care can be provided in the least restrictive environment. In addition, it is important to remember that, with the consent of the service user, we will involve the service user's carer or family in treatment and support during an assessment. The elements of a mental health assessment are broadly organised around the following areas:

- diagnostic assessment
- behavioural assessment
- psycho-social assessment
- humanistic assessment
- holistic assessment

See 'The Roadmap for National Mental Health Reform 2012-2022' at <http://www.coag. gov.au>.

CASE STUDY

Rebecca has been in detention now for over two months. At first she had tried to explain in Gaelic what she was doing at the airport when she was interviewed about her old passport, but now she has given up. No one has asked her about her new passport—the one she received when getting her citizenship. To be fair, though, Rebecca had forgotten about the new passport too, and her visions and voices suggested it was best to keep quiet now in case she got hurt.

Critical thinking

- What sort of environment would be most helpful to begin the assessment process with Rebecca?
- What priorities might you consider in the assessment partnership process for Rebecca?

MENTAL STATUS

The initial focus of assessment in mental health care is logically a person's mental status if there are no physically urgent problems or issues. While a number of health professionals will assess the service user's mental state, the perspective of assessment will vary, as will the frequency of the assessment. Initially, a full and in-depth Mental State Examination (MSE) will be conducted, probably by a psychiatrist. It is important to assess often because a person's mental status may be in a state of change—either because of illness or ongoing crises, or in response to some form of treatment or environmental issues.

The most common method used to assess a person's mental status is an interview. The interview is often conducted between two or more people: the assessor(s) and the service user. In order to minimise distractions, it is usually held in a quiet room away from the mainstream traffic of a ward or community centre. Sometimes it may be important to include others in an interview—for example, if the assessor is a male and the female service user expresses concerns, or vice versa. In the case of a minor (persons under the age of sixteen), a parent or guardian may also be required to attend the mental status assessment.

The mental status assessment usually is based on observations and questions asked during an interview, which might also be used to gain information about other aspects of the person's life or history. The mental status part is usually written up to reflect how a person presented at a given point in time and follows typical headings (see Table 11.1). While it is tempting to use jargon, it is much more informative to readers to use concrete examples of what the person said and to describe how they behaved in as rich an amount of detail as possible.

Table 11.1 Mental state examination categories and descriptors

Category	Descriptors
Appearance	Overall and specific assessment of a person's physical appearance. Overall impressions include their age and gender, grooming, clothing, poise and posture, whereas specific impressions can include hairstyle, use of makeup, state, combination and repair of clothing, complexion and any signs of anxiety or drug and alcohol usage such as tense posture, wide eyes and unusual amount of perspiration.
General behaviour	The type and amount of motor movement—such as specific mannerisms and gestures—are involved here. These might include facial expressions such as grimacing, tremors, twitches, tics, impaired gait, agitation or motor retardation. In addition, this category can include attitudes of friendliness, embarrassment, anxiety, fear, anger, resentment, negativity and impulsiveness. These behaviours may be purposeful and even over-active, disorganised or stereotyped, or controlled and consistent.

Category	Descriptors
Speech	Characteristics of speech descriptors include quantity, production and quality. These may include talkative, verbose, garrulous or chatty and taciturn, restrained and reserved for quantity; rapid or slow, pressured, dramatic, emotional, slurred, mumbled and mutterings for production; and stuttered, hesitant, stammered or faltering.
Mood	A description of mood here includes a comprehensive and persistent emotion that affects a person's perspective on life. The depth, duration, fluctuations and intensity of feelings are relevant, and are often assessed in two broad paths. Affect means responsiveness and may be described as blunt, flat, normal. Facial expressions and body language may be of assistance. Assessing relationship of mood to the topic being discussed is also helpful. Mood may be described as congruent or incongruent, appropriate or inappropriate, expansive, elated, euphoric, euthymic, dysphoria, depressed or labile.
Thinking	There are two areas for assessment here: form and content. Form includes excess or absence of thoughts—for example, rapid thoughts (flight of ideas) or slow, hesitant, ponderous thoughts are useful categories of descriptors. May also be described as vague and vacuous (empty) and as lacking direction and apparent relevance. Association between thoughts may be described as loose or the cause and effect (chain of ideas) as lacking. Tangential, circumstantial and circuitous (going around and around in circles) thoughts may be described, as well as thinking being described as evasive, rambling or confabulatory (storytelling, fables). Content includes delusions (fixed but false ideas), ideas of reference, ideas of influence, preoccupation with an idea and/or belief, intrusive or obsessional beliefs and ideas. Delusions that are more common may be classified as paranoid, persecutory, grandiose, somatic or nihilistic in content.
Perception	This includes hallucinations (visions or images that are not real), illusions, depersonalisation (feelings of not being oneself), detachment from self and environment, fantasies and waking daydreams. Hallucinations are often described by the senses they affect, such as auditory, visual, tactile, olfactory or gustatory.
Sensorium and cognition	Included here are descriptors of mental functioning through sensory input. These include levels of consciousness and awareness, memory such as immediate retention and recall, recent past and remote memory; orientation such as awareness of time, place and person; concentration and attention, such as an ability to calculate and maintain mental focus; and lastly in this category, the ability to reason in abstract terms, such as comprehending concepts.

continued

Category	Descriptors
Insight and judgement	Insight is a person's ability to comprehend and acknowledge their current situation, or reveal an awareness and understanding of their own illness and/or health. Judgement includes comprehending and understanding the most likely outcomes from past or current behaviours and the ability to predict what these behaviours may lead to.

CASE STUDY

You have just arrived at the mental health unit for the afternoon shift. You can hear loud voices coming from one of the bedrooms. Someone is yelling out, 'Don't touch my stuff, don't touch my stuff!' repeatedly. You head towards the source of the shouting.

In one of the single bedrooms, two of the nursing staff confront a service user. One of the nurses leans over and whispers to you, 'Don't worry. It's just Melissa going off because someone went through her wardrobe. She must be quite manic at the moment, because she is not normally so loud. Maybe you should get her some PRN medication to settle her down.'

As you walk back towards the staff office and clinic room, you think about what your reactions would be if someone went through your belongings without your permission.

Critical thinking

• How would you proceed in order to de-escalate this situation?
• How would you begin to assess Melissa's current state of mind?

Meeting immediate needs

Imagine you are rushed off to hospital at this very moment. Are there things in your life that would suffer? Who will feed your dog or water your plants, and do you have children to pick up after school or a workplace to notify? Meeting a person's immediate needs is about dealing with what is most important for the service user at that particular point in time. While these aims are not limited to times of assessment, it is important that, rather than focusing only on information-gathering, we need to respect a person's life and the manner in which they live it by focusing on what is important to them at the time.

The immediate need may be something simple, such as a missed meal, the need to make contact with family and or friends, or distress over someone rummaging through their belongings, as in the previous scenario. Even if the immediate needs are more complex, you can use a collaborative problem-solving approach to assist in most situations. The following points provide some ideas that can help:

- Regularly consult with service users and identify immediate and ongoing concerns.
- Listen to the service user for ideas on how to meet immediate needs, and what needs to be changed and improved.
- Clarify the service user perspective by talking through what is of immediate concern.
- Provide information and plan together for how to manage immediate situations.
- Work in partnership with service users, mental health-care professionals and all other health-care providers.

TOOLS FOR MENTAL HEALTH ASSESSMENT

In order to assess a person's mental health, a variety of tools will be required. These include a detailed psychiatric history, a mental state examination, psycho-social history and current life events, as well as a neurological and psychological examination (Shives 2011). Probably the most important tool is the relationship established between nurse and service user in the assessment (Coombs, Curtis & Crookes 2011, p. 368).

Interviewing skills in assessment

Although your skills at interviewing will be used in many areas of nursing, it is most important to use your best and most sensitive interviewing skills in a mental health assessment. The interview is a vehicle for gathering information that may be particularly important to ongoing treatment or service networking. It may clarify—even refute— some initial ideas and impressions. What type of questions you ask during the interview will affect the type and quality of information you receive and share, so careful consideration should be given not just to the areas for assessment such as cognition and mood, but also to how questions are phrased and structured.

Open questions

It is useful and respectful to begin an interview with open questions. These questions cannot be answered properly with a simple yes or no, and often lead to more expansive information. Initial open questions can relate to the nature of the presenting issue generally, and can be followed up by more specific open questions that aim to clarify, evolve and uncover issues of concern. Open questions help to encourage a person to talk and to concentrate on the present situation. In addition, open questions help to further a developing relationship, find common ground and establish a rapport.

Closed questions

While open questions should take place in the initial part of the interview, closed questions can also help to form a clearer outline of issues. A definition of a closed question is one where the expected answer is brief and does not generally allow for further probing or spontaneous discussions. An example of a closed question may be 'How old are you?' and the elicited response is brief and self-limiting: 'Thirty-two.' Another example might be: 'Are you comfortable?' 'Yes, thank you.' Closed questions are often useful to complete an assessment form or checklist.

Multiple-choice questions

Another form of questioning that may be useful—particularly if the person who is being assessed is having some difficulty in responding to open questions—is the multiple-choice question. In this case, the 'choice' question may be more useful. This question provides a range of possible answers to the person, but also allows for replies outside the suggested range: 'Do you feel . . . or . . . or something else?'

Communicating openly

Communication is not just the start of a relationship between the nurse and the service user, but is also the central tool for assisting the service user. Consider what the issues are for communication in the mental health-care setting:

* Communication should be focused on the service user as the priority.
* Honesty should be the general aim in all communications and should be sensitively managed.
* Limits and boundaries in the directions of communication should aim to protect the best interests of the service user and yourself as well as being culturally, age and gender appropriate.
* Information overload potential should be monitored carefully.
* It is important to avoid negativity in communication and highlight positive themes and attitudes where appropriate, but not at the expense of honesty and openness.
* Keeping communication simple and concentrating on central issues can assist in avoiding confusion and mixed messages.
* Communication helps to create a bond that may last for a long time, so it is worth spending time and thought on deciding how to begin.
* Communication should always be in the spirit of respect and professionalism, and be health directed.
* A mixture of body language, presentation—such as dress—and environment all make valuable contributions to communication.
* Time and timing are elements in communication that may be of particular relevance for the person experiencing mood or thought disorders.

How you introduce yourself is crucial

Apart from visually observing, one of the first things you should do when meeting a new service user for the first time is start talking by introducing yourself. What you say and how you say it is the first critical step towards creating a working relationship that could last for many years. Therefore, it is important to get it right from the beginning, and present a positive and warm manner that can allow a service user to recognise and feel that your presence is unconditional, non-judgemental and accepting.

The relationship between yourself and the service user is a unique one that centres on caring, so you might start by greeting the service user and sharing your name. Permission to use first names in some cultures may help to form a bond, and from here you can respect the service user's wishes to be addressed in their preferred manner.

MENTAL STATE EXAMINATION

A mental state examination (MSE) is a report containing details of thoughts and actions as well as descriptions of appearance and speech from an interview (Zuckerman 2010). Table 11.1 (above) lists the main categories of an MSE and provides some descriptors for each category.

Conducting an MSE can be time-consuming, and may be disconcerting for the service user. When assessing cognition more deeply for service users with dementia, it may be more appropriate and helpful to perform a mini-MSE (a smaller version of the MSE) that focuses on specific areas such as orientation, memory, attention, recall, language and content (Sadock & Sadock 2007). A mini-MSE can be utilised more frequently, particularly if there are ongoing cognitive issues for assessment.

It is important to remember that whatever MSE is used, your goal should be to allow for more emphasis within the assessment process for working from the service user's thoughts and goals, and for incorporating a shared relationship between assessment and the service user's perspectives.

PSYCHO-SOCIAL HISTORY

To understand the person in a specific situation, the collection and assessment of relevant information become an essential part of the psycho-social therapeutic process. This does not mean that 'the more the merrier' concept applies. It simply means gathering information that is relevant to the service user. The service user, the setting and the service required will ultimately dictate the amount of information needed for assessment.

A service user's psycho-social assessment should be viewed in total rather than as separate parts. This touches on the fundamentals of psycho-social health care (see Chapter 2). The key feature is that the individual is more than the sum of their individual parts. Therefore, a good understanding of their health patterns can only be determined by taking a broad view.

Information gathered from service users includes how service users view and understand themselves, their history, their world, their aims, concerns and future aspirations. Often the very task of clarifying and reviewing areas of understanding and perception with service users is part of the therapeutic process, and may become the content of the process itself. Other sources may need to be followed up, such as family/friends, social network, documentation and other professionals.

PSYCHO-SOCIAL ASSESSMENT

Often, the reason why our response to illness is a unique and individual experience is because our responses are affected at every point by a combination of our biological, psychological and social development. Physical illness is a stressor that constitutes a crisis particularly in combination with other psycho-social issues. In order to provide good psycho-social nursing care, accurate and ongoing nursing assessment is vital. A nursing assessment of psycho-social health is a fundamental aspect of the development of any nursing diagnosis and nursing intervention. There are two processes involved: the decision concerning which data to use and that related to what judgement to use. According to Newell and Gournay (2009, p. 107), a psycho-social assessment should include the following categories:

- biological, psychological and social details
- functional (behavioural performance)
- self-efficacy
- family relationships
- relationships with the wider social environment
- interpersonal communication
- social resources and networks.

Once an understanding of service users, their potential and limitations, the sources of strengths and stress, the resources for change and the barriers to desired change are established, the process of assessment (formulation of a professional judgement) can be made. The following information should be included in your psycho-social assessment:

- the service user's lifestyle, family and social network
- what the service user understands about their current illness
- the service user's usual coping mechanisms
- health priorities and personal development issues that you have determined in your discussion.

Psycho-social assessment aims to uncover how a service user responds to their current circumstances through a detailed understanding of their personal and social history. The emphasis of the psycho-social assessment is on working from the service user's thoughts and goals, and the way these will fit together for optimal mental health. In order to access this information, the mental health nurse will need to use advanced communication skills. These will specifically involve a number of therapeutic communication tools, including the following:

CASE STUDY

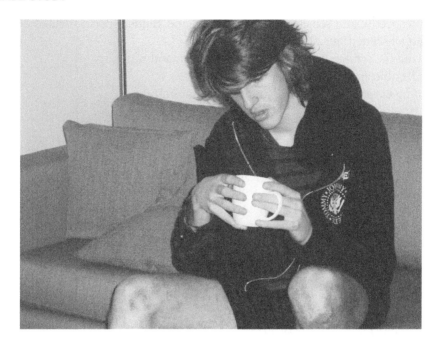

Over the weekend, Joseph presented at the Accident and Emergency Department of your hospital stating that he needed to talk to the 'head doctor' because he felt he was becoming unwell again; it was difficult to concentrate on his personal needs now, and 'the voices' were saying awful and distressing things to him. Although the weather is very hot outside, Joseph has on a long, thick, woollen overcoat and his shirt is torn and bloodstained. It is now Monday morning, and the psychiatrist has asked whether you would sit in on an interview with Joseph. The psychiatrist has a thick file that includes notes from Joseph's previous admissions—the last being nine months ago. Joseph's hands appear to tremble as he tries to hold a cup of tea you have given him.

Critical thinking

- Make a list of information that should be shared during the MSE in order to provide a thorough assessment of Joseph. Use the categories and descriptors in Table 11.1 to create your list.
- What information should you gain from Joseph regarding his psycho-social and physical assessment?

- active listening through eye contact, body and verbal response
- proceeding from general details to the specific
- open and positive voice tone, facial expression and body language
- being respectful and sensitive to age, cultural and gender-specific details
- using open-ended questions
- following the service user's cues using reflection and restating
- being flexible and using humour as appropriate
- providing empathetic feedback and touch as appropriate.

BUILDING ON STRENGTHS

Mental health assessment relates not only to recognising what might be wrong and why, but also recognising what is right and healthy and, even more importantly, being able to assess that there is nothing wrong. Psycho-social stressors will vary enormously from person to person (see Table 11.2). Assessing in order to distinguish the most important psychological and psycho-social issues can then lead directly into the process of goal-setting. This is where mental health nurses can facilitate the articulation and establishing of the service user's goals. The establishment and maintenance of therapeutic relationships here is vital because the most powerful agent in bringing about change is the influence of interpersonal communication and relationships.

Table 11.2 Severity of Psycho-social Stressors Scale: adults

| | | **Examples of stressors** | |
Code	Term	Acute events	Enduring circumstances
1	None	No acute events that may be relevant to the disorder	No enduring circumstances that may be relevant to the disorder
2	Mild	Broke up with boyfriend or girlfriend; started or graduated from school; child left home	Family arguments; job dissatisfaction; residence in high-crime neighbourhood
3	Moderate	Marriage; marital separation; loss of job; retirement; miscarriage	Marital discord; serious financial problems; trouble with boss; being a single parent
4	Severe	Divorce; birth of first child	Unemployment and poverty
5	Extreme	Death of spouse; serious physical illness diagnosed; victim of rape	Serious chronic illness in self or child; ongoing physical or sexual abuse
6	Catastrophic	Death of a child; suicide of spouse; devastating natural disaster	Captivity as hostage; concentration camp experience

Source: Adapted from Newell & Gournay (2009, p. 107).

CASE STUDY

You have been employed in the Adolescent Acute Care Unit for a couple of years now, and every day brings new challenges. A new service user named Jarli has arrived from Central Australia, where he has developed a paint sniffing ('chroming') habit over the past eighteen months, which is now causing a significant impact on his cognitive and physical functioning. Jarli has just turned fifteen years of age, and claims he has no parents: 'They are dead to me,' he tells you. As you complete your nursing care assessment, you become aware of the multiple physical, psychological and social challenges he faces.

Critical thinking

Write a list of the issues that come to mind that you would need to assess in developing a comprehensive care plan for Jarli. You can revisit your list at the end of this chapter and compare your answers.

You are aware that the behaviour known as 'chroming' is where a person inhales the airborne vapours released from certain household and paint chemicals in order to achieve an altered state of consciousness ('getting high'). Unfortunately, Jarli has been chroming with a substance most likely to cause a rapid deterioration in his physical and mental health. Furthermore, the psychological withdrawal symptoms may be severe, and include anxiety, depression, loss of appetite, irritation, aggressive behaviour, dizziness, tremors and nausea.

Recently, Jarli has lost a substantial amount of weight, has muscle tremors and is unable to recall many details of his life prior to coming into hospital. In addition, he is found to have moderate anaemia and is showing some signs of multiple organ damage due to this deliberate chemical poisoning. Despite his now obvious poor health, Jarli tells you that if he cannot get 'high', life is not worth living and he will find a way to get out and get high as soon as possible.

Critical thinking

- How might you respond to and assess Jarli's revelations?
- What particular communication skills will be of assistance to you?
- Can you recognise any particular psycho-social development stage from Jarli's narrative? How will this information assist you in making a nursing risk assessment?

SUBSTANCE USE ASSESSMENT

Taking an accurate substance use history and assessment involves a number of aspects, including current medication use, knowledge and practices, illicit drug use, past and current use, potential interactions of current and future medications as well as potential withdrawal issues. Again, collaboration between the nurse and service user will be vital in gathering information. Being transparent and open about the reasons for needing to perform this assessment may assist you to work with the service user, and will also help you to understand the effects of such probing on an individual. It is also important to remain non-judgemental, and to remember the confidential nature of any information within the assessment process.

Many health-care services will use a standardised form that can assist you and the service user to gather this information. There is currently no national standardised form—instead, they vary from state to state. Specific details may include the generic name of the medication used, the reason for the medication, the dose, frequency and route of the medication, the duration of the medication and the prescribing doctor's name and contact details. It is important that all drug use is included, even alternative and complementary medicines (see Chapter 10 for details about these). In your drug assessment, you may wish to include information about the current or previous prescriber of medication for the service user; whether the service user has any known allergies; and the service user's usual medication regime. The issues of self-medication, pain medication and management and knowledge/understanding of drugs including psycho-pharmacology are further points to assess.

An increasing issue in Australian society is the misuse of alcohol and drugs. Further details and discussion on this topic can be found in Chapter 8 and dual diagnosis is discussed in Chapter 7. The increase in drug use within our society as an emerging problem includes even those drugs that may have been prescribed and considered for physical conditions only, where they are involved in so-called 'recreational use' rather than used solely for medicinal purposes.

The following questions might assist you to assess for potential substance misuse:

- Does this person fit into the demographic characteristics of concurrent substance misuse (age, socio-economics, employment and education)?
- Is there a past history of drug and/or alcohol misuse?
- Have I asked and probed for information about the type, quantity, route and pattern of substance use?
- Can any current or previous case manager or other health service provide further relevant information?
- What information can friends, family and carers provide?
- Does the person cite reasons for their drug and/or alcohol misuse?
- Should I maintain a high 'index of suspicion', particularly when unsupervised or unobserved visitations from friends and or family occur?

- Can I use a clinical rating scale to assess drug and/or alcohol misuse?
- Should blood or urine samples be collected and tested?
- Is the person showing any signs or feeling any symptoms of current intoxication or withdrawal?

PHYSICAL AND MEDICAL ASSESSMENT

Assessing a person's physical state forms a central part of the MSE, so it is important not to simply focus on one aspect—such as mental health—and thereby miss important information on physical health. Sometimes signs and symptoms that have a physical basis can be mistaken for psychological or cognitive disorders. It is not unusual for a medical condition to be preceded by non-specific psychiatric signs and symptoms, and toxicity is one of the most common situations (Sadock & Sadock 2007). This is a drug-induced psychotic state where all signs and symptoms of psychosis disappear once the causative drug has cleared the system. Another example may be the service user who is assessed as having a psychiatric diagnosis, but on examination is found to have a space-occupying lesion (brain tumour) that is causing problems with cognition. Probably one of the most common situations for confusion is the mentally altered state of a person suffering from a high fever.

According to Sadock and Sadock (2007), associated physical disorders can be as high as 60 per cent in identified sufferers of mental illness. Appropriate referrals, keeping an open mind and follow-up on physical signs and symptoms can help to lower this high figure.

The following breakdown of physical systems may demonstrate psychiatric signs and symptoms:

- *Endocrine*: thyroid conditions (an excess or underproduction of thyroxin), diabetes and hormonal disturbances.
- *Metabolic*: electrolyte and fluid imbalances, hypoxemia.
- *Neurologic*: head trauma, dementia (Alzheimer's type) and brain neoplasms.
- *Toxic*: alcohol and drug withdrawal or intoxication, hydrocarbons, organophosphates and heavy metals.
- *Autoimmune*: systemic lupus erythemotosus (SLE).
- *Nutritional*: vitamin deficiencies (thiamine, nicotinic acid and folate deficiencies), trace elements (zinc and magnesium) and malnutrition.
- *Infections*: virus (hepatitis, encephalopathies, AIDS, herpes), bacteria (streptococcal and staphylococcal infections and abscesses), neurosyphilis and tuberculosis.
- *Cancer*: some primary and metastatic tumours, endocrine and pancreatic tumours. (Adapted from Sadock & Sadock 2007, p. 261)

Assessing and recording information relating to a person's physical state of health and details of their past health history will greatly assist in clarifying whether a physical condition underlies a mental state or contributes to a person's mental well-being. Areas that you may document and monitor include the following:

- vital signs (temperature, pulse and respiration rate and blood pressure)
- current and past history of sleep patterns
- urinalysis for general purposes, but noting specifically issues such as blood, protein, sugar and ketones
- skin integument, looking for any bruising, rashes, breaks in the skin, swellings or lumps
- headaches, sensory changes (vision, hearing, smell and touch)
- immunisation status and any history of conditions such as hepatitis (B and C), HIV and sexually transmitted diseases
- current weight and any past history of weight loss or gain
- any recent or past history of dietary abnormalities and food allergies
- any notable family history of possibly inherited diseases or conditions
- current medications and possible interactions between medications and with current diet
- date of the last physical check-up, including details of any recent illnesses, changes in bodily functions or pain and discomfort.

CASE STUDY

Shu Min Yang (Lucy) has been in your mental health unit for three days now, with little change in her mental status. Lucy's husband spends much of his time at her side, and often acts as her interpreter. Lucy was very frightened by the entire admission process and appears very nervous around the other service users in the mental health unit. In Lucy's initial assessment, she struggled to remember specific details about her home address, the 40th birthday of her twin sons and why she was now in hospital. Lucy's husband claims that for a few months now Lucy has been talking to a voice that only she seems to be able to hear, and her memory has been getting worse—she even forgot her own birthday two weeks ago. Apart from the increasing memory lapses and the auditory hallucinations, Lucy seems to be in good health for her age (65). Her admission to your unit occurred when the family's GP became concerned at Lucy talking to the voice in her head instead of her husband and children.

Lucy has four children who are all adults now, and apart from their births she has not been in a hospital for any illnesses. You discover from talking with Lucy's husband that, prior to their marriage in China, Lucy had been forced to work as a 'comfort girl' to Japanese soldiers in her home village in Jilin province, which borders North Korea. It is only after you have documented these details from Lucy's past that the medical officer orders a specific blood test for neurosyphilis.

> **Critical thinking**
>
> • Why was this information so relevant to Lucy's current health state?
> • How might positive blood results affect Lucy and her husband?

SUICIDE RISK AND AGGRESSION OR VIOLENCE ASSESSMENT

An important aspect of initial and ongoing nursing assessment includes determining what risk factors and events may be present and the estimated extent of these risks. When we talk about risks, we mean what dangers, hazards or threats to a person's safety may be assessed. Risks can arise because of self-induced dangerous actions and behaviour, but might also arise because of a temporary lack of judgement, understanding or self-control.

Appropriate and timely risk assessment can mean the difference between hope, care and recovery, or physical, emotional and spiritual harm—even death. How a risk assessment is performed is equally important. For example, is the risk assessment occurring simply from the perspective of harm minimisation or is it your overall aim to work collaboratively with the service user and build on recovery and optimism? It is important to remember that risk assessment should focus on strengths and positives as well as potential risks.

The general principle you might consider is to continuously assess the potential for risks while at the same time preserving the service user's dignity, rights to self-determination and best health care in the least restrictive environment possible. You might think this is quite a balancing act, and you can now see why many of the issues already discussed in this chapter are vital to the assessment process, such as communication and mental status assessment.

Risks to others and environment may include:

- aggression and violence (potential and/or actual)
- harm to others (physical and/or psychological)
- fire
- sexual threat to or from others
- drug and/or alcohol (substance abuse)
- withdrawal from substance abuse
- absconding (from a place of safety).

Risks to self may include:

- self-harm (physical and/or psychological)
- suicide.

While standardised tests for assessing the risk of suicide are relatively commonplace throughout the world and in Australia, it should be recognised that suicide continues throughout the history of 'humankind', and will probably continue despite our best intentions to recognise and render assistance to those at the greatest risk. The very act of wanting to take one's own life may be so covert and hidden that no amount of risk assessment will uncover that which a person does not wish to be uncovered. The same caution can exist for the risk of self-harm in that, for some individuals, the risk is hidden from carers and nursing staff, and sometimes even careful vigilance and ongoing assessment can fail to prevent an act of self-harm.

The risk assessment that you may complete will consider a person's potential to cause harm to themselves and/or other people. In addition to evidence of potential self-harm behaviour from the interview and your observation, there are other factors that can be considered in determining the possibility of such behaviour. These can include a history of dangerous behaviours, access to objects that can cause harm and an ability to use these objects. A good example of standardised assessment tools is the NSW Suicide Risk Assessment and Management Protocols, which can be accessed at: <www.health. nsw.gov.au/pubs/2005/suicide_risk.html>.

Ongoing research continues to highlight the relationship between aggression and violence, and the use of substances such as illicit drugs and alcohol (Butler et al. 2003). The excessive use of alcohol and illicit drugs may substantially increase the risk of violent behaviour and the risk of self-harm and suicide. A dual diagnosis (such as a mental illness and a dependence disorder—see Chapter 6) is an important factor to consider within the assessment of risk.

Table 11.3 lists four potential categories for an assessment of risk. The use of these categories can assist in determining the type of nursing interventions as well as potential outcomes of your nursing care.

ASSESSING FOR TRAUMA

Estimates of the prevalence of childhood trauma in the lives of women who come to the attention of mental health services are between 50 and 80 per cent (Read et al. 2005). There is a strong link between people who have experienced trauma and mental health service use. Given these statistics, it might be surprising to find that service users are not routinely assessed for information about prior trauma—type, duration and severity. This means that mental health services are not necessarily prepared to respond to the impact of that trauma in the lives of these service users. This is particularly significant because presenting symptoms may be connected to experience of trauma. For example, psychoses, self-harm, excessive use of drugs and alcohol, and eating disorders can be indicative of experienced trauma (Read et al. 2005).

In the United States, the National Association of State Mental Health Program Directors (NASMHPD), in conjunction with the National Technical Assistance Center

Table 11.3 Risk assessment levels and descriptors

Level of risk	Descriptors
No risk	This category may indicate to the nurse that there are currently no indications of suicidal ideas or thoughts of harming others. This includes any impulses. There is no prior history of suicidal or homicidal ideation, and no current indication of distress.
Low risk	In this category, a person may have had fleeting or brief thoughts of either suicide or harming others previously, but there is no current ideation, plan, intention or significant distress. There may be a history of substance use and of self-neglect, but without any history of disinhibition or behaviour having caused any harm.
Moderate or medium risk	In this category, there may be significant and current suicidal thoughts or wish to harm others, but no actual intent or conscious plan. In addition, there is no history of suicidal thoughts or wishes to harm others. Equally, though, there may be feelings of distress but without active suicidal or harm to others ideation; however, there is a history of suicidal or harm to others behaviour. For example, there may be a history of impulsive behaviour that includes suicidal intent or harming others, actions or threats, but these do not represent any current change in the person's conduct. There may be a history of previous substance use resulting in aggressive and disinhibited behaviour, as well as previous and current evidence of self-neglect.
Substantial or significant risk	This category includes those persons with current suicidal ideation or intent to harm others and/or a history of acting out such behaviour. There may be no current means for committing these behaviours, or the person may be currently opposed to these actions; however, the person's history reveals impulsive, threatening, harmful actions. Equally, a person may have escalated from previous inaction to active potential. There may be a pattern of past and recent substance use, resulting in aggression or inability to judge personal safety and the person is currently unable to care for his or her own health and the safety of others.
Serious or acute risk	For this category, a person is currently deemed at risk of suicide or of harming others. This means that the person has a plan as well as the means with which to carry out the suicide or harming others behaviour. There may also be a history of serious attempts or attacks that have been planned and not impulsive. There may be a pattern of violence or violent acts towards self and/or others when using substances, and there is strong physical evidence of an inability to care for oneself.

for State Mental Health Planning (NTAC), has developed a training program on the provision of trauma-informed care in mental health services. This model relies on a whole-of-organisation approach that includes routine assessment for trauma and a range of supports and responses that are trauma-informed. For further information about this model, see <http://www.nasmhpd.org/index.aspx>.

CASE STUDY

Debbie has extensive wounds to both her wrists, including tendon and vascular damage from attempting suicide 24 hours ago. Debbie seems very quiet—almost withdrawn—and answers most of your questions in simple monosyllables. Before you attempt to complete a nursing assessment, you need to learn more about Debbie's life prior to this admission.

Critical thinking

- How might you properly engage Debbie in conversation so that you can accurately assess any risk for further self-harm?
- Why might suicide risk rather than self-harm risk be important for someone in Debbie's situation?
- If you do deem Debbie to be at ongoing risk of suicide, safety issues become paramount. Should you continue to care for Debbie in a surgical unit, and what might be the ramifications of moving her to a mental health unit?

Debbie reports that she is the middle child in a family of three. Her middle-class parents are now retired, and her brother and sister are in Melbourne. Although Debbie claims her schooling years were unremarkable, she talks about several occasions where she was bullied, taunted and physically beaten by gangs of older adolescents. It seems that Debbie graduated from Sydney University's School of Veterinary Sciences and began a highly successful and very busy practice employing five other veterinarians. Despite her apparent success in life, Debbie has continued to question her self-worth from early childhood. Plagued by worries and depression that have increased over the past few years, Debbie wrote a note indicating that she now realised what a failure she was and proceeded to slash both her forearms with a sharp razor. (Adapted from Wilkinson & Van Leuven 2011)

Critical thinking

- It seems difficult to understand why someone in Debbie's position should not have developed a strong sense of self-worth. An apparently sound childhood, a good career, a position of power and influence and apparent good health prior to admission—why is Debbie struggling to survive?
- Is it possible that we perceive only certain socio-economic and cultural groups as being at risk of low self-concept?
- What are important indicators here for Debbie's psycho-social assessment?

RECORDING MENTAL HEALTH ASSESSMENT

Every encounter with a service user will contain potential assessment components. Consequently, written or verbal reporting on the mental status of service users is the work of every nurse on every shift in an in-patient unit, and every encounter in a community setting.

Nursing notes

The recording of a mental health assessment is an ongoing process. However, the initial recording may be substantial to provide as clear an understanding as possible of the issues for the service user's need for mental health services. Many of the assessment areas we have discussed in this chapter have been standardised onto admission and assessment forms. This means that, in many instances, you will simply be filling in the blank spots within a form.

In some respects, the standardised form is a limitation in the mental health assessment process, as it often leaves little room for clarification or elaboration on specific aspects relevant to the service user. The standardised form may also lessen the opportunity to cover assessment details not listed or cited within the form.

The use of documentation must relate to your nursing care and to that of health-care professionals. This will assist with the rationale of mental health care services, assessing changes and compliance/concordance issues (Kneisl & Trigoboff 2012; Stuart 2013). The principles that should be covered in your nursing notes relate to issues of:

- confidentiality and privacy
- non-disclosure of assessment details
- legality nature of documentation
- clinical relevance of documentation
- service user response and participation.

The writing up of your assessment details should be logical in flow and concise, and you should only elaborate in order to clarify specific examples (Stuart 2013). You should complete all categories of the assessment and explain if any are not completed. You will document significant events, actions and outcomes in a factual, non-judgemental manner (Antai-Otong 2008). Your recordings will guide and help structure other health professionals' care and approach. As the use of computer-based documentation increases, it may be that you enter assessment details and your nursing notes directly into a computer-based hospital or health-care service record. The principles as stated above apply to handwritten and computer records.

Some aspects of your nursing notes may include the use of quotations (Antai-Otong 2008). This is particularly relevant in the writing up of assessment details where a quote allows for the reader to gain a better understanding of the context of what was said and how it was said. The use of quotes in nursing notes must be managed carefully in order to preserve their true meaning by the service user.

Sometimes, taking a quote out of context may confuse or even misdirect the reader. The description of non-verbal responses may also be used to clarify the factual documentation (Antai-Otong 2008).

CASE STUDY
In the first week of your secondment to the Adolescent Acute Care Unit, you have been allocated a new service user named Danielle, who is suffering from extensive deep burns to over 30 per cent of her body from a motor vehicle accident. As you complete your nursing care assessment, you become aware of the multiple physical, psychological and social challenges she faces.

Critical thinking
Write a list of issues that come to mind that you would need to assess in developing a comprehensive care plan for Danielle. You can revisit your list at the end of this chapter and compare your answers.

It appears that at the age of thirteen, Danielle had become caught up with a group of adolescents who were involved in alcohol, drugs and criminal behaviour. As a part of the initiation to this group, Danielle was encouraged to steal and drive a motor vehicle. Unfortunately, Danielle crashed the car into a power pole and suffered burns as the car exploded into flames. Luckily, a passer-by reported the accident and police and ambulance officers were able to save Danielle's life. She is now suffering from a moderate amount of shock and pain, and appears despondent; this alternates with outbursts of anger and self-directed sarcasm. Danielle tells you that her life is now over, she has always hated herself, she has no real friends and now she will be permanently scarred from the burns and skin grafts. As she picks at the bandages, Danielle claims that no one will love her looking as she does, and that no one has ever loved her. Danielle tells you that her parents have never cared what happened to her.

Critical thinking
- How might you respond to and assess Danielle's revelations?
- What particular communication skills will be of assistance to you?
- Can you recognise any psycho-social development stage from Danielle's narrative, and how will this information assist you in determining a nursing risk assessment?

Developing assessment skills

Your documentation of a Mental State Examination should include a description of each relevant MSE category and should avoid the use of labels, judgements and terms. Re-read Danielle's story and the following example of one MSE category. You can practise writing other categories by using the headings from Table 11.1, making notes from the story and using the style of description below.

Brief notes that you may consider relevant in your documentation include:

- hates herself
- states that life is over
- worried about being permanently scarred
- continually picking at bandages
- states no one will love her or has ever loved her—feeling rejected, isolated, lonely or even unlovable
- states that her parents don't care
- currently in pain from her injuries
- looks and feels despondent—sad
- angry and sarcastic responses to some questioning.

Mental state examination assessment of mood

An assessment of Danielle's mood and affect reveals that she feels unhappy, sad and angry at her current situation. This could be described as a dysphoric (unpleasant) and irritable mood. Affect noted in our conversation while conducting a nursing admission is deemed appropriate to the circumstances of Danielle's admission; however, some evidence of a labile affect was noted when Danielle became angry and sarcastic, stating 'my parents never cared for me'.

Mental health team notes

Each profession within the mental health-care team brings a different perspective to the assessment process. Consequently, written and verbally communicated assessment details from the mental health team will vary greatly. For example, a social worker's assessment may focus on aspects such as lifestyle, employment, housing and supportive networks, whereas a psychological assessment might focus on memory, family relationships and intellectual assessment.

While the same legal requirements apply to all written records (name, date, designation and signatures), the details from the various mental health team members will contribute to the broader assessment profile. It is important for information to be recorded that has immediate and longer-term effects for the provision of nursing care such as changes from more restrictive status to less restrictive, and changes to and reasons for treatment approach.

CONCLUSION

Assessment in mental health care is an ongoing and even evolving process. Assessment settings and approach continue to change and be informed by our understanding of mental illness and the human condition. The initial mental health assessment is an important part of creating care directions, and should include assessment of strengths as well as highlight concerns. Throughout this chapter, we have stressed the need for collaboration between service providers and service users, families and carers as an important and emerging issue in contemporary mental health care. Your assessment skills will increase by observing, sharing, discussing and reflecting on the assessment process with experienced and competent mental health nurses. How you go about the assessment process will contribute to your goals of continuing therapeutic relationships.

REFERENCES

Antai-Otong, D. (2008). *Psychiatric Nursing: biological & behavioral concepts* (2nd edn). New York: Thomson Delmar Learning.

Barker, P.J. (2004). *Assessment in Psychiatric and Mental Health Nursing: in search of the whole person* (2nd edn). Cheltenham: Nelson Thornes.

Butler, T., Levy, M., Dolan, K. & Kaldor, J. (2003). Drug use and its correlates in an Australian prisoner population. *Addiction Research & Theory*, 11(2), 89–101.

Coombs, T., Curtis, J. & Crookes, P. (2011). What is a comprehensive mental health nursing assessment? A review of the literature. *International Journal of Mental Health Nursing*, 20, 364–70.

Frisch, N.C. & Frisch, L.E. (2011). *Psychiatric Mental Health Nursing* (4th edn). New York: Delmar Thomson Learning.

Hamilton, B., Manias, E., Maude, P., Marjoribanks, T. & Cook, K. (2004). Perspectives of a nurse, a social worker and a psychiatrist regarding patient assessment in acute inpatient psychiatry settings: a case study approach. *Journal of Psychiatric and Mental Health Nursing*, 11, 683–9.

Keltner, N.L., Bostrom, C. E. & McGuinness, T. (2011). *Psychiatric Nursing* (6th edn). St Louis: Mosby.

Kneisl, C.A. & Trigoboff, E. (2012). *Contemporary Psychiatric–Mental Health Nursing* (3rd ed.). Englewood Cliffs, NJ: Pearson Education.

Matthias, M.S., Salyers, M.P., Rollins, A.L. & Frankel, R.M. (2012). Decision making in recovery-oriented mental health care. *Psychiatric Rehabilitation Journal*, 35(4), 305–14.

Newell, R. & Gournay, K. (eds) (2009). *Mental Health Nursing: an evidence-based approach* (2nd edn). Philadelphia: Churchill Livingstone Elsevier.

Read, J., Vam, P.J., Morrison, A.P. & Ross, C.A. (2005). Childhood trauma, psychosis and schizophrenia: a literature review with theoretical and clinical implications. *Acta Psychiatrica Scandinavica*, 112, 330–50.

Sadock, B.J. & Sadock, V.A. (2007). *Kaplan & Sadock's Synopsis of Psychiatry: behavioral sciences/clinical psychiatry* (10th edn). Philadelphia, PA: Wolters Kluwer/Lippincott Williams & Wilkins.

Shives, L.R. (2011). *Basic Concepts of Psychiatric–Mental Health Nursing* (8th edn). Philadelphia, PA: Wolters Kluwer/Lippincott Williams & Wilkins.

Stuart, G.W. (2013). *Principles and Practice of Psychiatric Nursing* (10th edn). St Louis, MO: Elsevier-Mosby.

Thapinta, D., Anders, R.L., Wiwatkunupakan, S., Kitsumban, V. & Vadtanapong, S. (2004). Assessment of patient satisfaction of mentally ill patients hospitalized in Thailand. *Nursing and Health Sciences*, 6, 271–7.

Varcarolis, E.M. & Halter, M.J. (2010). *Foundations of Psychiatric Mental Health Nursing: a clinical approach* (6th edn). St Louis, MO: Saunders Elsevier.

Wilkinson, J.M. & Van Leuven, K. (2011). *Fundamentals of Nursing: theory, concepts & applications* (2nd ed). Philadelphia, PA: FA Davis.

Zuckerman, E.L. (2010). *Clinician's Thesaurus: the guide to conducting interviews and writing psychological reports* (7th edn). New York: Guilford Press.

12

Nursing care in mental health

Main points

- The role and function of the mental health nurse centres on providing health care that is collaborative and sensitive to needs, and that builds on existing strengths.
- The therapeutic relationship, therapeutic communication and use of self have become the most important goals for mental health nurses.
- The importance of caring for a person's physical health can be overlooked in mental health services.
- Working collaboratively with service users and carers aims to empower and connect service provision.
- Intimacy in mental health nursing includes physical, psychological and spiritual professional associations that are responsive to service user needs and recognise contemporary barriers.
- The issues of privacy and confidentiality are important in nursing care, but hold specific relevance in all mental health care.

Definitions

Interpersonal relationship: A connection and association between two people in order to interact and transact.

Reciprocity: A mutual exchange of dependence, action and influence.

INTRODUCTION

Providing nursing care to people experiencing a mental illness is very different from other types of nursing. The foundation of mental health nursing is the nurse–consumer relationship. This chapter will explore the care that is provided by the mental health nurse, and discuss specific features of the role and function of the contemporary mental health nurse. The emphasis throughout is on the therapeutic relationships the mental health nurse initiates and utilises as their 'tool of trade'.

Nurses aim to provide care by working collaboratively with service users and carers, and this chapter explores key aspects to achieving this goal. The notion of collaboration is compared with that of coercion. The aim of nursing care is to build upon the existing strengths of the person who is diagnosed with a mental illness and to respect his or her preferences when planning and developing therapeutic relationships. Finally, this chapter examines the important issues of privacy and confidentiality in the context of providing safe, responsible and therapeutic nursing care.

ROLES AND FUNCTIONS OF THE MENTAL HEALTH NURSE

The role of the mental health nurse is not easy to define or to distinguish from that of other mental health-care workers (see Chapter 4 for more detail on roles in mental health care). This is due in part to the diversification of mental health care in contemporary society and in part to a perceived lack of understanding about what a mental health nurse does. It is also true to state that the role of the mental health nurse is dynamic (changing) (Lakeman 2012). The politics of changes in mental health nursing roles are beyond the scope of this introductory book, so it is probably enough to claim here that not all change has developed or furthered the nurse's role. The fate of the mental health nursing profession often seems to be tied to the popularity (or unpopularity) of mental health care, and as Rydon (2005, p. 78) claims, 'if mental health nurses cannot practise in a therapeutic way, then they will struggle to find a way in which to articulate both the characteristics and distinctiveness of their practice'.

Role can be defined as an expected performance or a set of behaviours that is linked to an occupation, profession or position. These performances help us to describe and clarify the features of the occupation, profession or position. While nursing more generally has its role origins of domestic servitude, the mental health nurse role begins in a non-nursing occupation in eighteenth-century asylums (Smith 2005).

The origins of mental health nursing begin with a predominantly custodial role where persons (usually male) were employed as attendants to people with a mental illness. The role of the psychiatric attendant centred on enforcing imprisonment, and sometimes this required physical force (Prebble & Bryder 2008), and the loss of personal freedom and liberty. The arrival of nurses into the care of people with a mental illness marks a substantial change to how people with a mental illness are cared for—and all this has occurred just in the last 100 years!

CRITICAL THINKING

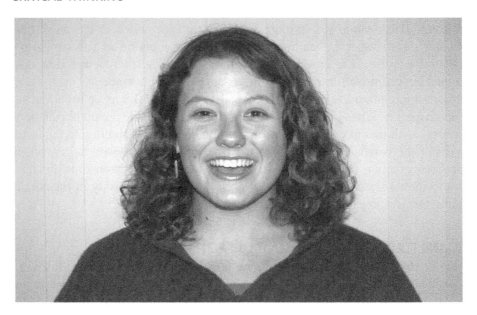

It was my first day in the mental health rehabilitation ward and I was full of worries. What would be expected of me? Would I be able to help people or was I just fooling myself? What would happen if people didn't like me and wouldn't talk to me? Everyone looked so different and they looked so unwell. I don't remember when I stopped seeing this and began to see the people behind the illness, but that is the point where I became a mental health nurse.

The role of the mental health nurse has emerged from those grim days of simply detaining and attending to the physical needs of people with a mental illness (Smith 2005). The idea that nursing care should be therapeutic and provide an environment where the carer and the cared for can develop their relationships helped to shape mental health nursing practice in such a profound way that the current role of the mental health nurse continues to centre on the therapeutic nurse–consumer relationship.

The distinction between the role of the medical–surgical general nurse and the mental health nurse begins with their tools of trade. While medical–surgical nurses might feel lost without a stethoscope, physical activity and ward routine, mental health nurses use therapeutic communication, relationship development and interpersonal skills as their daily tools. Figure 12.1 portrays a sense of overlap between the person, the general nurse and the mental health nurse.

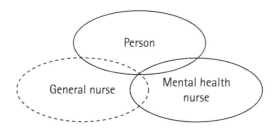

Figure 12.1 Overlap between nurse and person

Function of the nurse

The function of the contemporary mental health nurse is substantially different from that of the general medical–surgical nurse, and has altered considerably over the past few decades. The key functions of the mental health nurse discussed in this chapter, and indeed throughout this book, include:

- individualising care
- use of self
- crisis and early intervention
- connecting and reconnecting with service user, families and significant others
- investigating and potentiating mental health.

Perhaps the most important function of the contemporary mental health nurse is to provide a therapeutic relationship, using therapeutic communication, in a beneficial and restorative setting—whether that environment is an acute care ward or within the home and community. All encounters are potentially therapeutic, and even brief interactions can influence how a service user thinks and feels.

The interpersonal relationship

The art and science of relationship building has been described by many mental health nursing authors, and in particular the nursing theorist Peplau (1952). The therapeutic relationship built through 'therapeutic use of self' is the central feature, and includes cognitive, emotional and psychological events. Developing a relationship through therapeutic use of self is unique in the nursing skills repertoire. It is the domain of mental health nurses, and it is where we excel. The opportunity to create and promote helpful and healing relationships lies primarily with the nurse within the mental health team, as we will often spend the longest and closest time with people experiencing a mental illness. The therapeutic relationship does not occur without considerable knowledge, skill and expertise—although, from the outsider's perspective, it may appear that way. The following section explores and discusses the dynamic interactive process of relationships in mental health nursing care.

THERAPEUTIC RELATIONSHIP THEORY

The shift of mental health nursing from a custodial and handmaiden role gathered momentum in the Western world during the 1960s. Major changes in care delivery included the provision of community mental health care and multidisciplinary teams. At times, the nursing process challenged and suppressed the medical model as a framework for providing mental health nursing care, and nurses were able to embrace caring practices that involved group therapies and therapeutic milieus. Psycho-social care became a nursing focus as opposed to the previous care attendant role within many Western institutions. From the 1960s through the 1970s, it even became fashionable to be a psychiatric (mental health) nurse, and the provision of group and individual therapies to service users was no longer just the domain of psychiatrists and psychologists.

The shift to a holistic and psycho-social approach to mental health care may now have left nurses isolated, as the current trends of the new century in mental health care focus once more on the biological causes of mental illness. New psychotropic medication (see Chapter 9) dominates the treatment landscape, and once again the essence of the nurse–consumer relationship in mental health care is in danger of being subsumed. Peplau's theoretical framework for interpersonal relationships in mental health care (see Chapter 2), which provides an ideal structure for therapeutic relationships, is at risk of becoming less important than psycho-pharmacology.

What is a therapeutic relationship?

A therapeutic relationship is defined as a 'close, helping relationship based on trust, which allows the nurse and client to work collaboratively' (Mohr 2013, p. 117). A more in-depth and precise definition is offered by Benner Carson (2000, p. 202) as a 'time-bound alliance between nurse and patient, consciously entered into and characterised by respect, acceptance, empathy, and genuineness. Therapeutic relationships build on the premise that the resources for healing reside within the patient' (see Chapter 3).

Therapeutic relationships aim to provide nurturing and non-discriminate acceptance, and to support interpersonal relationships. The ability to form meaningful interpersonal relationships can be adversely affected by mental illness. People with a mental illness may be at risk of becoming socially isolated if they are unable to communicate and are unable to build or maintain lasting relationships (Aiyegbusi & Kelly 2012). One useful way of thinking about the therapeutic relationship is to compare your social relationships with those relationships that are of a therapeutic nature. The elements that are similar to both include:

* acceptance
* respect
* genuineness
* mutual appreciation

- honesty
- regard.
  (Adapted from Benner Carson 2000, p. 202)

A key difference between the social and therapeutic relationships is that the regard for each other in a social relationship is usually dependent on specific aspects within the broader social sphere, such as status, power and influence. The therapeutic relationship, however, begins with the premise of regard without any conditions. This means that, irrespective of social, cultural, economic or political details, the mental health nurse will begin with regard for the service user.

The term 'regard' is specific to the therapeutic relationship, and the psychologist Carl Rogers famously termed it 'unconditional positive regard' (see Chapter 2). Rogers states that unconditional positive regard is essential in the development of our therapeutic relationships, particularly for change. It is defined as communication that is 'deep and genuine' in caring for the service user 'as a person with human potentialities' and as 'uncontaminated by evaluations of thoughts, feelings or behaviours' (Rogers 1967, cited in Rogers 1990, p. 102). You might think about this type of regard, and wonder how to have unconditional positive regard regardless of what your service user may have done or said. This can be achieved by separating the behaviour from the person, in that someone's behaviour when diagnosed with a mental illness is separate to the strengths and qualities of the person.

Other elements that may differ between a therapeutic and social relationship include the purpose and focus, the degree of self-disclosure and personal involvement, and the responsibility for the relationship (Aiyegbusi & Kelly 2012).

What is therapeutic use of self?
The therapeutic relationship is a helpful and healing activity that aims to assist the service user to achieve and maintain mental health. Nurses will use their own personal life skills, knowledge and identity in order to actualise personal healing potentials. The nurse is the instrument of therapy rather than an external procedure such as a bandage or a medication. The nurse responds to interaction with service users by role modelling his or her optimal adjusted coping skills, and by recognising, promoting and building on service users' strengths.

SKILLS REQUIRED FOR DEVELOPING THERAPEUTIC RELATIONSHIPS
In order to enter into any therapeutic relationship, the mental health nurse first requires an in-depth understanding of the 'self'. This includes self-awareness, self-understanding, self-acceptance and self-knowledge. Non-therapeutic interactions here will include reacting in a spontaneous manner without deliberate thought by the nurse as to how the interaction can be therapeutic to the service user. The self-consciousness areas in

CASE STUDY

Sara is nineteen years of age, and rings the crisis hot line at least once a week—although sometimes it is every day. Sara describes herself as anorexic, and says she is surrounded by people who don't care about her. She describes her family as a 'bunch of losers' who hold her back from reaching her potential and who make her sick through their poor diet. Sara says she wants to move out of home, but she feels too weak from the anorexia and lacks the confidence required to live her own life. Last month, Sara took an overdose of 20 Panadol tablets then reconsidered the act and asked her parents to drive her to the emergency department, where her stomach was pumped.

Critical thinking

- What might be some of the potential obstacles to establishing a therapeutic relationship with Sara?
- What possible attitudes from a nurse's personal and cultural background might interfere with the nurse's ability to convey an accepting, non-judgmental approach to Sara?
- What specific actions would be most helpful to establish rapport with Sara, define the parameters of the relationship and reduce anxiety?
- What are Sara's strengths, and how can you help her to build upon these?

which the mental health nurse will benefit from exploring prior to developing therapeutic relationships can include:

- self-awareness (insight)
- self-acceptance (I'm okay)
- self-identity (distinctiveness, uniqueness)
- self-knowledge (self-assessment)
- self-preservation (self-intervention)
- self-understanding (values and attitudes)
- self-esteem (I feel good about myself).

An in-depth understanding of 'self' can help put you in a position to engender trust and acceptance with your colleagues and with service users. The above introspective self-consciousness can form the basis of skills for developing beneficial and healing therapeutic relationships. Self-understanding is your responsibility in the nurse–consumer relationship, and is an ongoing process (see Chapter 15 for methods to support self-consciousness, such as clinical supervision, mentoring and preceptoring).

The following questions may help you to clarify your capacity and development for self-understanding:

- Can I be in some way that will be perceived by others as trustworthy, dependable or consistent?
- Can I be expressive enough as a person so that what I am will be communicated unambiguously?
- Can I let myself experience positive attitudes towards this other person (attitudes of warmth, caring, liking, interest and respect)?
- Can I be strong enough as a person to be separate from the other?
- Am I secure enough within myself to permit the other person's separateness?
- Can I let myself enter fully into their world of feelings and personal meaning, and see these as they do?
- Can I receive a person as they are?
- Can I act with sufficient sensitivity in the relationship so that my behaviour will not be perceived as a threat?
- Can I free the service user from the threat of my external judgmental evaluation?
- Can I meet the service user as a person who is bound by their past and my past? (Adapted from Mohr 2013)

Creating a therapeutic relationship

A road map or framework for the development of therapeutic relationships in nursing now exists, thanks to the thoroughness and creativity of nursing theorists such as Peplau (1952). The stages of a therapeutic relationship are given a variety of titles by nursing theorists and authors; however, they can be summed up as an introductory beginning phase, a middle working phase and a termination phase (Mohr 2013). The overall broad elements within the therapeutic relationship should include that:

- therapeutic relationships are planned in order to meet the needs of the service user
- the basic tool of the therapeutic relationship is communication
- the mental health nurse uses their own personality as an integral tool
- the mental health nurse uses involvement such as 'being there' as a tool to develop the relationship.

A more in-depth description within the stages or phases of therapeutic relationships may include details from Table 12.1.

During the *introductory stage* of a planned therapeutic interaction, consideration can be given to timing. Examples here include assessing how to communicate and provide therapy or assistance in the time available. This is particularly important when you and the service user are getting to know each other for the first time. You might imagine meeting a new service user and beginning to discuss mental health issues when you are late for a case management meeting, due to give a shift handover or needing to help organise another service user's discharge or follow-up.

Table 12.1 Phases of therapeutic relationships and their definitions

Phase	Definition
Designing	Establishing the practical details of the therapeutic encounter
Warm-up	Beginning the therapeutic relationship, building rapport and engaging each other in the therapeutic process
Agreement	Mutually negotiating a contract or plan that states outcomes of the therapeutic relationship; assessing individual strengths and planning on how to build upon these
Rehabilitation	Working to facilitate movement towards mutually set goals through negotiation of defences, transference and counter-transference.
Finishing	Terminating and evaluating the therapeutic relationship at a mutually negotiated end time while maintaining openness to future therapeutic contracts to allow the service user 'time up' to reconsider the direction of their life goals.

Source: Adapted from Mohr (2013).

Timing is important for the service user as well in the introductory stage. A therapeutic interaction with the nurse (particularly if the nurse is new or not known) may be overwhelming at first. The service user may be shy, tired or unwell, and the introductions or expected responses of a therapeutic interaction may intrude on delusional and/or hallucinatory thoughts.

Another consideration is the physical setting. Where is the most appropriate place for a therapeutic relationship to begin in a busy, often overcrowded mental health unit? An ideal location to begin therapeutic interactions is a quiet place such as an interview room or another quiet spot within the environment of the health-care facility, where both the nurse and service user can relax and feel comfortable and safe without invading each other's personal space.

Cultural and gender issues are particularly important during the introductory phase of a therapeutic relationship. Ongoing assessments should be made regarding issues of taboo subjects, eye contact, body language, body space, religion and cultural codes of conduct (Benner Carson 2000). Stereotypical responses such as 'I know how you feel' or 'you will be okay' should be avoided where possible. Interpreter services may be of value at first to both the nurse and the service user, in order to gain an understanding of a service user's specific characteristics and behaviours.

During the introductory phase of a therapeutic relationship, the foundations can be prepared for ongoing care and mutual goals can be explored. The aims at this beginning stage of the therapeutic relationship may include specific details such as:

- introductions—getting to know each other's names
- finding some common ground
- dealing with any preliminary concerns, questions or issues
- structuring the boundaries for the therapeutic relationship
- exploring strengths and past success
- assessing needs and gathering information
- finding priorities, setting goals and outlining future possible interventions
- raising goodwill, hope and decreasing anxieties.

The *middle stage* or working phase is where the work within the therapeutic relationship is achieved. Peplau (1952) called this the exploitation stage, where service users draw from the therapeutic relationship those items that are most likely to improve their health or be of assistance, such as access to specific services and psycho-therapeutic support. During the middle or working phase, feedback and support from the mental health nurse to the service user is critical to maintain the momentum of change and the therapeutic nature of the relationship. Recovery and changes in quality of life are potential indications that the therapeutic relationship may be integral to mental health care.

The aims of the middle phase may include:

- recognition of previous triggers and challenges to a person's mental health, including behaviours and thought processes that have been detrimental
- implementing or re-establishing strategies for recovery and health maintenance
- unfolding of new ideas and approaches to mental health through psycho-education and changes in understanding
- strengthening individuals by promoting coping skills, and investigating and increasing personal resilience
- building upon strengths and working towards recovery
- reducing barriers to mental health and increasing safety, education, meaningful employment and suitable housing
- developing and testing independence and hope for the future.

The *final stage*, or termination phase, of the therapeutic relationship tends not to exist in social relationships, or is often not acknowledged or planned. However, it is a crucial part of the caring relationship—particularly as the length of admissions to mental health care facilities grows shorter. The aims of the introductory stage may not yet be complete before the service user is discharged. A lack of time and resources may have significantly shortened the middle stage of the therapeutic relationship, and community services may be unable to actualise and support ongoing improvements and change. The termination stage may represent loss, rejection and fear for some service users. How the termination phase of a therapeutic relationship is managed may determine the difference between ongoing improvements and health maintenance or future relapses (Fragkiadaki1 & Strauss 2012).

The aims within the termination phase may include any of the following:

- a decrease in contact, communication and support for the service user, and an increase in encouraging independence
- establishing and revisiting outcomes and goals achieved throughout the therapeutic relationship
- expression of mutually acceptable grieving for loss and change
- introduction of a more light-hearted and less intense style of communication—less purpose-driven
- discussion of future plans, hopes and goals
- declining or avoiding involvement in the service user's new challenges and issues
- assistance to create and forge strong links to new networks, including family supports, community liaisons and other rehabilitative services.

Some specific therapeutic techniques that you might consider helpful within these phases are shown in Table 12.2.

Table 12.2 Therapeutic techniques and examples

Title	Example
Using silence	
Accepting	Yes. That must have been difficult for you.
Acknowledging	I noticed that you're showered and ready.
Offering self	I'll come with you.
Open-ended questioning	How can I be of help to you here?
Leading into	Please go on . . . you were saying?
Time stamping	When did the voices begin?
Observations as lead-in	You seem to be very angry . . .

CRITICAL THINKING

- How do you start a therapeutic relationship
- What aspects of the therapeutic relationship would you find most challenging?
- How do you feel when discussing your personal issues with another person?

THERAPEUTIC COMMUNICATION SKILLS

As stated in Chapter 13, 'therapeutic communication' is the name and aim for a style of communicating that you specifically plan to be of benefit to a person. It is a face-to-face interpersonal interaction between you and the service user, during which you can focus on any specific needs that will promote the exchange of information.

The deliberate and skilled use of therapeutic communications within the therapeutic relationship can help you to gain an understanding of and insight into the service user's experience and perspective. In order to gain these understandings, it is important that both people within the therapeutic communication situation be aware of the potential sensitive and confidential nature of the information being communicated, and that a therapeutic goal drives the process.

Encounters using therapeutic communication can be brief—for example, using a person's name and acknowledging their presence. Other potential therapeutic communication examples may include greetings such as hello, goodbye, good morning and good evening. Opportunities for therapeutic communication and building upon therapeutic relationships continually arise, such as starting conversations with service users, carers and visitors, or even simply picking up where a conversation left off previously.

Therapeutic communication can be used to gather information from the service user to determine mental health problems and concerns, as well as to assist in assessing and changing behaviour. It can also be useful to assess and provide health-care education and create collaborative (joint) approaches to ongoing alliances with mental health care services.

Therapeutic communication within the therapeutic relationship is useful in all of the following situations:

*   guidance on the service user's perception of his or her mental health problem; this can include thoughts and feelings about the current situation and clarifying aims and goals
*   creation and ongoing maintenance of therapeutic relationships
*   an opportunity to safely express and acknowledge emotions and thoughts
*   recognition of the service user's needs, desires and concerns as they evolve
*   identification and clarification of important concerns for the service user in any setting
*   implementation of interventions aimed at assisting the service user to meet their needs.

THERAPEUTIC OPTIMISM

A new direction springing from therapeutic communication strategy is that of thera-peutic optimism. This is defined as hopeful positive expectations for treatment and

CASE STUDY

Maggie has finished her graduate year and has just started work in the acute care mental health unit. This is the first time Maggie has worked in mental health since her clinical placement as a student, and she is quite nervous about meeting and communicating with the service users. Maggie was somewhat timid and shy during her orientation to the unit, and showed concern regarding locked doors and the psychiatric intensive care area. She seems quite relieved to find that her first assigned consumer, Sarah, is of similar age, and feels she will be able to establish a therapeutic relationship with her.

Sarah was brought to the emergency department two days ago by her father after a suicide attempt. At the shift handover, the nursing staff stated that Sarah had been admitted to the unit on previous occasions and had once accused her father of raping her. Sarah's father is the current mayor of a nearby council area. Her mother died when Sarah was nine years old. During the last admission, Sarah rescinded her previous claim of her father's behaviour and was subsequently discharged by the consultant psychiatrist into her father's care. This was despite the fact that Sarah is over eighteen years of age. She returned to university and was reported by the community mental health team to be doing well until just before Christmas.

Over the weekend, Sarah was often found standing in the middle of the room looking as if she were lost. She repeated over and over that 'he did it again'. Maggie gave Sarah PRN medication on top of her prescribed anti-depressant medication. After visiting the magistrate, an order of two weeks' hospitalisation was made and Sarah's father requested guardianship rights.

Maggie attempts a therapeutic interaction, but Sarah is vague and non-responsive. She appears to be actively hallucinating. Maggie realises that communication will probably not be successful because of Sarah's symptoms, but continues to try. Maggie continues to feel inadequate as a mental health nurse, and can sense her anxiety increasing.

After about five minutes of receiving only stares in response to her inquiries, Maggie asks whether what the other nursing staff are saying is true—that Sarah was raped by her father. Sarah does not verbally respond at first, but is incontinent of urine while sitting in the chair. When Maggie is assisting to clean and redress her, Sarah begins speaking. She tells Maggie, 'The only one that can help me is my mother. This all started when she died. My father smothered me. He killed me.'

Critical thinking

- What reactions are you experiencing about Sarah?
- What self-assessment questions would be appropriate for Maggie to ask herself about her initial feelings towards Sarah?
- How would you interpret Sarah's incontinence and disclosure about her father?

- What are Sarah's strengths, and how can you help Sarah to build upon these and increase her communication with you?
- What therapeutic relationship and therapeutic communication strategies would you use during an initial encounter with Sarah?

rehabilitation outcomes (Cleary et al. 2012), and while hope and positivity might seem to be what all care should include, this is not always the case.

How to encourage therapeutic optimism

- Create and maintain a service user-focused environment.
- Be flexible and responsive at all times.
- Be respectful, positive and empathetic and use good communication skills.
- Advocate for the service user and mental health care wherever possible.
- Create achievable goals for self and others.
- Take personal responsibility as well as work as a team. (Adapted from Cleary et al. 2012)

PHYSICAL HEALTH CARE

Just as we plan to provide nursing care in the medical–surgical area from a multiple perspective of physical, mental and spiritual care, the same should apply in mental health-care services. There is an ongoing inherent danger that physical health may be less of a focus in the mental health-care setting, as attention and perhaps even expertise are focused on mental health status. Recent statistics of morbidity and mortality in mental illness (AIHW 2012) provide evidence that physical health care for people diagnosed with a mental illness is often lacking, and can lead to a substantially reduced lifespan. Neglect of any perspective in health-care services can be avoided by keeping in mind that health and well-being are dependent on a balance between mind, body and spirit.

In a similar manner to the evidence that women will live longer than men and Indigenous persons have an average lifespan ten to 20 years less than Caucasian Australians (AIHW 2012), people who suffer from a mental illness are more likely to die at least ten years earlier than those without any episodes of mental illness—and according to Lawrence, Kisely & Pais (2011), this gap is increasing rather than decreasing. An episode of serious mental illness such as schizophrenia and bipolar conditions carries specific physical health risks such as cardiovascular disease, respiratory disease and type II diabetes ((Lawrence, Kisely & Pais 2011). Communicable diseases such as hepatitis B and C, and HIV infection, are also more prevalent, although cancer is not.

The possible reasons for neglect of physical health can include access to physical health services—particularly when a person is suffering from a diagnosed episode of mental illness. Once within the health care services, the focus of the health-care staff may be on mental health, or staff may consider physical complaints psychosomatic (imagined physical illness), thereby missing vital physical health indicators.

Other important, and perhaps more pervasive, reasons might include poverty, lifestyle and habits. For example:

- a higher incidence of smoking
- a higher incidence of obesity
- a higher incidence of nutritionally deficient diet
- higher risk-taking activities such as unsafe sex and unsafe drug-taking behaviours
- less impact from health and lifestyle education and fewer avenues for penetration
- more toxicity and health-damage risks from psycho-pharmacology
- less health-care empowerment and greater marginalisation, meaning fewer self-initiated physical health checks.

CRITICAL THINKING
Consider the list of reasons for increased physical health problems and devise possible ways to improve each of these. You may want to consider creative and collaborative interventions and consult service user groups for assistance.

WORKING COLLABORATIVELY WITH SERVICE USERS AND CARERS

Previous models of mental health care historically have tended to disempower or inhibit both providers of care and service users of mental health care. Often, the person most distant to the mental illness would formulate the type of care while nurses and carers may have a limited say in how the care would be provided and managed.

Fortunately, many changes and reforms have occurred since the days of large asylums and institutional care. One of the most important changes has been the notion of 'working together with people', or collaborating with service users and carers. The current National Mental Health Strategy aims to:

- promote the mental health of the Australian community
- where possible, prevent the development of mental disorder
- reduce the impact of mental disorders on individuals, families and the community
- assure the rights of people with mental illness.

Consumer consultancy is another more recent inclusion into joint participation in mental health care. Terms used to describe this role of 'education and training, peer support, leadership and advocacy' include 'consumer advocate', 'consumer representative', 'consumer worker', 'peer support worker' and 'service user' (Bennetts, Cross & Bloomer 2011). Despite increasing support for collaboration between service providers and service users, barriers continue to persist in the shape of a lack of support, information, commitment to empower and attitudinal issues such as patronising and blocking by some mental health professionals (Bennetts, Cross & Bloomer 2011).

Community-based services—rather than the previous large institutional model of care—provide much greater scope for us to work collaboratively with service users and carers. The principles for models of care that incorporate the goals of collaboration between mental health service providers and service users are supported by the Mental Health Council of Australia (2011) and include the following:

- the notion that the rights of service users and carers are paramount
- service user participation in choosing, planning, evaluating and changing their service provision
- where appropriate, carer participation in choosing, planning, evaluating and changing the service provision for the person for whom they provide care
- locally based flexible community support services that consider the needs of all social and cultural groups within a particular community
- services designed to prevent illness, to provide early intervention support once the illness presents and to prevent relapse following recovery
- services designed to assist people to live independently in their homes
- services designed to assist people living with mental illness to safely participate in education, employment and the social life of their community
- services that respect the privacy and confidentiality of service users while facilitating the appropriate use of data for learning
- a collaborative approach to supporting people living with mental illness.

Providing collaborative care in circumstances where the service user does not have legal power to refuse treatment, or where the service user is being detained in hospital without their consent, can be a challenge. If service users are coerced into nursing care, they may be powerless to really collaborate with you. In such circumstances, it may be helpful to be reminded of the following points. Nurses can:

- take every opportunity to encourage service users to make their own choices
- highlight and attempt to facilitate the preferences of the service user wherever possible
- advocate for the preferences of the service user where possible
- be knowledgeable about what other resources/agencies exist for referral purposes.

In order to maintain collaborative care, it is important to be transparent about the duty of care that you have to the person, and to explain the grounds upon which decisions are being made so that the service user remains informed about their care—even if there are aspects of their care over which they have little control.

It is important to remain vigilant against the potential for coercive care, including attitudes such as 'I know what is best for my service user', which do not facilitate working with service users. Such attitudes must be examined carefully and often.

PLACING THE SERVICE USER AT THE CENTRE: ADVANCE DIRECTIVES

Psychiatric advance directives (PAD), also known as 'advance agreements', 'living wills' or 'Ulysses agreements', are documents that state the service user's instructions/ preferences for treatment and life decisions (Nicaise, Lorant & Dubois 2013). They are increasingly being used in the United States, and are in the early stages of use in the United Kingdom, but have yet to become a common feature in Australian mental health policy or services. Service users welcome the opportunity to make decisions about what should happen if there is a crisis in the future. They can cover a breadth of life issues such as care of family, pets, plants and bill payments, and can nominate a person trusted by the service user who can help carry out these preferences and wishes. Although they are not legally binding, advance directives are a useful tool for the service user and provider when there is a crisis because if wishes are already specified and documented, it is easier to facilitate them. More information can be found at <www.nrc-pad.org>.

CASE STUDY

Julie has been in the mental health acute care unit for nearly a week. Each day, Julie has felt a little better about making her way around the unit and being around people. However, Julie still finds herself visibly trembling when she is forced to go to the dining room to eat her meals with the other service users and the nursing staff. No one seems to understand how scared she feels when she is around other people, and she knows these are not her normal thoughts, as the fear came on just recently when she began hearing voices again. Julie had tried to explain her fear to her nurse, but she could tell the nurse had no real idea of what this fear was like. Today was going to be a nightmare as the nurse informed Julie that a group of service users and nurses were going to the shopping mall. Julie tries to tell her nurse that she is not ready to be among so many people, but instead is told that such an outing will be good for her. In a way, Julie feels sorry for her nurse because, although the nurse tries hard, she really has no idea what is good for Julie.

Critical thinking

- What is coercive about Julie's situation, and why do you think this has occurred?
- How might you work collaboratively with Julie?

WORKING WITH FAMILY AND CARERS

As discussed in Chapter 1, the process of deinstitutionalisation over the past few decades has seen the care of service users shift increasingly from psychiatric hospitals out into the community. This has meant that families and carers now provide much of the vital day-to-day support for service users who, without this support, are likely to have a lower quality of life and a much greater risk of homelessness.

Families and carers can often be unprepared for their caregiving role, and can experience a significant burden in supporting their partner, child, sibling, parent, other family member or friend (Trondsen 2012). This can include subjective burdens such as:

- feeling emotionally exhausted (burnout)
- feeling lonely and isolated
- feeling distressed and having emotional problems.

It can also include objective burdens such as:

- difficulty understanding and coping with the person's mental health problem
- difficulty supervising the person's behaviour
- difficulty attending to other family members' needs
- difficulty juggling financial and household responsibilities and/or paid work.

Family carers have also reported difficulty in getting enough social support for themselves and the service user, difficulty finding other carers to share information with and feeling the need for respite from their caring role from time to time (Grant & Westhues 2012). Carers can also experience grief relating to the impact of the mental health problem on them, their family and the service user (Trondsen 2012). The stress and burden relating to the caring role can affect carers' own health and well-being.

A recent Australian survey of family carers found that 56 per cent reported that their mental and physical health had been affected by their role as a carer of a person with a mental health problem. Many of them (55 per cent) had also experienced a lack of information and support from mental health professionals, while 70 per cent had not received any education or training in how to understand and manage mental health problems that might help them in carrying out their caring role (SANE Australia 2007). Yet carers can often cope well with the impact of their family member's/friend's mental health problem, and demonstrate significant resilience and a strong relationship with the service user—particularly if they receive adequate information and support from health and other professionals (Trondsen 2012).

For these reasons, it is very important that nurses and other mental health professionals who work collaboratively with service users also recognise and support the family and/or carers. Ways in which nurses and other professionals can do this include:

- acknowledging in an empathetic and non-judgemental way family carers' own issues and needs

- providing families and carers with written information on mental health problems and treatments
- providing education and strategies on how to manage the service user's symptoms
- referring family carers to relevant websites, resources, organisations and carer support and respite programs
- listening to and respecting family carers' experiences and views concerning the service user's symptoms
- including family carers in collaborative care for the service user (with the service user's agreement).

Websites with further information and resources on family and carer issues include:

- Carers Australia <www.carersaustralia.com.au>
- Children of Parents with Mental Illness <www.copmi.net.au>.

INTIMACY AND THE MENTAL HEALTH NURSE

Nursing intimacy is generally defined as a professional relationship characterised by commitment, closeness and involvement: caring for and caring about service users (Stavropoulou et al. 2012). Other general characteristics of nursing intimacy include spending time with service users and families, 'being with' the service user and attempting to demonstrate an understanding of the service user's experience (past, present and future). Three types of intimacy discussed here include physical, emotional (psychological) and spiritual. The following table includes examples from all three types. You will notice that many of these are vital to the development of therapeutic relationships, communication and use of self.

Nursing intimacy is a relatively new direction in nursing care, although it would be reasonable to argue that it has always been a core attribute of therapeutic care. Throughout most of the twentieth century, the biomedical model has dominated our health-care provision and prescribed our nursing actions (see Chapter 2). Previously, nurses were taught that emotional distance and detachment was the ideal model for nursing care provision (Group & Roberts 2001). This may have stemmed from Nightingale's model of nursing care, where the focus initially was on providing an environment suited to health improvements, which became a major value of nursing education throughout the twentieth century. As a female-dominated profession, nurses were encouraged to obey, serve and conceptualise the patient as a biological entity in need of care but not necessarily understanding (Simpson et al. 2012). Some senior nurses warned of dire consequences if 'over-involvement' occurred. Consequently, nurse–consumer relationships remained an enigma in both image and expectations for the new nurse.

Task allocation (the need/wish to keep physically doing things) provides a protection for nurses against the stress of close relationships (intimacy with service users) (Williams

2001). However, case management and primary nursing care utilise an increasing amount of intimacy. Case management nursing increases the opportunity for intimacy with service users, and therefore increases the likelihood of stress. Changing the way we practise nursing—from task allocation to case management—may increase the vulnerability of the unprepared nurse. Previous management of this has been to regularly rotate nurses throughout health-care areas, concentrate on tasks rather than service user management and split workloads routinely (Williams 2001). However, such reaction from nursing management is more likely to increase stress and anxiety for some nurses, as it may create depersonalisation (a disconnection and distance between nurse and service user).

Table 12.3 Examples of nursing intimacy

Reciprocity	Understanding
Partnership	Acceptance
Closeness—physical, psychological, spiritual	Trusting
Connectedness	Shared worries and concerns
Unity between self and other	Mutual seeking of appropriate solutions
Being there	Compassion
Potential contact with another	Empathy
Emotional contact	Attachment
Self-disclosure	Transference

If the nurse acts as a 'therapeutic instrument', stresses and strains can surface because of conflict between being a professional and being intimate. In fact, being professional and being human—or being distant and being close—is a finely tuned balance that develops with expertise in mental health nursing.

Why, then, is intimacy important in mental health nursing? A therapeutic effect is intrinsically related to the type and degree of intimacy in the relationship between the nurse and the service user (therapeutic intimacy). For example, the health outcomes have been assessed as higher in those circumstances where nurse and service user intimacy is higher (Williams 2001). Therefore, intimacy appears to be a valuable nursing approach for increased health outcomes and for supporting service user health determination. A positive correlation exists between the degree of nurse and service user intimacy and better recovery and health outcomes (Stavropoulou et al. 2012).

Contemporary barriers to intimacy in mental health nursing

It is clear that nursing intimacy within a framework of holistic nursing practice is an ideal situation for the growth of therapeutic relationships. In working together with the service user, the nurse is in an excellent position to assist with health-care decisions. We might ask here, though, just how much intimacy is reasonable and helpful. This is particularly relevant in the mental health field, where physical, emotional and spiritual boundaries (including body space) are different from those of general nursing, and over- or under-involvement may become a life-threatening issue (Videbech 2010).

If the risk of high involvement can lead to burnout, stress and emotional costs, but low involvement leads to distancing and a poor therapeutic relationship, how can you find the right measure of involvement that is tailored to each service user's needs and your current experience level? As stated earlier, maintenance of a professional role balance with good use of therapeutic intimacy is an ongoing skill and it is developed and supported through good role models from experienced mental health nurses.

Specific barriers to mental health nursing therapeutic intimacy may include any of the following:

- staff shortages
- skill and expertise issues
- cultural and gender differences
- policies and procedural directives
- management issues
- medical directives
- coercive requirements of the nursing role
- aggression and/or violence issues
- medication issues
- safety issues
- personality issues.

NON-THERAPEUTIC RELATIONSHIPS

Not all interactions in mental health care will mould themselves neatly into a therapeutic relationship, no matter how hard we try. Some nursing interactions are not wanted by the service user, and in cases where the service user cannot withhold consent, it is easy to see how this might interfere with the maintenance of a therapeutic relationship. In fact, a few interactions may turn out to be non-therapeutic—they may even be destructive and dangerous. There are various reasons why this might occur. The key features may include:

- an abrogation (loss or change) of the service user's best interests
- a betrayal of trust the service user places on the nurse
- a replacement of therapeutic goals with exploitative or non-therapeutic goals (sexual or otherwise).

Each nurse brings a personal set of beliefs, values, knowledge and skills to the relationship, and it may be that these aspects cause friction, leading to adverse reactions with service users (Mohr 2013). In other words, sometimes a clash of beliefs and values may occur between the service user, family carers and even other staff. In addition, there are a number of possible attitudes and approaches to therapeutic relationships that may prevent their development or reduce their effectiveness. These can include:

- *Judgemental attitudes and moralising*: These could include expressing approval/ disapproval of service users' thoughts and actions. An overly critical attitude can prevent acceptance and unconditional positive regard, which are central to the development of therapeutic intimacy and relationships. An example here may be the nurse who is critical of the service user's suicide attempt: 'She is attention-seeking (suicide attempt)—she can wait until I've seen my other service users and taken all my meal/ tea breaks.'
- *Excessive probing and faulty assumptions*: These can include a lack of appropriate assessment, invading a service user's privacy, personal space and freedoms when it is not warranted. Jumping to conclusions regarding a service user's meanings and health status can derail any goals and outcomes from therapeutic relationships. For example, probing questions to a person suffering from memory loss may lead to a variety of false and misleading information because the person feels under pressure to provide elaborate histories and background.
- *Rescuing and giving advice*: These can include making service users feel that you are able to save them from their current problems and that you are the source of dependency for future problems. The act of rescuing is not about supporting a therapeutic relationship with a service user, but rather about power, control, authority and legitimacy. It is presumptuous to give advice when self-actualisation, insight and independence may be the service user's goals. For example, directing a service user to avoid contact with a family member while in hospital on the basis that it will save face for the service user may prevent long-term family cohesion and support.

THERAPEUTIC RELATIONSHIP BOUNDARIES

There is a 'symbolic separation' that exists between people, and this is an important consideration to take into account when you are establishing and managing therapeutic relationships (Benner Carson 2000, p. 215). There are boundaries within which our therapeutic relationships should occur, and such boundaries offer expectations and structure to nurses and service users.

A breach or violation of boundaries can sometimes arise in mental health care. For example, if the distance between a commonly held reality, fantasy and illusion is narrowed and interferes with our interactions, then clear, tangible and manageable boundaries are vital. These boundaries may include negotiations on time and effort, physical and personal space and the possibility of gratuities (money or gifts given).

CASE STUDY

During a home visit, you discover that 35-year-old Mrs Zorka has decided she does not want to take her Risperidone any longer (see Chapter 9 for more information about this medication) again, and is now experiencing psychosis. Mrs Zorka has two children under the age of five, and both are at home with her during the daytime. Mrs Zorka has initially refused to open her front door to you on your visit, and she eventually tells you that it is much safer for her and the children if they do not 'touch the outside world'. Mrs Zorka also tells you that God is telling her to stay in her home and pray for the end of the world, which is happening soon. In the background, you can hear the children crying. Mrs Zorka does not appear to have showered in over a week and she fears that you are trying to harm her and her children.

Critical thinking

- What possible attitudes from your personal and cultural background might interfere with your ability to convey an accepting, non-judgemental approach to Mrs Zorka?
- What specific actions would be most helpful in establishing rapport with Mrs Zorka, to define the parameters of the relationship, build upon her strengths and help her to reduce her anxiety?

The *Nurses Act* in each state determines legal and professional boundaries. For example, the New South Wales *Nurses and Midwives Act 1991* sets out legal boundaries for the nurse when providing professional nursing care. Further reading includes the Australian Nursing and Midwifery Council's document, *A Nurse's Guide to Professional Boundaries* (ANMC 2010).

Mental health nursing care is based on establishing and maintaining a therapeutic relationship, not a social one. Even so, nurses and service users are often together in informal situations that may test boundaries, such as shared dining rooms or in the service user's home. While the service user usually has limited access to information about the nurse, the nurse has privileged professional information about the service user. The potential exists for this to be unwisely used to influence and determine service user outcomes, such as ward leave, discharge decisions and service/resource provisions. The nurse has significant power over the service user, who is vulnerable in the power relationship (Baca 2011).

It is useful to consider all service user interaction as potentially a therapeutic event. This is true even if the contact appears to be a social activity (a trip to the shops or the cinema). For example, having a cup of coffee with a service user may not start as a social activity, but for the service user this may be a good opportunity to chat in surroundings that are less threatening and more private than an interview room or the unit environment. You can consider how this interaction opportunity may help (be therapeutic) to the service user. Generally, mental health nurses are reluctant to consider or perceive other nursing staff's therapeutic relationship actions as boundary violations. There are steps to take when therapeutic relationships have violated professional boundaries. This is particularly critical for sexual misconduct, but it is also important for other aspects of nurse–consumer relationship breaches:

- Immediate reporting should occur, to the nursing unit manager as well as the clinical nurse consultant.
- Discussion may also take place with nursing supervisors, directors of nursing and area directors of nursing.
- An official report should be submitted to the state Nurses Registration Board.
- Complaints may be lodged with either the Australian Health Practitioner Regulatory Authority (AHPRA) or in New South Wales the New South Wales Health Care Complaints Commission. See <www.ahpra.gov.au/Notifications-and-Outcomes/Conduct-Health-and-Performance/Make-a-Notification.aspx>.

GETTING ASSISTANCE

Support, advice and assistance for non-therapeutic relationships and interactions may be readily available for individual situations. For example, clinical supervision is one method of professional support for the nurse, along with mentorship and preceptorship (see Chapter 15. In some circumstances, a more experienced nurse may be of assistance to the service user; however, assistance and support can also be provided from a psychiatrist, psychologist or counsellor. It is important to keep in mind that the nature of therapeutic relationships can overwhelm even the most experienced mental health nurse and service user.

Maintaining professional and therapeutic standards for the nurse–consumer relationship can include any of the following guidelines:

- Set firm and reasonable therapeutic limits with service users.
- Dress professionally—flamboyant or seductive clothing is not acceptable; nurses who expect to be treated professionally should dress accordingly.
- Use language that conveys caring and respect. Sexually explicit or vulgar language violates boundaries. Use of first or full names should be mutually negotiated by the service user and nurse, and should reflect the custom of the place where treatment takes place.
- Use self-disclosure discriminately. Some self-disclosure can be appropriate when its purpose is to model or educate, foster the therapeutic alliance or validate a service user's reality.

PRIVACY AND CONFIDENTIALITY

The issue of privacy and confidentiality is important in all nursing care; however, the case of mental health care has specific considerations that are discussed in more detail here but also throughout this book. Confidentiality forms a part of privacy; however, privacy is a much broader concept that includes a person's right to know how their health information is managed, stored and accessed, as well as issues of self-access to health information. In the same manner as all nursing care, any discussion of a service user's personal life, and in particular their health status, must occur only with those directly involved in a person's care (Wilkinson & Van Leuven 2011). Generally, confidentiality is considered to be of paramount importance except in cases of possible harm to self and/or others (Treatment Protocol Project 2000). For example, it is not a reasonable expectation to be told something in confidence that will have an adverse effect on a person's health and safety, even though interpersonal relationships are often built on a foundation of trust and confidentiality.

In special circumstances such as personal or public safety, criminal activities and terrorism, confidential information may be sought and released:

- to the police
- to the coroner
- to other health services
- when ordered by a court of law.

CASE STUDY

You knew that Matthew was very keen on taking his weekend leave from the mental health acute care unit. He had been talking about visiting his friend James for days. Matthew's depression had lifted so substantially that the mental health treating team had agreed that he could spend the weekend away from the hospital as a stepping stone towards discharge in the coming weeks. As you help Matthew pack an overnight bag, he tells you that his friend owns a farm and he is looking forward to the fresh air, peace and quiet of country living. Matthew looks down at his bag and quietly tells you that his friend James also has ammunition. You quickly ask him what he means by this, but Matthew refuses to say anything further about his comment.

Critical thinking

- Although you feel comfortable talking to the mental health care team about Matthew's comment, do you (or the team) release this confidentiality to Matthew's friend James as well?
- What are the implications of your decision?

The following section from the Mental Health Council of Australia's Privacy Kit provides some sense of direction for the example:

> Discharging someone from a facility without a plan in place for his or her treatment and care could pose a serious threat to the person's life or health, or to that of some other person. Thus, disclosure of a person's health information in the course of making appropriate care plans for them is not contrary to the privacy legislation. The privacy legislation should not be used to justify the lack of inquiry being made about the availability of family or community support. Further, carers may have responsibility but they also have rights, and their health and safety might also be an issue. Therefore, privacy and confidentiality concerns have to be dealt with thoughtfully. Even though formal consent mechanisms are usually not required of a tribunal, before discharging a patient from a facility, a mental health board or tribunal should ideally obtain the patient's understanding that their family, or carer(s) will be informed so that they can be properly prepared to fulfil their responsibilities. (Mental Health Council of Australia 2004, p. 18)

Broadly, confidentiality of information in mental health care is governed by state legislation. The new national board (AHPRA) sets policy and professional standards, whereas the state and territory boards make individual notification and registration decisions. Regular updates of policies and guidelines flow from the Health Departments through to individual local health services and non-government services, and become protocols at the service delivery end.

You may find that although the protocols on the issue of confidentiality are clear in the workplace, there are some circumstances where information regarding a service user is requested, such as a telephone inquiry from an employer or a visitor inquiry from a close friend or neighbour. The principle of safeguarding confidentiality should be upheld at all times when information regarding a service user's health status is sought without the service user's consent. This may include not confirming a person's admission to mental health services and any other details (Treatment Protocol Project 2000). In all such circumstances, you should discuss each situation with a senior mental health professional. Ensure that you check all documentation such as case files, nursing records and protocols before any course of action is determined.

The rights of people with mental illness include the issue of privacy and, as with confidentiality, this right should be upheld at all times while providing the best clinical practice. The Commonwealth *Privacy Act 1988* (amended 2012) covers issues such as mental health care with an overriding caveat of not hindering or impeding clinical decision-making and clinical practice (Mental Health Council of Australia 2004). Important issues relate to the following:

* privacy standards in the conduct of human medical research in Australia
* the collection, use and disclosure of personal medical information in relation to the conduct of research, and the compilation and analysis of statistics relevant to public health, safety or health service management activities.

We need to gather information about service users, and sometimes this may be understood as an invasion of privacy. However, without the 'information-gathering process', determinations regarding health care, status and progression cannot accurately be made (Mohr 2013). Care and consideration of a person's rights to privacy and the confidential nature of health status information should form the basis for decision-making. There are many circumstances where issues are not so clear cut; however, health service policy and more senior experienced mental health professionals offer guidance and direction.

CRITICAL THINKING

- Why are therapeutic relationships so critical in mental health nursing?
- What was the contribution to therapeutic relationships theory from Peplau, and is it still relevant today?
- What is therapeutic use of self?
- What skills are required for good therapeutic communication?
- What does intimacy in mental health nursing entail?
- If a nurse–consumer relationship is non-therapeutic, what problems might arise?
- How can you heal (redress) a violated therapeutic relationship?

CONCLUSION

The role and function of the contemporary mental health nurse have been discussed briefly in light of the changing health-care setting as well as therapeutic relationships and interactions from a theoretical and practical perspective. The special relationship developed by the mental health nurse is compared with social relationships as well as other nursing relationships. Therapeutic use of self and reflection of our self-consciousness as central building blocks for the nurse–consumer relationship have been highlighted, and a number of case stories help to add context to these concepts. The creation, development and termination of the therapeutic relationship are discussed and therapeutic communication is evaluated as a fundamental aspect of the therapeutic relationship. Barriers, boundaries and violations of the therapeutic relationship are often difficult to confront and discuss; however, each of these issues has been explored from the professional, cultural and socio-political perspective. Finally, the contemporary aims of building on strengths and creating therapeutic alliances, confidentially and privacy complete this chapter.

REFERENCES

Aiyegbusi, A. & Kelly, G. (eds) (2012). *Professional and Therapeutic Boundaries in Forensic Mental Health Practice*. London: Jessica Kingsley.

Australian Institute of Health and Welfare (AIHW) (2012). *Australia's Health 2012*. Australia's health series no. 13. Canberra: AIHW.

Australian Nursing and Midwifery Council (ANMC) (2010). *A Nurse's Guide to Professional Boundaries*. Canberra: Australian Nursing and Midwifery Council.

Baca, M. (2011). Professional boundaries and dual relationships in clinical practice. *The Journal for Nurse Practitioners*, 7(3), 195–200.

Benner Carson, V. (ed.) (2000). *Mental Health Nursing: the nurse–patient journey* (2nd edn). Philadelphia, PA: WB Saunders.

Bennetts, W., Cross, W. & Bloomer, M. (2011). Understanding consumer participation in mental health: issues of power and change, *International Journal of Mental Health Nursing*, 20(3), 155–64.

Cleary, M., Horsfall, J., O'Hara-Aarons, M. & Hunt G.E. (2012). Mental health nurses' views on therapeutic optimism. *International Journal of Mental Health Nursing*, 21, 497–503.

Fragkiadaki1, E. & Strauss, S.M. (2012). Termination of psychotherapy: the journey of 10 psycho-analytic and psychodynamic therapists. *Psychology and Psychotherapy: Theory, Research and Practice*, 85, 335–50.

Grant, J.G. & Westhues, A. (2012). Mental health crisis/respite service: a process evaluation. *Social Work in Mental Health*, 10(1): 34–52.

Group, T.M. & Roberts, J.I. (2001). *Nursing, Physician Control and the Medical Monopoly*. Bloomington, IN: Indiana University Press.

Lakeman, R. (2012). What is good mental health nursing? A survey of Irish nurses. *Archives of Psychiatric Nursing*, 26(3), 225–31.

Lawrence, D., Kisely, S. & Pais, P. (2011). The epidemiology of excess mortality in people with mental illness. *Canadian Journal of Psychiatry*. 55(12), 752–60.

Mental Health Council of Australia (2004). *Privacy Kit—for private sector mental health service providers*. Viewed 8 July 2007, < www.ama.com.au/web.nsf/doc/WEEN–5XU7LM>.

—— (2011). *Ten Year Roadmap Workshop: Report of Key Issues and Themes*. Canberra: MHCA.

Mohr, W.K. (2013). *Johnson's Psychiatric–Mental Health Nursing* (6th edn). Philadelphia, PA: Lippincott Williams & Wilkins.

Nicaise, P., Lorant, V. & Dubois, V. (2013). Psychiatric advance directives as a complex and multistage intervention: a realist systematic review. *Health and Social Care in the Community*, 21(1), 1–14.

Peplau, H.E. (1952). *Interpersonal Relations in Nursing*. New York: G.P. Putnam's Sons.

Prebble, K. & Bryder, L (2008). Gender and class tensions between psychiatric nurses and the general nursing profession in mid-twentieth century New Zealand. *Contemporary Nurse*, 30, 181–95.

Rogers, C.R. (1990). *The Carl Rogers Reader* (edited by Howard Kirschenbaum and Valerie Land). London: Constable.

Rydon, S.E. (2005). The attitudes, knowledge and skills needed in mental health nurses: The perspective of users of mental health services. *International Journal of Mental Health Nursing*, 14, 78–87.

SANE Australia (2007). Family carers and mental illness. *Research Bulletin 5*. Viewed 28 January 2013, <www.sane.org>.

Simpson, R., Slutskaya, N., Lewis, P. & Höpfl, H. (eds) (2012). *Dirty Work Concepts and Identities*. Basingstoke: Palgrave Macmillan.

Smith, T. (2005). 'With tact, intelligence and a special acquaintance with the insane': a history of the development of mental health care (nursing) in New South Wales, Australia, Colonisation to Federation 1788–1901. Unpublished PhD thesis, University of Western Sydney.

Stavropoulou, A., Kaba, E., Obamwonyi, A.V., Adeosun, I., Rovithis, M., Zidianakis, Z. (2012). Defining nursing intimacy: nurses' perceptions of intimacy. *Health Science Journal*, 6(3), 479–95.

Treatment Protocol Project (2000). *Acute Inpatient Psychiatric Care: a source book*. World Health Organization and the Centre for Mental Health and Substance Abuse, Sydney: Brown Prior & Anderson.

Trondsen, M.V. (2012). Living with a mentally ill parent: exploring adolescents' experiences and perspectives. *Qualitative Health Research*, 22(2) 174– 88.

Videbech, S.L. (2010). *Psychiatric Mental Health Nursing* (5th edn). Philadelphia, PA: Wolters Kluwer/ Lippincott Williams & Wilkins.

Wilkinson, J.M. & Van Leuven, K. (2011). *Fundamentals of Nursing: theory, concepts & applications*. Philadelphia, PA: FA Davis.

Williams, A. (2001). A study of practising nurses' perceptions and experiences of intimacy within the nurse–patient relationship. *Journal of Advanced Nursing*, 35(2), 188–96.

13

Therapeutic roles in mental health

Main points
- The provision of counselling is an important role for nurses.
- Different schools of psychotherapy or counselling explain personality development and mental distress in different ways, and suggest different approaches to addressing problems.
- The therapeutic alliance is one of the most important contributors to therapeutic outcomes.

Definitions
Psychotherapy/counselling: Psychotherapy and counselling are professional activities that utilise an interpersonal relationship to enable people to develop self-understanding and to make changes in their lives.

INTRODUCTION
Counselling and psychotherapy utilise a professional relationship to enable people to develop self-understanding and make changes in their lives (PACFA 2012). The distinction between counselling and psychotherapy is blurry. Both require specific training and ongoing supervision, emotional intelligence and specific skills on the part of the practitioner. Counselling tends to be considered shorter term, and focuses on solving specific problems, resolving crises and working through developmental issues such as grief and loss. Psychotherapy, on the other hand, tends to focus on self-understanding and insight, is longer term in nature and may even assist in helping people restructure aspects of their personality. This chapter provides a brief overview of some of the main

branches of psychotherapy, and then describes in a little more detail several brief forms of therapy that may be used in mental health nursing.

The term 'psychotherapy' is derived from the Greek *psyche*, meaning soul, and *therapeia*, meaning healing. The focus in both counselling and psychotherapies is on helping the person heal from psychological problems they are experiencing. There are hundreds of different schools of psychotherapy distinguished by different theories of how problems develop and are resolved, as well as specific techniques employed by the therapist. Some nurses practise psychotherapy, and will see people for contracted therapy at specified times one or more times a week. However, Peplau (1952) proposed that nurses cannot usually provide counselling in the same manner as a psychotherapist because of differing role demands and round-the-clock relationships with service users. She suggested that nurses more often assume counselling roles. All nurses ought to learn and practise communication skills, which are the foundational skills of psychotherapy. Furthermore, training in psychotherapy can be very helpful in developing formulations to explain and guide nursing practice (Crowe, Carlyle & Farmar 2008).

CRITICAL THINKING
Consider someone who has helped you through talking together. What qualities did they have that contributed to the conversation being helpful? What did they say and do? Which of their behaviours or qualities would you like to cultivate and use in your professional roles as a nurse?

MODELS, THEORIES AND SCHOOLS OF PSYCHOTHERAPY

While people have obtained solace, healing and been assisted to solve problems by talking with others since language evolved, professional psychotherapy was invented by Sigmund Freud and his associates. Psychoanalysis was the most dominant model of therapy in the twentieth century, and most therapies have been influenced by its tenets (Wachtel 2000).

Psychoanalysis and the unconscious

Freud, his colleagues, students and family (such as Carl Jung, Harry Stack Sullivan and Anna Freud) proposed and elaborated on theories of personality, human development and therapeutic techniques that have influenced the development of almost every talking therapy. They suggested that a person's development is greatly affected by experiences in early childhood, and that much human behaviour is determined by various drives, which are largely unconscious. They proposed a structure or typography of personality that is composed of the *id*, which operates on the *pleasure principle*, seeking to fulfil all basic needs and wants; the *superego*, which is the critical, self-observing, idealistic and moral aspect of the personality; and the *ego*, which is the part of the personality that deals with reality, develops slowly and must mediate between the conflicting demands of the id and superego. In the 1930s, Anna Freud first described in detail how defence mechanisms work as a tactic developed by the ego and employed unconsciously to protect against anxiety (see Table 13.1). Defences, as Anna Freud (1993, p. 69) notes, assist the ego in its struggle with instinctual life, and are motivated by instinctual anxiety, objective anxiety and anxiety of conscience.

Table 13.1 Ego defence mechanisms

Repression	Pushing unacceptable impulses out of awareness, e.g. a traumatised or abused individual is unable to remember anything about an experience.
Denial	Refusing to accept the truth, reality or facts of the matter, e.g. a person who has repeatedly been convicted for drink driving denies having an alcohol problem.
Displacement	The transferral of feelings from an unacceptable object towards another, safer object, e.g. a person is angry with their boss but can't express this safely so goes home and yells at the children.
Projection	Personal shortcomings, problems or unacceptable impulses are not recognised but are instead attributed to others, e.g. a heterosexual person who may have repressed homosexual impulses accuses others of the same gender of 'hitting on them'.
Regression	When faced with stress, reverting to an earlier stage of development, e.g. a person sucks their thumb when stressed.
Reaction formation	The transformation of an unacceptable motive into its opposite, e.g. a person may be sexually attracted to another person but they express bitter hatred towards them.
Rationalisation	The replacement of an unacceptable motive with a more acceptable one, e.g. a person who has not worked hard all semester blames his poor exam technique for a poor grade.
Sublimation	The replacement of an unacceptable impulse with a socially more acceptable one, e.g. a person wrestles with violent impulses and becomes an accomplished rugby league player.
Intellectualisation	Neutralising feelings of anxiety, anger or insecurity by thinking away the problem, e.g. a person loses a cherished intimate relationship but deals with the sense of loss by reasoning that they will save considerable money by not going out.

> **CRITICAL THINKING**
>
> - For each of the defence mechanisms introduced in Table 13.1, think of a situation when you, a friend or colleague might have unconsciously employed this defence.
> - For each defence mechanism, consider an example a nurse might observe in the course of their work with service users.

The process of psychoanalysis and its adaptations stressed creating a comfortable physical and accepting social environment in which the person was able to *free associate*—that is, to express whatever came to mind. Over time, the person's unconscious or repressed material would be revealed to the analyst in different ways, such as *transference* (or the way that old conflicts are played out in the relationship between the person and the analyst) or in the interpretation of dreams or slips of the tongue. The analyst's feeling responses to the person might include *counter-transference*, which can be explained as the analyst responding to the person's projected transference feelings. Therapy proceeded at least once a week (often more frequently) for long periods (often years). Variations of classical psychoanalysis are still undertaken today, and are a feature of public mental health service provision in much of Europe. However, it is expensive and time consuming, and in much of the English-speaking world it has been usurped by brief kinds of therapies aimed principally at reducing symptoms, such as cognitive behavioural therapy (discussed later). Over the course of the twentieth century, many different approaches and theories stressing the interplay between conscious and unconscious motivation were derived from psychoanalytic schools. These broad schools of thought and practice are called 'psycho-dynamic'.

Peplau (1952), arguably the first nurse theorist, entitled her book *Interpersonal Relations in Nursing: A Conceptual Frame of reference for Psychodynamic Nursing*. In it, she stressed many psycho-dynamic concepts which still prove important to the everyday work of nurses today. She emphasised the importance of understanding anxiety in its various forms, how it is manifested in the context of interpersonal relationships and how it might be understood psycho-dynamically. She noted that anxiety arises when people's goals or expectations are frustrated. People may 'dissociate' experiences that cannot be permitted or remembered in awareness; in particular, she suggested that people commonly repress emotions associated with traumatic events while being able to remember the event itself. Peplau viewed the counselling role as very important for nurses:

> Counseling in nursing has to do with helping the patient to remember and to understand fully what is happening to him [sic] in the present situation, so that the experience can be integrated with rather than dissociated from other experiences of life. (Peplau 1952, p. 64)

CRITICAL THINKING

Think about an occasion when you met someone for the first time (perhaps a service user), and had a strong emotional response to them (perhaps you liked or disliked them). Did the person remind you of somebody else in your life? Could this have been a transference reaction? It is not uncommon for this dynamic to work in the other direction when the service user responds to the nurse or other helper in a way that they have responded to other relationships. The nurse, for example, might remind the service user of a close relative, friend or confidant. The service user experiences feelings as though the nurse is their remembered person, and can induce corresponding feeling responses in the nurse. When the nurse begins to respond to the service user in this role, this is called counter-transference. Can you think of occasions when you have felt like a mother, father, sibling or friend to a service user? Could this be an example of counter-transference? These dynamics are natural, but can become problematic if people are not aware of what is going on.

Behaviourism

A criticism of psycho-analytic theory and practice has been the difficulty of subjecting theory to testing outside of the therapy situation (which tended to be characterised by a long-term relationship not easily replicated or reduced to a set of procedures for testing). Behaviourism in the early twentieth century evolved as a radical alternative to psycho-analytic theory. Early behavioural theorists stressed the objective study of behaviour and experimental methods. The theories emphasised environmental factors in shaping personality. For example, in Pavlov's classical conditioning experiments, paired stimuli were presented to a dog (a bell followed by food). The food elicited salivation and after repeatedly exposing the dog to the bell–food pairings, the bell alone could cause the dog to salivate. The idea of *reinforcement* of particular behaviour through reward is a behavioural concept that remains relevant today.

Systematic desensitisation (or *graded exposure*) consists of a group of behavioural strategies that were developed by Joseph Wolpe and are used to treat fears, phobias and social anxiety. This involves firstly teaching people ways to cope with anxiety (for example, through meditation, relaxation training or *cognitive reframing*—changing one's internal dialogue about the situation). The person then creates a hierarchy of situations relating to the fear from least fearful to most fearful. For example, if someone has a fear of talking in public, greeting a shop attendant may be rated a 1, whereas delivering a speech in class may be ranked a 10. The person then practises exposure to their fears interspersed with relaxation or coping techniques, and often a talk with the therapist about what they are thinking and feeling. As the person progresses through the hierarchy, their anxiety or fear usually diminishes.

CRITICAL THINKING

Consider a fear that you have that you would like to overcome. Create and write down an exposure hierarchy, beginning with the least-feared and ending with the most-feared situation. Also write down a list of activities that help you feel calm or relaxed when you have been feeling anxious. Share your exposure hierarchy plan with a trusted friend or colleague. You will gain confidence helping others if you can work through your exposure hierarchy, using your calming techniques and talking to your trusted friend/colleague to manage your anxious feelings as you attempt each progressive step, until you reach your goal.

Cognitive approaches

Almost everyone has heard of cognitive behavioural therapy (CBT). The central premise of CBT is that a person's responses to events (feelings and behaviour) are mediated by their beliefs, images, inferences and evaluations. Cognitive behavioural therapy was developed in the mid- and late twentieth century, and developed from three major sources of influence:

- *The 'phenomenological' approach to psychology:* This arose particularly from Greek Stoic philosophy, which emphasised that one's view of self and one's personal world largely determine behaviour.
- *Structural theory and depth psychology:* Particularly Freud's conceptualisation of cognitions being hierarchically arranged into primary (rigid, primitive cognitive processing that is utilised during distress) and secondary-process thinking (characterised by greater flexibility and finer discrimination).
- *Cognitive psychology:* Particularly the idea of 'personal constructs' and the role of beliefs in behavioural change.

There are several schools of cognitive behavioural therapy, the most significant being Rational Emotive Behavioural Therapy (REBT), founded by Albert Ellis, and Cognitive Therapy, founded by Aaron Beck. These vary more in technique than underlying theory, and today there are many versions of CBT that address specific mental health problems or symptoms.

Cognitive therapy was reportedly developed out of research examining the cognitions of people with clinical depression (Beck & Greenberg 1984; Beck & Weishaar 1989; Dobson & Block 1988). The cognitive model hypothesises that negative thinking characterises depression. Depression is defined in terms of a cognitive triad, in which the client thinks of him or herself as helpless or hopeless, interprets most events unfavourably and believes the future to be hopeless (Akiskal 1995). Beck and Weishaar (1989) make it clear that cognitions do not cause depression, or any other psychopathological disorder, but that they are intrinsic to mental disorder. During psychological distress, there is a shift to a more primitive information-processing system in which there are apparent systematic errors of reasoning or cognitive distortions that include the following:

- *Arbitrary inferences:* A person quickly draws a conclusion without the necessary evidence—'I didn't get invited to the party because nobody likes me.'
- *Selective abstraction:* Taking detail out of context and ignoring the context, such as focusing only on negative information—for example, a person got four As on their report card and concluded they were a complete failure because they also got one C.
- *Over-generalisation:* Taking one instance in the here and now and imposing it on all other situations—for example, 'I dropped a plate. I am a complete klutz and always will be.'
- *Magnification and minimisation:* Seeing negative aspects of a situation as bigger and more positive aspects of a situation as less significant; or seeing risks or problems as greater than they really are ('Catastrophising')—for example, where an airline has had some maintenance issues, 'My plane is sure to crash and I will die.'
- *Personalisation:* The attribution of blame or personal responsibility for events to someone (including oneself) over which the person has no control—for example, 'My friend is unhappy; it must be my fault.'
- *Dichotomous or black-and-white thinking:* Seeing things as all good or all bad—for example, 'If you are not with us you are against us.'

The shift to primitive information processing is triggered by an interaction of personal and environmental factors. Each individual has unique vulnerabilities that appear to be related to personality structure and fundamental or core beliefs about the world. Previous negative events are thought to be coded in the form of 'schema' that are activated when similar events are experienced, influencing the interpretation of those events (Brewin 1988). Beck suggests that schemata develop early in life from personal experience and identification with significant others, and that these early conceptualisations are reinforced by further learning experiences, and in turn influence the formation of other beliefs, values and attitudes (Beck & Weishaar 1989).

Adverse life events and early life experiences

All approaches to therapy discussed thus far emphasise how life experiences—particularly childhood experiences—affect personality development through different mechanisms. There is considerable evidence that adverse experiences in childhood cause subsequent mental health problems in adulthood. Some of the most impressive and disturbing findings are from the Adverse Childhood Experiences (ACE) study, in which over 17 000 people underwent a physical examination and provided details about their childhood experience of abuse (physical, psychological or sexual), neglect (emotional or physical) and family dysfunction (household substance abuse, mental illness and incarceration; and parental domestic violence, separation or divorce) (see <www.cdc.gov/ace/index.htm>; Felitti et al. 1998). The prevalence of adverse childhood events was very high, with almost two-thirds of people experiencing at least one event and 12.5 per cent of people experiencing four or more adverse events. As the number of adverse childhood events increased, so did the risk of experiencing many health problems. The number of adverse childhood events experienced was correlated with the occurrence of the following health issues:

- alcoholism and alcohol abuse
- chronic obstructive pulmonary disease (COPD)
- depression
- foetal death
- health-related quality of life
- illicit drug use
- ischemic heart disease (IHD)
- liver disease
- risk of intimate partner violence
- multiple sexual partners
- sexually transmitted diseases (STDs)
- smoking
- suicide attempts
- unintended pregnancies
- early initiation of smoking
- early initiation of sexual activity
- adolescent pregnancy.

Childhood adversity has also been found to be strongly associated with an increased risk of subsequent psychosis (Varese et al. 2012). The theoretical orientations discussed thus far provide different explanations for why adverse life events might have such a profound impact on people's health. Behaviourists might argue that particular patterns of behaviour are learned or reinforced. Cognitive behavioural therapists might argue that the person constructs a relatively enduring cognitive schema made up of beliefs about one's self and the world in childhood.

A dominant idea that bridges belief systems is that of attachment (Bowlby 1977). The quality of our attachment to our caregivers as infants and children has a great bearing on how safe and secure we feel, and how at ease we are in exploring the world. Anything that interferes with the emotional bond between infants and their caregivers (e.g. abuse, neglect or inconsistent caregiver responses) may impact on personality development, and how people experience and respond to themselves and others. This has obvious and clear implications for *primary prevention* in mental health (e.g. reducing financial and social stressors for families with young children and providing resources to help them parent well), but it raises questions about the most therapeutic ways to address these problems.

CRITICAL THINKING

- Visit the ACE study website at <http://acestudy.org> and complete the ACE study questionnaire. Consider how your experience of adversity might have contributed to your personality development or the way you relate to people.
- Complete an attachment-style questionnaire (e.g. <http://internal.psychology. illinois.edu/~rcfraley/links.htm>) and consider how you have acquired this way of being with people.

Humanism and the importance of relationship

An important development from the mid-twentieth century was the rise in humanistic psychology and humanistic approaches to psychotherapy. You were introduced to some of the main theorists in Chapter 2: Abraham Maslow and Carl Rogers. These approaches view the individual as essentially good, with tendencies towards growth or actualisation. They stress the provision of warmth, compassion, empathy and understanding on the part of the therapist. Indeed, Rogers (1957, p. 95) suggested that the necessary conditions for constructive personality change to occur were:

- Two persons are in psychological contact.
- The first—whom we shall term the client—is in a state of incongruence, being vulnerable or anxious.
- The second person—whom we shall term the therapist—is congruent or integrated in the relationship.
- The therapist experiences unconditional positive regard for the client.
- The therapist experiences an empathic understanding of the client's internal frame of reference, and endeavours to communicate this experience to the client.
- The communication to the client of the therapist's empathic understanding and unconditional positive regard is achieved to a minimal degree.

Rogers went further, suggesting that if these conditions exist and continue over time, constructive personality change will occur. Demonstrating honesty, unconditional regard and communicating empathic understanding towards the client over time are the critical ingredients of therapy. These thoughts have to a large extent been confirmed in research looking at psychotherapy outcomes. When different kinds of therapies are compared, no one approach has been found to be superior for most mental health problems. The factors that appear to make the most difference in terms of outcomes are common to most therapies (such as warmth and empathy), and the quality of the relationship (sometimes called the therapeutic alliance) (Lambert & Barley 2001; Horvath et al. 2011).

The therapeutic alliance is a complex idea and process. Howgego et al. (2003) suggest that it is a concept comprising three main elements:

- *Tasks:* A shared understanding between the service user and therapist about who does what in therapy.
- *Goals:* Mutual agreement and valuing of the outcomes of therapy; and
- *Bonds:* Elements of attachment between service user and therapist, including a sense of trust, empathy, valuing and warmth.

The quality of the therapeutic alliance also appears to be the most important factor in mental health case management outcomes and even in service users adhering to prescribed medication (Howgego et al. 2003; Weiss et al. 2002). In the treatment of depression, therapeutic alliance relates directly to positive outcome, regardless of the treatment provided (Zuroff & Blatt 2006), and in bipolar disorder it has been described as a 'mood stabilizer' (Havens & Ghaemi 2005).

Empathy, or conveying or communicating understanding of the other's experience, is pivotal to a good relationship and to psychotherapy. Indeed, many of the communication techniques outlined in Chapter 12 are selected to convey warmth and empathy. Egan (1998, p. 83) suggests that if attending and listening are skills that enable helpers to get in touch with the service user's world, then empathy is the skill that enables them to communicate their understanding of that world. A simple formula is helpful to thinking about how to convey empathy (Egan 1998):

> You feel . . . [here name the correct emotion and intensity of emotion expressed by the service user] . . . Because (or when) . . . [here indicate the correct experiences and behaviours that give rise to these feelings] . . . eg 'you feel really angry because I forgot to return your phone message yesterday'.

This formula can even be adapted to respond therapeutically to people who might be expressing delusional ideas, providing it is expressed tentatively and carefully (Lakeman 2006). Communicating an understanding of how a person feels, and linking those feelings to a cause, is more than active listening or summarising: it is a form of interpretation. This in itself might assist the person to see their problems or situation differently.

CRITICAL THINKING

Ask a colleague to share a brief story about an occasion that evoked a strong emotion. After listening carefully, summarise the story by using the empathy formula ('You felt . . . because/when . . . '). Clarify whether your statement really captured the intensity of the feelings and the most important aspect of the event.

Finding meaning

At much the same time as humanistic or person centred therapy was being developed and infusing the practice of therapy with warmth, a range of other therapists and researchers, influenced by existential philosophy and phenomenology, developed practices of therapy that might be called existential. As the name suggests, these are concerned with existential concerns that are an inevitable part of living, and are concerned with death, freedom, isolation and meaning. Victor Frankl, a psychiatrist and Holocaust survivor, suggested that finding meaning, even in the most dehumanising or painful situations is fundamental to people's survival (Frankl 2006). Many people seek therapy because they feel that life is meaningless, empty and lacking purpose, or they are terrified of dying or of annihilation. These represent existential crises, which therapy seeks to resolve. The differences between existential therapy and humanistic psychotherapy may be subtle but for what counts as important material to discuss. Spinelli (2006, p. 1), an existential psychotherapist, states:

> [T]herapy, at its most fundamental level, involves the act of revealing and reassessing the 'life stories' that clients tell themselves in order to establish, or maintain, meaning in their lives. The role of the therapist is not only that of an engaged listener but also of 'attendant' (the original meaning of therapist) in that he or she is also involved in the explication and reconstruction of the client's narrative via various forms of clarification and challenging input. It is, therefore, the very relationship that develops between therapist and client that is the central constituent of the therapeutic enterprise.

Existential phenomenology is concerned with how people experience themselves in the world. One school of psychotherapy, called Gestalt (founded by Fritz Perls), also draws on existential philosophy—particularly how people are in the present moment. Additionally, it draws on systems theory (the theoretical platform for systemic family therapy), viewing the individual as embedded in a web of relationships, and change as occurring within a system.

CRITICAL THINKING

In 1964, Everett Shostrom created a film in which the most famous psychotherapists of the time demonstrated how they might work with a woman called Gloria. The psychotherapists were Albert Ellis (rational emotive behavioural therapy), Fritz Pearls (Gestalt) and Carl Rogers (person-centred). The videos are available on YouTube (simply enter 'Gloria' and the name of the psychotherapist). Watch the videos and consider the following questions:

* Who would you prefer to see for therapy and why?
* How did the therapists convey empathy and understanding?
* How were the ways in which the therapists approached Gloria similar or different?

Social constructionism

Arising largely from family therapy traditions, a range of contemporary therapists now view the world largely as socially constructed (at least in theory). This is most pronounced in an approach developed largely in Australia and New Zealand called narrative therapy. This holds a view that we construct our identities through narratives, or the stories that we tell each other and ourselves. Often these stories are saturated with problems, and a goal of therapy is the construction (or re-authoring) of a different kind of narrative. Psychotherapy and counselling also tend to be constructed, and experienced therapists often integrate techniques and ideas from a range of sources into their practice. The following section illustrates in a little more detail some forms of therapy that may readily be adapted by nurses in routine practice.

PLANNED SHORT-TERM PSYCHOTHERAPIES

Planned short-term—or brief—psychotherapies are a group of therapies that aim to manage problems as they are in the present, rather than emphasising past experiences or influences. As their name suggests, they are usually offered over a short length of time rather than extending for long periods. Planned short-term psychotherapies include solution-focused approaches, cognitive behavioural therapies, narrative therapy and interpersonal psychotherapy. You will notice that the assumptions and techniques used in these therapies share many similarities, and that the importance of relationships with others, the constructive use of language and an emphasis on empowering the person and recognising their strengths are common themes throughout the following explanations. These therapies have been used for a range of mental health problems and issues, including depression, the psychological sequelae of grief, stress and low self-esteem, as well as being helpful for service users recovering from psychotic episodes.

Solution-focused therapy

Solution-focused therapy (SFT) was introduced in Chapter 2. As the name implies, solution-focused therapists work with people in an active way to resolve issues or problems through finding solutions to them that are situated in the present, rather than looking for causes from the past. SFT is an approach that is used widely and with a variety of people and settings, including with children and adults, in schools and organisations, as well as in health care.

Solution-focused therapy was first developed by the therapists de Shazer, Berg and colleagues in the 1980s, and is based on Milton Erickson's work (Corcoran & Walsh 2005). The approach emphasises the strengths and resources that people have, which can be used to address their issues, and service users rather than therapists are viewed as being the experts on the solutions to their problems (Stevenson, Jackson & Barker 2003). Theoretically, SFT is influenced by social constructionism, which considers that 'reality' does not exist in an objective sense, but rather is a construction based on the assumptions people make of their interactions with others in their social world (Corcoran & Walsh 2005). In SFT, the person's concerns are therefore commonly addressed within the context of their relationships with others. In mental health, although SFT is usually considered a short-term psycho-therapy, it has also been used very effectively with service users who require longer-term support and/or have a number of problems, including psychosis (Webster & Vaughn 2003).

SFT is a language-based approach where service users are assisted to retell their experiences in ways that can provide positive opportunities for change (Webster & Vaughn 2003). The emphasis is on a collaborative and interactive process between the therapist and the person undergoing therapy, and SFT is useful for both individual as well as group settings (Lethem 2002).

There are a number of assumptions or ideas that underpin a solution-focused approach, including the following:

- The person's strengths, abilities and resources are the focus of therapy (rather than their deficits or vulnerabilities).
- Change occurs within the context of a system, so small changes made by the person can lead to others in their environment responding differently to them, which in turn may encourage the person to make further changes.
- No single person holds the objective truth of a situation. Every person has the right to their own perspective and the person is encouraged to find solutions that match their own views of their situation.
- The therapist works in partnership with the person to build their awareness of their strengths, which are activated and then applied to their problems (Corcoran & Walsh 2005).

Techniques used in SFT

According to Lethem (2002), solution-focused therapeutic techniques include the following:

- *Goals are set for each session*, with the person asked what they want to talk about to help them feel their session has been worthwhile for them.
- *Problem-free talk is included*, with the person talking about other aspects of their life that do not include the problem for which they have sought help. This provides a more comprehensive picture of their life and situation.
- The session includes a strategy known as *building a preferred future*, where the person is asked how they would like their life to be without the problem they are currently experiencing. This includes asking various types of question, such as the *miracle question*, which is worded something like this:

Suppose tonight, while you're asleep, a miracle happens and the problem sorts itself out. What would you see tomorrow that would let you know the miracle had happened? What would you find yourself doing the day after this miracle? What would others notice you doing?

- *Other questions* are phrased in a way that is designed to gain information about the interactions between people, such as:
    - 'What do you think your mother would like to get out of this meeting?'
    - 'What is she hoping you may get out of it, do you think?'
- Questioning is also used to find examples of *exceptions to the problem*—for instance:
    - 'When are the times it's easier to resist the temptation to lose your temper?'
    - 'When did you last have a holiday from obsessive-compulsive disorder?'
- *Ending the session* includes giving *compliments* about the person's strengths, resources and personal qualities, and *acknowledging the problem* in a non-blaming way. *Tasks* may also be given so the person can carry on the solution-focused work until the next session.

CRITICAL THINKING

Think about a common problem or issue you have experienced (e.g. becoming anxious before exams; getting annoyed with a friend because they are often late for appointments). Using your understandings of the principles of SFT, develop some questions you could ask yourself to help find solutions to your problem. After you have done this and applied the questions to yourself, respond to the following:

- How did answering these questions impact on the way you thought about the problem?
- Were they helpful?
- How could you use the principles of SFT in your work with service users?

For nurses, using a solution-focused approach when working with service users offers a variety of benefits and challenges. It can provide an opportunity to enhance service users' resilience, assist them in finding solutions to problems and encourage a focus on using the therapeutic relationship to enhance both service users' and nurses' sense of self-efficacy. SFT may also be challenging, as it can be difficult to move away from a problem or deficit-focused approach, and usually involves relinquishing some control and power within the therapeutic relationship. Yet this type of approach to working with service users can be seen as particularly aligned to nursing's focus on therapeutic engagement, and building and maintaining health and well-being (McAllister 2003).

COGNITIVE BEHAVIOURAL THERAPY/COGNITIVE THERAPY

As mentioned previously, cognitive behavioural therapy (CBT), another well-known and commonly used therapy in mental health, focuses on the person's cognitive (thoughts) and behavioural (actions) aspects of functioning, and works to help people think about things differently. The emphasis is on challenging faulty assumptions or self-defeating beliefs that the person holds, and teaching them coping skills that may be helpful in addressing their problems. A self-defeating belief is one that distorts reality, involves illogical ways of evaluating oneself, others or the world, blocks achievement of goals, creates extremes of emotions that persist and cause distress, and leads to behaviours that are harmful.

Cognitive behavioural therapy is educative. That is, people are taught about different and common ways in which their thinking may be distorting things and then to learn to catch and correct themselves. One of the major techniques used in cognitive therapy is 'Socratic questioning', which involves asking questions that help to clarify a person's assumptions, thinking and motivations. The service user is introduced to models of cognition in some way. For example, the basic model illustrated in Figure 13.1 can be helpful for explaining that events trigger us to make inferences about what is going on, which in turn has meaning for us. It is these interpretations and evaluations that lead us to feel and behave in particular ways. Our feelings and behaviour, or other people's responses to us, can in turn be activating events.

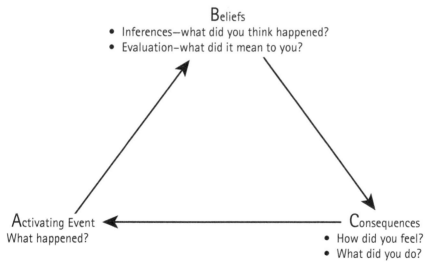

Figure 13.1 A basic cognitive model in CBT

The following case study presents an example of some techniques used in cognitive behavioural therapy.

CASE STUDY

Jim is a 46-year-old man who has experienced strong feelings of depression. He has recently separated from a long-standing partner, and feels listless, sad and direction-less. He works casually as a forestry labourer but recently the weather has been poor and he has not been called into work. Outside of his relationship, working has been an important part of his identity. Jim has been introduced to a basic CBT model and is aware of some of the ways he jumps to conclusions or evaluates things catastrophically. The following is some of the dialogue with his therapist.

Therapist: How have things been for you over the last couple of days?

Jim: Awful . . . everything is going wrong!

Therapist: Everything?

Jim: Not everything . . . I mean . . . Roger didn't call me in for work. He knows I really need it . . . He's got it in for me . . .

Therapist: You are feeling angry and despondent because you think Roger has treated you unfairly? [Jim nods] . . . What happened to trigger these thoughts?

Jim: He didn't ring me yesterday . . . If there is work on he usually rings me on a Monday . . .

Therapist: Roger did not ring you . . . and you thought that he deliberately denied you the opportunity to work . . . that he doesn't like you and that confirmed that you are no good? How did that lead you to feel and what did you do?

Jim: I felt awful . . . the worst ever . . . I did nothing useful with my day . . . I just waited for the phone to ring.

Therapist: On a scale of 1 to 10 . . . 1 being the worst you've ever been . . . how did you feel?

Jim: A 4 I suppose . . . it wasn't as bad as last week.

Therapist: It seems to me you jumped to some quick conclusions about Roger's motivations . . . Can we explore other possible reasons for Roger not ringing you?

Jim: Well it was torrential rain . . . there were roads closed everywhere . . . he might have just thought, 'It is obvious there is no work today'.

Therapist: Let's suppose that was true . . . it sounds plausible to me . . . How might you have felt?

Jim: I would have been disappointed . . . about a 6 . . . but I wouldn't have been devastated.

Critical thinking

After reading Jim's story, consider and discuss the following issues:

- How has the therapist worked collaboratively with Jim?
- Where can you see examples of the use of Socratic questioning?
- What communication skills were used and for what purpose?

The person who uses cognitive behavioural therapy principles in their practice is likely to be careful with their use of language, being sure to take care to differentiate between thoughts and feelings. People often narrate their stories in a manner that suggests their inferences or best guess about what has happened or will happen is a fact and people behave accordingly. The CBT-informed nurse will help the person tease out and name their inferences and evaluations, and clarify the triggering event. They are likely to use selective reflection to point out people's tendency to exaggerate, over-generalise or catastrophise. Asking people to rate the intensity of a feeling or compulsion can be helpful in reducing people's tendencies to see things as black or white, all good or all bad. CBT often involves homework tasks such as keeping thought diaries, undertaking exposure to anxiety-provoking events or other behavioural experiments to test out new cognitions.

INTERPERSONAL PSYCHOTHERAPY

Interpersonal psychotherapy (IPT) is another therapy designed to encourage the service user to address current life events and assist them to make changes to interpersonal problems such as low self-esteem and difficulty trusting others. It is also a time-limited or short-term approach, which is initiated within the context of an interpersonal relationship. This therapeutic approach has been found to be particularly effective with mood disorders such as depression, eating disorders and anxiety disorders, including post-traumatic stress disorder (Bleiberg & Markowitz 2005; Crowe & Luty 2005).

IPT can be a particularly useful therapy for nurses in the mental health setting, as it provides a structured framework within which nurses can intervene with service users and use their interpersonal skills to help them recover from their particular mental health problem (Crowe & Luty 2005). The main premises of IPT are that mental health problems such as depression develop and continue within the context of interpersonal relationships. Therapy focuses on addressing the person's relationships with others, and links these to changes in their mood, identifying problem areas such as role transitions, interpersonal deficits, grief and interpersonal role disputes. The person is assisted by the therapist/nurse to develop and implement new ways of being in a relationship with others (Crowe & Luty 2005).

Consider the following case study of how IPT may be useful for someone experiencing depression.

NARRATIVE THERAPY

Narrative therapy is a relatively recent psycho-therapeutic approach, which came to prominence when Michael White and David Epson published their seminal book *Narrative Means to Therapeutic Ends* in 1990. The focus of narrative therapy, as the name

CASE STUDY

Before starting therapy, Dolores was assessed as having moderate depression. She then participated in a series of twelve IPT sessions. By the end of these sessions, she was not experiencing depressive symptoms.

In the first stage of IPT, Dolores was asked to identify all the significant people in her life, and was then prompted with the following questions:

- What is s/he like as a person?
- How often do you see him/her?
- What kind of things do you do together?
- Do you ever clash at all?
- Would you want the relationship to be different?

Dolores then described her relationships with family and friends, and identified a pattern of avoidance whenever she experienced conflicts with them. She avoided expressing anger, and this became increasingly difficult for her the more she tried to suppress her expression of it.

Following the initial assessment phase, the therapist negotiated with Dolores regarding which IPT problem area would be the focus of treatment (for example, interpersonal disputes, role transitions, grief or interpersonal deficits). They agreed that interpersonal disputes would be the focus, as this was having the most impact on her mood symptoms.

In the early phases of the treatment, Dolores experienced a sense of struggling to survive, but this began to shift as she was encouraged to explore her feelings and make connections between these and her relationships with other people. During the middle phases of treatment, Dolores also identified trust as an important issue, and identified that if she couldn't trust herself, it was difficult to trust others. With a commitment to the therapy, Dolores was able to recognise that change was possible. This more optimistic approach also assisted her to address other relationship issues with which she had previously felt unable to deal.

As Dolores began to reconstruct her sense of self, her mood began to improve and she was able to express her needs more effectively with her partner, and was able to consider other options and have a sense of hope for her future. She described therapy as having helped her to see things more clearly, and used the metaphor of IPT being the 'guide dog' that enabled her to see other opportunities in her life. (Adapted from Crowe & Luty 2005, pp. 127–31) implies, is on how people express the experiences in their life through the stories they tell about them. Like solution-focused therapy, the theoretical foundation of narrative therapy is social constructionism, and it draws heavily on techniques from family therapy. Language is important, as it is the basis from which a person may reframe problems and negative life experiences—contained in their 'dominant story'—through using various narrative strategies and techniques. In this way, the person may come to understand and 're-author' their lives through developing an 'alternate' or competing story that attends to previously neglected aspects of their experiences.

Narrative therapy techniques, which rely on the use of written and spoken language in various forms, include:

- *Externalising the problem*: The person is encouraged to objectify the problem they experience as being difficult. The problem becomes a separate entity, and therefore becomes external to the person or the relationship that was considered to be the problem. 'Relative influence questioning' is used to help people to externalise their problems because this encourages the person to map out how the problem has influenced their life and relationships, and is used to map how *the individual* concerned has influenced the life of the problem (see the case study below for an example of how this technique was used with a family where a young boy was experiencing the problem of encopresis).
- *Using letters*: Narrative therapists often use the writing of a variety of types of letter as another therapeutic technique. For instance, 'letters of invitation' may be written to invite service users to engage in therapy.
- *Counter-documents*: These include certificates and declarations, often produced at the end of therapy and presented to the service user. They 'certify' service users to be free of their problem, and affirm them as having successfully managed their experiences (White & Epston 1990).

Narrative therapy has a variety of applications and uses. It is often utilised with families and for working with children (White & Epston 1990). It has also been used to address substance abuse and dependence, and to help people come to terms with the effects of trauma and loss. In mental health nursing, narrative therapy has been considered useful for a range of psycho-social issues, including working with children and adolescents who are experiencing problems of living, such as Asperger's disorder (Cashin 2008; DeSocio 2005). As with the previous therapies that have been discussed, nurses—like other health professionals—need to engage in specialised education and training in order to provide effective narrative therapy.

CASE STUDY

In this engaging story, White & Epston (1990) recount a young child's problem with encopresis (soiling himself) so as to illustrate 'mapping the influence of the problem' and how the family managed to overcome the problem using narrative therapeutic techniques.

The problem

Nick was six years old, and had been brought in for therapy by his parents. Nick had a long history of encopresis and, despite various attempts to solve it, it had remained a daily issue for him. Nick had also made friends with the 'poo' and it had become his playmate. He would streak it down walls, smear it in drawers, roll it into balls and even plaster it under the kitchen table!

In response to questioning about the influence of the poo in the lives of all the family, the family and therapist discovered:

- The poo was making a mess of Nick's life by isolating him from other kids and interfering with his school work.
- The poo was driving Sue, Nick's mother, to despair, and forcing her to question her ability to be a good mother as well as her general capability as a person. She felt overwhelmed and on the verge of giving up.
- The poo was very embarrassing for Ron, Nick's father, and had isolated him from his friends and relatives. It was difficult to have family and friends to stay overnight due to Nick's 'accidents'.
- The poo affected all the relationships in the family. It created a wedge between Nick and his parents, and a lot of the fun had been driven out of their relationships.

Mapping the influence of 'Sneaky Poo'

They decided to call the problem 'Sneaky Poo' (an example of externalising the problem). In 'mapping the influence' of Sneaky Poo in the family's lives, they discovered:

- Although Sneaky Poo tried to trick Nick into being his playmate, Nick had sometimes outsmarted him and declined to play with him. He had declined to be tricked.
- Recently, Sue could have been made miserable by an incident with Sneaky Poo, but had resisted and turned on some music instead.
- Ron was interested in defying Sneaky Poo's requirements, and not allowing his embarrassment about Sneaky Poo to isolate him from others, and said he might try telling a workmate about Sneaky Poo.
- In discussion, Sue realised there was an aspect of her relationship with Nick that she still enjoyed, and Ron was still trying to persevere in his relationship with Nick. Nick thought that perhaps Sneaky Poo had not yet destroyed all the love in his relationship with his parents.

- Nick, Sue and Ron were then encouraged by the therapist to use questions that might help them to 're-author' their lives and relationships:
  - How had they managed to be effective against the problem in this way?
  - How did this reflect on them as people and on their relationships?
  - What personal and relationship attributes were they relying on in these achievements?
  - Did this success give them any ideas about further steps they might take to reclaim their lives from the problem?
  - What difference would knowing what they now knew about themselves make to their future relationship with the problem?

Re-authoring their lives

Two weeks later, the family met with the therapist again. Nick had had only one small accident (a light 'smudging'). Sneaky Poo had tried to win him back after nine days, but Nick had resisted. He had taught Sneaky Poo a lesson—he wouldn't let it mess up his life anymore. He believed his life was no longer coated with Sneaky Poo, and that he was now shining through. Sneaky Poo had been tricky, but Nick had done well to get his life back for himself. He was more talkative, happier, felt stronger and was more active.

Both Sue and Ron had also decided not to cooperate with the requirements of Sneaky Poo and had started to take actions that resisted the problems presented by Sneaky Poo.

The whole family was encouraged to reflect on their successes and looked at other ways to decline to support Sneaky Poo.

The family then met with the therapist twice more, and at their six-month follow-up were doing well, with only one or two occasions of slight 'smudging'. Nick was doing well with his friends and at school. Everyone was happy with his progress. (Adapted from White & Epston 1990, pp. 43–8)

GROUP THERAPY

Most of the therapies are discussed in this chapter as individual or one-to-one approaches, but they can also be offered in the form of groups. Research on many different types of groups has found that group therapy can be just as, if not more, effective than individual therapy (McDermott 2003). It provides a number of advantages compared with individual therapy, including being more time- and cost-effective and offering support for individuals provided by others with similar issues. This approach has the benefit of including a number of perspectives on issues rather than simply those of the therapist and service user.

Groups often include a combination of therapeutic and educational aspects that involve helping people to make changes to their ways of thinking, feeling and behaving, as well as giving them new understandings of their issues and teaching them new coping skills (Corey 2004). Like individual therapy, group therapy can be short term (i.e. extend for six months or less) or longer term (McDermott 2003) and can be offered for all types of mental health problems.

Types of group

There are a variety of groups commonly run in in-patient units, community mental health settings and in residential and day programs. Groups generally are classified as being either open or closed. The membership of open groups changes over time (e.g. psycho-education groups in a mental health unit), whereas closed groups are those where members initially are selected by the group leader/s and then remain the same for the duration of the group. If a member leaves the group, they are not replaced. Psycho-therapeutic groups (such as those addressing a particular issue—for example, being diagnosed with borderline personality disorder or an experience of sexual assault) are generally closed groups.

Groups are also classified as being homogenous or heterogeneous. Homogenous groups are composed of members with the same issue (e.g. substance misuse), the same gender (e.g. women who have been sexually assaulted) and/or the same age (e.g. adolescent groups where members are between thirteen and eighteen years old). Heterogeneous groups, on the other hand, include members with a range of issues, ages and genders, such as a daily communication group or morning ward meeting in a mental health unit.

Common types of groups you are likely to see used in mental health include:

- *Psycho-education groups*: Often run by one or more health professionals on specific issues such as psychotropic medications, men's issues, nutrition, cooking, smoking and budgeting, to name a few. As the name suggests, these groups are educational, and aim to develop members' understanding and skills in particular areas, as well as providing an opportunity for social interaction.
- *Counselling groups*: This is a broad term describing groups that usually have treatment and often preventative aims. They involve an interpersonal focus and are often problem- as well as growth-oriented. As noted, narrative, solution-focused and cognitive behavioural therapy can be offered in the form of groups.
- *Self-help groups*: Groups such as Alcoholics Anonymous (AA), Narcotics Anonymous (NA), Overeaters Anonymous (OA), Gamblers Anonymous (GA) and Grow are well-known examples of groups that are run by members rather than a health professional. Many address a specific problem using a twelve-step approach, which recognises the problem as being an addiction or dependence over which the person

is powerless unless they seek help. Others primarily offer education and support, or seek practical change.

- *Relaxation groups*: These groups include the use of music and verbal techniques such as guided imagery to assist in developing mindfulness skills and in facilitating mental and physical relaxation and reduction of stress. They are often used in day programs, in-patient settings and alcohol and other drug programs.

Leading groups

Although there are groups that do not have or need a leader, you will find that most groups in mental health use the direction of a group leader or leaders. The roles of a group leader (in the mental health setting, the leader is often a nurse or occupational therapist) include facilitating interaction among group members, helping members to learn from each other, assisting them to establish and reach personal goals and encouraging them to develop strategies that involve taking action with problems in their everyday lives (Corey 2004).

Depending on the size and characteristics of the group, it may have a single leader or be co-led by two leaders. As you might imagine, being a group leader requires considerable attention to both the content and the dynamics between people. The group leaders may agree on specific roles they will assume within the group and will often discuss the process and content afterwards. Nurses can develop their group facilitation skills by working with and observing skilled facilitators. Corey (2004) outlines some important personal qualities and skills for group leaders (see Table 13.2).

CRITICAL THINKING

Think about situations in which you have found yourself—perhaps on clinical placement—where you have been in a group. Consider the following:

- What sort of group was it?
- Was the group leader effective, in your view?
- If so, what was it about them that made the group run effectively?
- If not, what do you think could have been done to improve the running of the group?
- If you were to lead a group in a mental health setting, what sorts of groups would you feel comfortable running?
- What would you need to do to prepare yourself to run it/them?

Table 13.2 Qualities and skills of group leaders

Personal qualities	Leadership skills
Be able to be emotionally available and present.	Have good active listening and attending skills, e.g. questioning, clarifying, summarising
Have self-confidence and a sense of one's own personal power	Be able to reflect feelings back to members and facilitate communication
Have courage, e.g. to take risks and admit mistakes	Be able to empathise with members
Be willing to confront and question oneself	Provide encouragement, support, protection and reinforcement for members, particularly when painful feelings are being disclosed. Be able to set productive goals with the group
Be sincere and authentic	Be able to give honest, constructive feedback to members
Have a clear sense of one's own identity	Provide role modelling of desired qualities/behaviours such as honesty, respect, assertiveness
Be enthusiastic and creative, and believe in the value of the group process	Be able to continually evaluate the group's progress, and know when and how to end the group's work

CONCLUSION

This chapter has sketched a very broad overview of some of the main psycho-therapeutic approaches. Examples of several brief therapies were provided, which share an emphasis on working collaboratively with service users to acknowledge their strengths and enhance their ability to adapt and cope. Nurses working in mental health need to be aware of the main psychotherapeutic schools and their underlying assumptions, partly so they can support service users making the right choice for themselves about the kind of therapy that might be most helpful. Training and supervision in psychotherapy and counselling are essential for any nurse who wishes to have a career in the mental health field, and are likely to be of benefit to nurses working in many areas, both professionally and personally.

REFERENCES

Akiskal, H.S. (1995). Mood disorders: introduction and overview. In H. I. Kaplan & B.J. Sadock (eds), *Comprehensive Textbook of Psychiatry* (6th edn), Vol. 1. Baltimore, MD: Williams & Wilkins, pp. 1067–79.

Beck, A.T. & Greenberg, R.L. (1984). Cognitive therapy in the treatment of depression. In N. Hoffman (ed.), *Foundations of Cognitive Therapy: theoretical methods and practical applications*. New York: Plenum Press, pp. 155–78.

Beck, A.T. & Weishaar, M.E. (1989). Cognitive therapy. In T. Freeman, K.M. Simon, L.E. Beutler & H. Arkowitz (eds), *Comprehensive Handbook of Cognitive Therapy*. New York: Plenum Press, pp. 21–36.

Bleiberg, K. & Markowitz, J.C. (2005). A pilot study of interpersonal psychotherapy for posttraumatic stress disorder. *American Journal of Psychiatry*, 162(1), 181–3.

Bowlby, J. (1977). The making and breaking of affectional bonds. I. Aetiology and psychopathology in the light of attachment theory. An expanded version of the Fiftieth Maudsley Lecture, delivered before the Royal College of Psychiatrists, 19 November 1976. *British Journal of Psychiatry*, 130(3), 201–10.

Brewin, C.R. (1988). *Cognitive Foundations of Clinical Psychology*. Hove: Lawrence Erlbaum.

Cashin, A. (2008). Narrative therapy: a psychotherapeutic approach of merit in the treatment of adolescents with Asperger's disorder. *Journal of Child and Adolescent Psychiatric Nursing*, 28(1), 48–56.

Corcoran, J. & Walsh, J. (2005). Solution-focused therapy. In J. Corcoran (ed.), *Building Strengths and Skills: a collaborative approach to working with clients*. Oxford: Oxford University Press, pp. 5–18.

Corey, G. (2004). *Theory & Practice of Group Counselling* (6th edn). Sydney: Thomson.

Crowe, M., Carlyle, D. & Farmar, R. (2008). Clinical formulation for mental health nursing practice. *Journal of Psychiatric and Mental Health Nursing*, 15(10), 800–7.

Crowe, M. & Luty, S. (2005). Interpersonal psychotherapy: an effective psychotherapeutic intervention for mental health nursing practice. *International Journal of Mental Health Nursing*, 14(2), 126–33.

DeSocio, J.E. (2005). Accessing self-development through narrative approaches in child and adolescent psychotherapy. *Journal of Child and Adolescent Psychiatric Nursing*, 18(2), 53–61.

Dobson, K.S. & Block, L. (1988). Historical and philosophical bases of the cognitive-behavioral therapies. In K.S. Dobson (ed.), *Handbook of Cognitive-Behavioural Therapy*. New York: The Guilford Press, pp. 3–38.

Egan, G. (1998). *The Skilled Helper: a problem-management approach to helping* (6th edn). Pacific Grove, CA: Brooks/Cole.

Felitti, V.J., Anda, R.F., Nordenberg, D., Williamson, D.F., Spitz, A.M., Edwards, V. et al. (1998). Relationship of childhood abuse and household dysfunction to many of the leading causes of death in adults. *American Journal of Preventive Medicine*, 14(4), 245–58.

Frankl, V. (2006). *Man's Search for Meaning: an introduction to logotherapy*. Boston, MA: Beacon Press.

Freud, A. (1993). *The ego and the mechanisms of defence* (Translated by Cecil Baines, 1937). London: Karnac Books.

Havens, L.L. & Ghaemi, S.N. (2005). Existential despair and bipolar disorder: the therapeutic alliance as a mood stabilizer. *American Journal of Psychotherapy*, 59(2), 137–47.

Horvath, A.O., Del Re, A.C., Flückiger, C. & Symonds, D. (2011). Alliance in individual psychotherapy. *Psychotherapy*, 48(1), 9.

Howgego, I.M., Yellowlees, P., Owen, C., Meldrum, L. & Dark, F. (2003). The therapeutic alliance: the key to effective patient outcome? A descriptive review of the evidence in community mental health case management. *Australian and New Zealand Journal of Psychiatry*, 37(2), 169–83.

Lakeman, R. (2006). Adapting psychotherapy to psychosis. *Australian e-Journal for the Advancement of Mental Health*, 5(1), 1–12.

Lambert, M.J. & Barley, D.E. (2001). Research summary on the therapeutic relationship and psychotherapy outcome. *Psychotherapy: Theory, Research, Practice, Training*, 38(4), 357–61.

Lethem, J. (2002). Brief solution focused therapy. *Child and Adolescent Mental Health*, 7(4), 189–92.

McAllister, M. (2003). Doing practice differently: solution-focused nursing. *Journal of Advanced Nursing*, 41(6), 528–35.

McDermott, F. (2003). Group work in the mental health field: researching outcome. *Australian Social Work*, 56(4), 352–63.

PACFA (2012). Definition of Counselling and Psychotherapy. Viewed 24 November 2012, <www.pacfa.org.au/resources/cid/41/parent/0/t/resources/l/layout>.

Peplau, H.E. (1952). *Interpersonal Relations in Nursing*. New York. G.P. Putnam's Sons.

Rogers, C.R. (1957). The necessary and sufficient conditions of therapeutic personality change. *Journal of Consulting Psychology*, 21, 95–102.

Spinelli, E. (2006). *Tales of Un-knowing: therapeutic encounters from an existential perspective*. Ross-on-Wye: PCCS Books.

Stevenson, C., Jackson, S. & Barker, P. (2003). Finding solutions through empowerment: A preliminary study of a solution-orientated approach to nursing in acute psychiatric settings. *Journal of Psychiatric and Mental Health Nursing*, 10(6), 688–96.

Varese, F., Smeets, F., Drukker, M., Lieverse, R., Lataster, T., Viechtbauer, W. et al. (2012). Childhood adversities increase the risk of psychosis: a meta-analysis of patient-control, prospective- and cross-sectional cohort studies. *Schizophrenia Bulletin*, 38(4), 661–71.

Wachtel, P.L. (2000). Psychotherapy in the twenty-first century. *American Journal of Psychotherapy*, 54(4), 441–50.

Webster, D.C. & Vaughn, K. (2003). Using solution-focused approaches. In P. Barker (ed.), *Psychiatric and Mental Health Nursing*. London: Arnold, pp. 187–93.

Weiss, K. A., Smith, T. E., Hull, J. W., Piper, A. C., & Huppert, J. D. (2002). Predictors of risk of non-adherence in outpatients with schizophrenia and other psychotic disorders. *Schizophrenia Bulletin*, 28(2), 341–9.

White, M. & Epston, D. (1990). *Narrative Means to Therapeutic Ends*. Adelaide: Dulwich Centre.

Wren, K. & Norred, C.L. (2003). *Complementary and Alternative Therapies*. Philadelphia, PA: Saunders.

Zuroff, D.C. & Blatt, S.J. (2006). The therapeutic relationship in the brief treatment of depression: contributions to clinical improvement and enhanced adaptive capacities. *Journal of Consulting & Clinical Psychology*, 74(1), 130–40.

14

Cultural safety

Main points
- An understanding of the relationship between culture and health care is crucial to skilled nursing care.
- Cultural safety is a philosophy of nursing developed in Aotearoa New Zealand by Māori scholar Irihapeti Ramsden.
- Cultural safety uses a particular definition of culture.
- Health-care systems and professions have cultural expectations of those who work in them, based on established worldviews and ways of doing business.
- Cultural safety recognises that all nursing encounters are bicultural, making it a useful approach to nursing care with any population and in all contexts.
- Cultural safety is strongly based on social justice principles—it has historical and socio-political dimensions.
- Cultural safety is based on the nurses' self-awareness as bearers of their own cultural identity and assumptions.
- Cultural safety requires nurses to be able to articulate their cultural position so that they can understand how their personal culture impacts on nursing care and assessment.

Definitions
Culture: Learned yet dynamic ways of being in everyday life, informed by attributes such as age, class, ability, ethnicity, gender and sexual orientation, which influence beliefs, values and attitudes, and how humans explain and respond to life's context and circumstances

Biculturalism: every interaction between a nurse and a client involves at least two cultures, that of the nurse and that of the client

---

INTRODUCTION

This chapter discusses the relationship between culture and nursing care and introduces readers to the philosophy of cultural safety and the steps towards becoming a culturally safe practitioner. We believe that cultural safety and the process that nurses need to undertake to achieve cultural safety could be powerful transformative factors in a mental health system that has long struggled to achieve social justice for mental health service users. We discuss why we think cultural safety is the most appropriate way to consider issues concerning culture and mental health nursing care; review the definitions and assumptions on which it is based and examine how this philosophy can be applied in your everyday nursing practice.

CULTURE AND HEALTH CARE

The authors' experience teaching undergraduate nursing students reveals that many students, especially those from an Anglo-Saxon, Anglo-Celtic or Caucasian background, struggle with accepting that issues of culture are highly relevant in nursing care in any context and with all populations. The problem here is twofold. First, those who view ethnicity and culture as characteristics of exotic 'others' may find it difficult to take issues concerning health care and culture seriously. In an Australian national review of how nursing educators dealt with issues of culture, Eisenbruch (2000) notes that in the social sciences, debates have advanced to include issues concerning race/racism and education—concerns that had not filtered into nursing education. Eisenbruch (2001, p. 21, citing Culley 1996) comments that: 'Here [in Australia] a cultural essentialism continues to dominate the debate, in which health educators use "culture" to maintain a separation between ethnic minority patients and those of the dominant white group.' From this perspective, as noted above, culture belongs to 'the exotic others' not to 'the dominant us'. The material discussed in this chapter decisively challenges this perspective. Second, among these students there is often the strong Australian ethos that everyone should be treated the same. No one would argue with the practice of treating everyone equally in terms of trust, respectful, non-judgemental and active communication. However, a cornerstone of cultural safety is that clients should be treated according to their unique needs and differences, and many Australians find this notion a challenge to their ingrained ideas about equality as sameness.

So, contrary to the views that some students bring to their studies at university, the nursing profession accepts that the interaction between culture and health care is something that nurses working in all fields of nursing must consider (see ANMC 2006; Eisenbruch 2001). The relationship between culture and health is important, as humans define health and conceptualise the necessary and sufficient conditions for health maintenance in various ways. Further, humans attach diverse meanings to the experience of becoming unwell, entertaining different ideas about why we become unwell, about how an illness will develop, its outcomes and useful treatments and interventions.

In Australia, the predominant model of health adhered to by health professions and health-care systems is a strict biomedical view that sees health as the absence of disease. This view—often part of the cultural perspective of health-care professions—tends to see the individual and their behaviours as the sole location and determinant of health and illness. Thus the culture of mainstream health-care systems in Australia has a strong focus on an individual's *lifestyle* as a health determinant, in both policy and practice, and in treatment and in prevention. Nurses who take this cultural perspective on health and illness bring related assumptions, values, beliefs and attitudes to their nursing care, which can have decisively negative impacts on the outcomes of their care. These issues are discussed further below when we ask you to identify the conceptual framework you are currently using to think about mental health issues.

A different model used to understand and define health is based on sociological perspectives (see Willis & Elmer 2011). It recognises that individuals are always enmeshed in social networks and societal contexts, which impact on their health and well-being. Thus health and illness have determinants far beyond the bodily boundaries of an individual, and illnesses also impact on an individual's family and social networks—not just on the person with the diagnosis. In keeping with these perspectives, in this book we take a sociological approach to health and illness—in other words, we have a strong focus on life chances, and so see good health care as a matter of social justice. Chapter 8 focuses exclusively on the social determinants of mental health and social and emotional well-being.

The recognition by the nursing profession that the dynamics between culture and nursing care are important is reflected in the fact that over the past few years new editions of the major texts used in Bachelor of Nursing Programs have included material about the issue of culture and nursing care (see Crisp et al. 2013; Jarvis 2012; Brown et al. 2012). Yet a quick look at these texts shows that the issues are far from straightforward. These texts reflect the different cultural understanding of health and illness we described above, and so they take various approaches to instructing nurses about culture and health care.

Some nursing texts see the importance of the relationship between culture and nursing care as located in the cultural diversity among users of health services, an approach that is known as transculturalism (Taylor & Guerin 2010, p. 11). This line of thinking focuses on cultural *groups*, and on the idea that nurses can become culturally competent by learning the cultural practices of various cultural groups (transcultural nursing) (see Brown et al. 2012). Other texts advocate for an alternative approach called *cultural safety*, accepting that it is the nurse's culture—and indeed the cultures of hospitals, medicine and nursing—that can be major impediments to good nursing care (see Cox & Taua 2013). It is outside the scope of this chapter to provide a thorough critique of transcultural approaches, and we refer readers to some of the excellent work available on this topic such as that by Seaton (2010). In this book, we also advocate for cultural safety, reviewing pertinent issues for mental health nursing practice; however, before discussing cultural safety itself, we first clarify the definition of culture that is used in cultural safety.

Relationship between culture and health

Diverse ideas exist about:

- what is considered healthy/normal
- what causes [mental] health issues/emotional/social problems
- the location of problems—the individual? The family? The community? The society? Global issues?
- what can help an individual, family or community experiencing mental health issues
- the impact of the culture of nurses and the health-care system on the treatment of clients in mental health settings.

CULTURE AND CULTURAL SAFETY

The culture concept is notoriously complex, and evades neat and precise definition (see Rapport & Overing 2007, pp. 109–19). Therefore, in any discussion about the inter-action between culture and health care, it is important to consider that definitions of culture vary, and we all have our own idea of what the term means. Some definitions of culture focus solely on the notion of worldview, and define culture as systems of beliefs, values and behaviours that are common to those who share a cultural identity. However, a moment's reflection on our own cultural experience will demonstrate that those who share a cultural identity are not homogeneous and express or identify with their culture in myriad ways.

Very often, nursing students approach culture in this commonsense fashion of capital 'C' Culture (or, as one of the author's mentors called it, 'the Opera House view of culture') in a way that focuses on visual and performing arts, customs, cere-monies and other highly structured human activities that are construed as static, 'traditional' and shared, and usually belong to 'others'. It is not surprising that those who approach culture from such a perspective find it difficult to see what it has to do with nursing care or health services in general.

However, in this text we focus on small 'c' culture: culture as ways of being in everyday life, as this approach has much more relevance in the context of health care. This approach to culture is based on a number of assumptions, including that cultures are constructed by humans, and ultimately refer to the human capacity to strategise and make meaning out of life experiences—culture is dynamic, and adapts to changing circumstances of our lives. Further, culture is developed intersubjectively, since humans and society are always in an open co-constituting relationship with each other. Our embrace of the culture/s into which we are born, and that we learn as children, changes. As we go through life, we exercise power, adapt, develop and refine our values and beliefs; we may try on, adopt and drop various cultural identities according to our current needs, and we rethink our cultural position based on experiences.

These limits to the shared nature of culture mean that even those who grow up in the same family can have vastly different values, beliefs and cultural practices from one another, as society and aspects of the personal lifeworld mould their cultural being and perspectives. As nurses, you will interact with people of all ages at a time of their life when they are dealing with profoundly distressing life events and problems. Therefore, mental health nurses in particular must have a sound grasp of Husserl's phenomenological concept of the lifeworld, referring to the world as it is experienced (Dahlberg & Drew 1997, p. 304). It is worth remembering that, although people may live in the same place and perhaps have the same cultural identity, we cannot assume that their lifeworld is the same as each others'. There will be variations in personal, social and cultural history, and in wealth, status, social connectedness, education and so on. To summarise, we all experience events, problems and social conditions that differ, even if we are members of the same society, ethnicity, profession, class, community or family, and these ways of being all influence the way we act in the world.

It is this level of cultural complexity and the historically specific nature of our cultural identity that has informed the development of cultural safety and the definition of culture as it is used in this approach. Some models of nursing care claim that culture and ethnicity are the same thing, and focus on exotic beliefs, values and customs. In contrast, cultural safety takes a very broad view of culture that has a strong focus on the context in which our lives are lived, which can be seen in the definition of cultural safety below.

The Nursing Council of New Zealand defines cultural safety as:

> The effective nursing of a person/family from another culture, and is determined by that person or family. Culture includes *but is not restricted to* age or generation; gender; sexual orientation; occupation and socioeconomic status; ethnic origin or migrant experience; religious or spiritual belief; and disability. The nurse delivering the service will have undertaken a process of reflection on [their] own cultural identity and will recognise the impact that [their] personal culture has on [their] professional practice. Unsafe cultural practice is any action, which diminishes, demeans or disempowers the cultural identity and well-being of an individual. (NCNZ 2011, p. 7, emphasis added)

The Australian Nursing and Midwifery Council's (ANMC) Registered Nurse Competency Standards also take a very broad view of the cultural issues that can impact on nursing care, which closely corresponds to the definition of cultural safety:

> The registered nurse recognises that *ethnicity, culture, gender, spiritual values, sexuality, age, disability and economic and social factors* have an impact on an individual's responses to, and beliefs about, health and illness, and plans and modifies nursing care appropriately. (ANMC 2006, p. 2, emphasis added)

If you look back at the definition of cultural safety above, you will notice that it aligns with the approach of Australia's national registration authority in other ways, as the current National Competency Standards for the Registered Nurse in Australia note that nurses must practise is a way that 'ensures that personal values and attitudes are not imposed on others' (ANMC 2006, p. 4). Clearly, nurses cannot give such an assurance unless they are fully aware of their personal cultural values and attitudes. We return to this issue of the need for a process of reflection on your personal culture, values and attitudes in mental health nursing below, after providing more information on the development of cultural safety.

The philosophy of cultural safety is based on attitude change, and was developed in the late 1980s in Aotearoa (NZ) by Māori scholar Irihapeti Ramsden. The philosophy is a strong underpinning of nursing practice and education in New Zealand, and has led to a global focus by health professions on culture and health and on the impacts of colonisation on health (Taylor & Guerin 2010, pp. 14–15). Cultural safety fits into what Eisenbruch calls a 'diversity model'. Eisenbruch (2000, p. 29) states:

> Cultural safety is not about cultural practices as such but seeks to recognise the position of certain groups in society, and how they are treated rather than how they are different. It is not based on multiculturalism, but on biculturalism, and focuses on the power and racism of the dominant over the native inhabitants.

In developing the model of cultural safety, Ramsden took seriously some Māori nursing students' concerns that anthropological approaches to cultural issues in their nursing education were an assault to their identity (Eckermann et al. 2010, p. 184). These approaches focused on notions of 'traditional' Māori culture, insinuating that those who did not strictly adhere to Māori traditions were not properly Māori. Seaton (2010) identifies that transcultural approaches to nursing practice are ahistorical, as they do not account for the issues of power and cultural dominance that allowed the genocidal practices which sought to destroy Indigenous cultures both in Australia and in Aotearoa New Zealand. As Coup states:

> Teaching nurses to be experts in Māori culture leads to further disempowerment of Māori, given that there are significant numbers who have been deprived of knowledge of their own identity and traditions. (Coup 1996, cited in Ramsden 2002, p. 113)

Australians will recognise how strongly identity policing such as this applies to Indigenous Australians, many of whom were dispossessed from their land and its resources, and as a consequence of other genocidal polices were deprived of access to law/lore, traditions, language and kin. The resultant inability of many to then fulfil their cultural responsibilities to country and family has had profound and ongoing impacts on the social and emotional well-being of Indigenous Australians, a topic discussed more fully in Chapter 8 of this text.

The Australian Nursing and Midwifery Council defines cultural safety as:

> a nurse or midwife's understanding of his or her own personal culture and how these personal cultural values may impact on the provision of care to the person . . . cultural safety incorporates cultural awareness and cultural sensitivity and is underpinned by good communication, recognition of the diversity of views nationally and internationally between ethnic groups and the impact of colonisation on Indigenous cultures around the world. (ANMC 2007, p. 1)

However, although cultural safety grew out of a colonial context, and certainly is applicable to the colonial context and history and the impacts on Indigenous peoples in Australia, we extend the concept and argue that all Australians are impacted by a shared history of colonisation, no matter where one is positioned in these dynamics of power, dominance and violence (Eckermann et al. 2010, p. 212). Concerns such as power, dominance and violence are especially important in the field of mental health care, which in itself is a culture with a long history of stereotyping, human rights abuses and poor community relations (for example, see Burdekin 1993; McSherry 2008).

Due to the history of cultural safety and its applicability to post-colonial contexts, the author has consistently found that many student nurses assume that cultural safety is only applicable to nursing Indigenous people. This is a misunderstanding of its potential and scope, and ironically contradicts its central tenet that the focus of cultural safety is *not* on the culture of so called 'exotic others' but rather on the mundane everyday cultural assumptions of dominant professions and systems, and how these impact on service users. Indeed, it is the circumstances concerning power, attitudes and poor relations with others that make another key aspect of cultural safety exceptionally important for mental health nursing practice with any client whatsoever. This concept is *biculturalism*, meaning that every time you are with a client there are at least two cultural perspectives at play: your cultural background and that of the client. As Eckermann et al. (2010 p. 188) clarify, these circumstances set up the dynamics for a power imbalance. Cultural safety education facilitates nurses to recognise such dynamics.

There are also broader cultural influences at play in your nursing care, as it takes place within the context of mental health nursing—yet another culture with traditions, practices, assumptions, values and understandings about the nature of mental health and illness, and the circumstances and conditions that can bring these about, as described earlier. Ramsden gives an example of the culture of nursing disempowering clients by serving the needs of the professionals rather than those of clients:

> I realised that the major right of patients was to information and that we health professionals were manipulating information for reasons that related more to our need for routine and control than they did to empowerment of the people we were there to serve. (Ramsden, 2002, p. 35)

But here too it would be misleading to assume that all mental health nurses embrace this culture to the same degree, or that they understand and experience it in the same way. The highly varied way in which each of us expresses and experiences our culture/s leads to the next aspect of cultural safety, concerning who is the cultural expert.

A cornerstone of cultural safety is that the client is the expert on their culture. Ramsden said of cultural safety:

> It is about the analysis of power and not the customs and habits of anybody. In the future it must be the patient who makes the final statement about the quality of care which they receive. Creating ways in which this commentary may happen is the next step in the cultural safety journey. (Ramsden 2002, p. 181)

Interestingly, this notion of the health service users being at the centre of care is a founding principle of mental health nursing by virtue of the integral role of the nurse–patient relationship that was established with Peplau's (1952) seminal work on nursing. In recent years, this principle has been extended even further in the mental health field due to the 'recent shift from "provider" as "expert" to provider as "partner" in a person's health concerns' (see Chapter 1). Cultural safety is therefore very well suited to mental health nursing care. As indicated above, part of your challenge is to bring your cultural assumptions to mind—an issue discussed further below.

Four key objectives of cultural safety education

1. To educate student nurses and midwives not to blame the victims of historical process for their current plights.
2. To educate student nurses and midwives to examine their own realities and the attitudes they bring to each new person they encounter in their practice.
3. To educate student nurses and midwives to be open-minded and flexible in their attitudes towards people who are different from themselves, to whom they offer and deliver service.
4. To produce a workforce of well-educated, self-aware registered nurses and midwives who are culturally safe to practise as defined by the people they serve.

CULTURAL SAFETY IN MENTAL HEALTH NURSING

As mentioned above, cultural safety is strongly committed to social justice, and it is underpinned by a wide definition of the cultural factors that can influence a person's mental health (Ramsden 2002, p. 5). Therefore, cultural safety is interested in promoting nursing care that contributes to a socially just society by not demeaning or discriminating against clients due to their cultural identity, their social situation or the nature of their needs. While important in all nursing contexts, these issues are especially important in the mental health field, due to the social stigma experienced by those with a diagnosed mental illness. It is imperative that those providing nursing care in the mental health field do not compound these social issues by bringing their own social and cultural biases to bear on their nursing work. Cultural safety education can play a pivotal role in preventing such dynamics in mental health settings.

Chapter 2 provided an overview of the various, and at times conflicting, conceptual frameworks underlying mental health, mental illness and mental health nursing. These theories or frameworks are tools that we use to think through the problems humans encounter; they are the ways in which we explain these issues to ourselves. Although you may not yet be familiar with these theories, you will have ways by which you explain issues of mental health and mental illness to yourself. There will be specific and identifiable ways in which you talk about mental health and mental illness, and of course the way you think and talk about those who experience mental illness. If you or your family have experienced a mental illness, your theories are likely to be well developed—or at the very least you will have strong opinions about some of the issues that we ask you to consider in the following exercise.

To take a beginning step in developing a culturally safe approach, it is important that you consider these issues and then undertake a process of reflection to determine which conceptual frameworks or theories are informing your work as a nurse. To assist you in this process, undertake the following critical thinking exercise.

CRITICAL THINKING

To prepare, have to hand your computer, or pen and paper, and make some time and space to quietly think and write about these issues. Alternatively, you could undertake these steps in a study group and share and discuss your responses.

- Complete the following statements:
    - Mental illnesses are located in a person's . . .
    - People with a mental illness are . . .
    - People develop a mental illness because . . .
    - I believe that the best way to assist those with a mental illness is . . .
    - Anyone can develop a mental illness if . . .

- Look at Chapter 2, on conceptual approaches, and see whether you can find where your responses fit within these.
  - Did your responses suggest that you believe that mental illnesses are biological disorders?
  - Or that they occur within a person's head—they are psychological disorders?
  - Or that they are largely behavioural—they are bad behaviours that can be changed by rewards and punishments?
  - Or that they are related to moral weakness or a failure to develop morally?
  - Or that they are related to the person's socio-cultural situation and context?
  - Or that they are largely to do with how the person interacts with others and their environment?

Your responses to these questions, and then locating the theory that best describes them, will assist you to articulate your cultural position and the related assumptions about your clients that you are bringing to your nursing care. For example, many of the nursing students with whom I have worked over the years indicate that they find it difficult to feel compassion towards anyone with mental health issues related to substance misuse. Some students explained that from their point of view (that is, according to their cultural values), the person chooses to misuse the substance, so any resulting issues are 'self-inflicted'. This, of course, is the moralistic position described above, where the person's problems are seen to be related to weaknesses in their character and morals—they are seen to be 'bad' rather than 'mad'. Such a position is known as 'victim blaming', and is a well-recognised dynamic in health care (see Eckermann et al. 2010, p. 71; Willis & Elmer 2011, p. 314). It is related to the strongly individualistic nature of biomedical cultural understandings of health and illness, as described earlier. As Fanany and Fanany & Fanany (2012, p. 13) note:

> This moral aspect of individual concern for health is still observable today. Those who do not smoke and who limit their consumption of alcohol, ride a bicycle instead of driving a car, eat a low-fat diet are often seen (and view themselves) as virtuous and morally superior to others whose choices are different. In some situations, engaging in behaviours viewed as high-risk in the context of health can result in social exclusion, stigma and even denial of treatment.

It is, of course, such health-care outcomes—of central concern to users of mental health services and their families—that cultural safety education seeks to avoid. We turn now to a consideration of how to apply cultural safety in your work.

CULTURAL SAFETY, ASSESSMENT AND MENTAL HEALTH NURSING

As discussed in detail in Chapter 11, a major part of mental health nursing work lies in undertaking a holistic assessment of the person's situation, including their presenting complaint and its duration; personal and social history; their work, financial and living situation; their significant relationships; their emotional and biological state; and current needs as the client and their family perceive them. Nurses also assess the person's strengths and access to social and other resources that might assist recovery. These aspects of assessment are crucial, as they seek to answer the questions of how this person, with this problem, came to be in this situation at this time, and to identify all the factors that led to this moment in time and those that can be mobilised in nursing care. Nurses also undertake another key assessment process called the Mental State Examination (MSE), which—as the name suggests—gives a detailed snapshot of the person's mental, behavioural and emotional state at the time of the assessment.

It is immediately obvious that successfully undertaking this work with someone who has reached some sort of crisis in their life requires considerable communication skills. This is especially so when we recall that under the *Mental Health Acts* of all states and territories in Australia, many mental health clients will be in hospital against their will, and those in the community may be taking medication under Community Treatment Orders, which they would rather not take. Even those who seek treatment voluntarily can quickly find themself under an involuntary order if the nurses and doctors decide that this is necessary. So, to avoid alienating mental health clients, nurses must recognise and take steps to lessen the power imbalances inherent in situations involving them and their clients.

Power-sharing is essential to cultural safety, so cultural safety is central to achieving this goal as, due to the process of reflection that characterises it, the nurse will have examined and thus be aware of how their own cultural position and background can influence outcomes for the client. Such a process translates into practical ways of power-sharing. For example, a client might decide where and when they would like the conversations described below to take place, and who they would like to be present. How the conversation will unfold can be based on the client's priorities and concerns not only what a nurse (or the system) says they have to get done. How the seating for the conversation is set up can also lessen power imbalances, and the nurse can take a relaxed, human and friendly attitude—as is taken when speaking with someone who is considered an equal. We give a detailed overview of how these issues play out in undertaking an MSE below; however, these steps immediately begin to address issues of power imbalances.

The approach described above facilitates the establishment of trust, which is common to both mental health nursing and cultural safety, because positive outcomes in mental health nursing are dependent on trust. Trust can be consolidated further by eliciting the information covered by an MSE using a conversational style, so that rapport can be established. In practice, it is often during the history-taking conversation (interview) that the MSE is undertaken in such a way that the client does not have a sense of being interrogated to a format. Sound observation and communication skills allow the nurse to gather this information and later record it in the standard MSE format as required.

However, the MSE is strongly culturally determined, being based on a white, Anglo-Saxon Protestant (WASP) understanding of what is normal and what might be considered a mental, social or emotional disturbance. That is to say, the items assessed in it are strongly informed by specific cultural assumptions that are far from universal. It is very easy for nurses to assess a client according to cultural assumptions of what is normal for the nurse or what is normal in the dominant society, rather than focusing on what is considered normal for that particular person in their socio-cultural context. In the following, we examine aspects of an MSE undertaken by nurses who have not undergone cultural safety education, allowing us to consider how nursing care and service to the client would be improved if nurses recognised and reflected on their own cultural position, values, beliefs, attitudes and assumptions.

These examples, based on MSEs, demonstrate how easy it is to judge someone as disordered when we have not reflected on how our own cultural identity, position, life-world and world-view might be influencing our clinical judgement. It should also be obvious that different people have vastly different communication styles, often based on differing priorities governing the interaction between them. These priorities are often culturally driven by a person's personal culture, combined with influences of the broader cultural context in which the encounter takes place.

To illustrate this point, imagine that you are observing the following scenario and then undertake the exercise at the end.

CRITICAL THINKING: DEVELOPING A CULTURALLY SAFE APPROACH IN MENTAL HEALTH NURSING

You can develop a culturally safe approach in your mental health nursing care by:

- reflecting, exploring, examining and then writing down in detail your cultural position, realities, values and beliefs
- reflecting, exploring, examining and then writing down in detail your attitudes towards those with mental health issues
- reflecting, exploring, examining and then writing down in detail your attitudes towards those who you perceive to be different to yourself
- using a flexible and open-minded approach towards people from cultures other than your own, and towards those from your own culture who may have different values, priorities, beliefs and experiences from you
- being aware that mental health problems frequently are related to the historical and social context of a person's life—they have social and emotional dimensions

SAMPLE MSE: CULTURAL ASSUMPTIONS IMPACTING ON CLINICAL JUDGEMENT

Appearance

An older nurse describes Nathan's (a young male) hairstyle as 'dirty and unkempt' when it is carefully styled with gel to appear that way (cultural assumption of middle-aged female).

In assessing Clive, who has been 'sleeping rough' for some weeks, a nurse writes that he is 'dirty and dishevelled'. Clive is judged as incapable of undertaking his activities of daily life (ADLs) due to mental issues, when the actual problem is that he doesn't have access to facilities (cultural assumption of housed nursing staff; social issues ignored).

Behaviour

Nineteen-year-old David snatches his backpack out of a nurse's hand, reacting against it being searched. The nurse did not ask permission or explain why it might be necessary to search it. David's behaviour is described as 'aggressive and uncooperative' (power imbalance and cultural assumption of superiority of an older person who is on staff over a younger person who is a client).

Speech form

A female nurse describes Kate's slurred speech and concludes that she is drunk (cultural assumption of an older able-bodied woman towards a younger woman with multiple sclerosis).

Mood

When asked by the nurse how he is today, Jed says he feels 'fully sick'. The older nurse writes down 'nauseous' but doesn't describe his emotional state—the client means he feels great (cultural misunderstanding based on language and generational difference).

Affect

The affect of Fabien, a young Indigenous client, is described by the nurse as 'unresponsive and blunt', based on his minimal facial expression—he has already sent a text to his brother saying he is scared of the nurses and urging him to 'tell Mum to come along soon' to support him (cultural misunderstanding due to nurse's cultural assumptions about the meaning of minimal facial expression).

Thinking

Thought Content

The nurse really can't get Fabien to say anything much apart from 'I am waiting for Mum to come. She's coming on the bus'. The nurse happens to know that the woman who gave birth to the teenager has passed away. The nurse writes in the notes that Fabien 'has a delusion that his mother is still alive'. The young person is waiting for his biological mother's sister, who he also calls Mum (cultural assumption of the nurse that only biological mothers are called Mum).

Thought form
Based on the above experiences the nurse also concludes that Fabien is suffering from 'poverty of thought' (cultural assumption of the nurse that a lack of conversation indicates a formal thought disorder).

Sensorium and cognition
Orientation
Marla, a client recently arrived in Australia from a context of torture and trauma, is judged as being disorientated by a nurse as Marla doesn't seem to know where she is or what she is doing there (cultural assumption by a nurse in her own cultural environment about a person who is not familiar with that environment and who is traumatised).

Cognition
Shamus's cognition is tested using 'serial 7s'. He is instructed to count backwards from 100 by 7. However, the young man dropped out of school at age thirteen and is innumerate. Using serial 7s in this case does not assess the degree to which his pre-morbid functioning has diminished—it only reinforces his established disability (cultural assumption by nurse that the young man was numerate—only 47 per cent of Australians are assessed as having numeracy skills sufficient to meet the complex demands of everyday life (ABS 2007)).

Insight and judgement
Insight
Gladys, an elderly woman, recently lost her husband of over 60 years. She regularly sees him around the house in the morning. The community nurse is concerned that she is developing a mental illness. The nurse tells Gladys that because of her hallucinations she needs to go to an appointment with the psychiatrist. She refuses, saying that there is nothing wrong with her at all and that she misses her husband (cultural assumption by the nurse that a 'lack of insight' as this is medically framed is a criterion for mental illness). See Bell (2008), who argues that hallucinations are a normal grief reaction and cites research showing that 80 per cent of elderly people in grief experience hallucinations of their loved one.

Judgement
Judy, a Filipino woman studying in Australia, has developed symptoms of depression and has been referred by university counselling services. She tells the assessing nurse that she has no money since she sent all her wages to her parents. (The nurse concludes that this decision shows very poor judgement, based on her own cultural assumptions.)

- thinking about how power is operating between you and your client:
  - How does the balance of power look? Are you in the more powerful position?
  - How can power sharing be negotiated? How can your client be 'empowered'?
  - How do you refer to your clients when talking to your colleagues? When addressing the clients?
  - Do you use terms that indicate respect for peoples' humanity? Do you use terms that demean or diminish your clients?
  - Can you identify a list of common insults used towards clients?
  - What does this everyday talk about clients between you and your colleagues tell you about power? About trust? About respect? About your capacity for cultural safety, given that it is judged by those who receive the service not by those who give it?

Imagine that you are a client or a member of a client's family or friendship network. How does your professional conduct look from this position?

CASE STUDY: FRIDAY NIGHT, AUGUST 2012, 11.00 P.M. AT A BUSY METROPOLITAN HOSPITAL EMERGENCY DEPARTMENT (ED)

The setting is a conversation between Eliza, a middle-aged Caucasian Australian mental health liaison nurse on intake, and Gerard, a middle-aged Caucasian Australian brought to the ED by the police following an attempt to jump off a city bridge.

You observe that Eliza has not long been on duty, and already has several people to see—she has to start with Gerard as he is at risk of harming himself. The young girl whose stomach has been pumped following an overdose and is now sleeping, the well-known client with schizophrenia with an acute cardiac condition who has had a shot of morphine and is now on the monitor, and the woman who had a panic attack at the ballet will all have to wait.

Eliza knows that by the time she finishes with Gerard there will almost certainly be a number of other clients vying for her attention. And she'd hoped to get some of the reading for her assignment done overnight. Eliza sets herself very high standards for her postgraduate studies in nursing—getting less than a High Distinction is not an option: 'Imagine the shame if I actually fail,' she thinks to herself.

Eliza goes into the cubicle where Gerard waits. Eliza is so flustered she doesn't introduce herself or say hello to Gerard, or ask him how he is going. Instead, she asks Gerard a number of questions in rapid succession.

E: What is your name?
G: Gerard Hyrst.
E: Age?
G: 51.

E: Address?
G: Um 402 Stringer St.
E: Where?
G: Stafford.
E: How did you get here?
G: Ah, um, the police brought me.
E: Have you been drinking? (Kind of leans forward a bit and sniffs the air. Gerard leans back.)
G: No.
E: What seems to be the problem? (Eliza's tone is impatient.)
G: Um . . . I, I . . . (Gerard starts crying.)
E: Come on what's up? (Gerard is convulsively sobbing now—he can't speak.)

Eliza keeps looking towards the door of the cubicle and scribbling on a piece of paper. She abruptly leaves the cubicle. She is away about five minutes and Gerard calms down a bit. Eliza comes back with a new pen and asks:

E: You married?
Gerard nods.
E: Children?
G: Three (Gerard whispers) two boys at uni and um, a girl at high school.
E: So tell me what seems to be the problem?
G: (replies softly) I got sacked today—been at that government job fifteen years. I got sacked today. (Shakes his head disbelievingly)

Eliza barely acknowledges Gerard's explanation as there is suddenly a loud argument between police, nurses and an intoxicated man in the next cubicle. Eliza rushes in there and joins the fray. Gerard gets up and quietly leaves unnoticed. Outside, he catches a taxi to the bridge.

Critical thinking
Review the NCNZ (2011, p. 7) definition of culture given above, then consider the following questions:

- What aspects of Eliza's personal culture influenced this outcome?
- Eliza and Gerard both identified with the 'same' culture. How did their culture differ?
- What aspects of Eliza's professional culture influenced this outcome?
- How do you think the culture of the ED influenced this outcome?
- If you were Gerard would you assess Eliza's nursing as culturally safe?

CRITICAL THINKING: STEPS TO UNDERTAKE A REFLECTION ON AN EVENT

Reflect on a nursing encounter where you felt unhappy or uncomfortable with your performance/attitude/actions/words.

- Write down what happened.
- What did you do/say?
- Are there values, attitudes or beliefs that you might need to challenge in yourself?
- Are there issues influencing this experience that are outside of your control?
- Were your actions/words influenced by others?
- Were your actions/words influenced by the system—for example, established ways of doing things in the culture of the place where the events took place?
- Were there priorities in the place of work that conflicted with your personal or professional priorities?
- What insights did this experience give you into yourself, and your cultural identity and position?
- If you had the chance to do it again, what would be different about your approach?

CONCLUSION

In this chapter, we provided an overview of the culture concept, and looked at the way it is defined in the philosophy of cultural safety, and how this definition aligns with professional nursing standards and the requirements of professional nursing registration authorities. We discussed how the philosophy of cultural safety developed and then how to apply it in your own professional development of cultural safety and in mental health nursing work. We showed that the key to cultural safety is self-awareness and reflection arising from the recognition that we are all cultural beings, and so each encounter with a client is bicultural. We argued that, especially in the field of mental health nursing, an approach such as cultural safety can lead to more just and humane outcomes for mental health clients by recognising the impact of nurses' and nursing culture on practice, by power-sharing and negotiation, and by putting the needs of the client and their families, as *they* have defined them, at the centre of our practice.

REFERENCES

Australian Bureau of Statistics (ABS) (2007). *Adult Literacy and Life Skills Survey: summary results, Australia*. Cat. no. 4228.0. Viewed 9 November 2012, <www.abs.gov.au/ausstats/abs@.nsf/Latest products/4228.0Media%20Release12006%20%28Reissue%29?opendocument&tabname=Summary &prodno=4228.0&issue=2006%20%28Reissue%29&num=&view>.

Australian Nursing and Midwifery Council (ANMC) (2006). *RN Competency Standards* (4th edn). Viewed 7 August 2012, <www.nursingmidwiferyboard.gov.au/Codes-Guidelines-Statements/Codes-Guidelines.aspx#codesofprofessionalconduct>.

—— (2007). *Inclusion of Aboriginal and Torres Strait Islander Peoples' Health and Cultural Issues in Courses leading to Registration or Enrolment.* Viewed 9 June 2011, <www.anmc.org.au/userfiles/file/guidelines_and_position_statements/Inclusion%20of%20Indigenous%20Health%20Issues%20in%20Undergraduate%20programs.pdf>.

Bell, V. (2008). Ghost stories: visits from the deceased. *Scientific American*, 2 December. Viewed 9 November 2012, <www.scientificamerican.com/article.cfm?id=ghost-stories-visits-from-the-deceased>.

Brown, D., Edwards, H., Lewis, S.L., Heitkemper, M.M., O'Brien, P.G., Bucher, L. & Camera, I. (eds) (2012). *Lewis's Medical-surgical Nursing: assessment, management of clinical problems.* Sydney: Elsevier.

Burdekin, B. (1993). *National Inquiry into the Human Rights of People with Mental Illness.* Sydney: HREOC. Viewed 27 August 2012, <www.humanrights.gov.au/disability_rights/inquiries/mental.htm>.

Cox, L. & Taua, C. (2013). Socio-cultural considerations and nursing practice. In J. Crisp, C. Taylor, C. Douglas & G. Rebeiro (eds), *Fundamentals of Nursing* (4th edn). Sydney: Elsevier.

Crisp, J., Taylor, C., Douglas, C. & Rebeiro, G. (2013). *Fundamentals of Nursing* (4th edn). Sydney: Elsevier.

Dahlberg, K. & Drew, N. (1997). A lifeworld paradigm for nursing research. *Journal of Holistic Nursing*, 15(3), 303–17.

Eckermann, A.K., Dowd, T., Chong, E., Nixon, L., Gray, R. & Johnson, S. (2010). *Binang Goonj: bridging cultures in Aboriginal health.* Sydney: Elsevier.

Eisenbruch, M. (2000). *National Review of Nursing Education*, Multicultural Nursing Education. Higher Education Division, Department of Education, Training and Youth Affairs. Canberra: Commonwealth of Australia. Viewed 15 August 2012, <www.google.com.au/url?sa=t&rct=j&q=&esrc=s&source=web&cd=1&cad=rja&ved=0CCQQFjAA&url=http%3A%2F%2Fvital.new.voced.edu.au%2Fvital%2Faccess%2Fservices%2FDownload%2Fngv%3A10272%2FSOURCE2&ei=qopNUK2CF8iyiQemiYGYAw&usg=AFQjCNFN05h0laUJchG9AsYe-ZQkPxxF9Q>.

Fanany, R. & Fanany, D. (2012). *Health as a Social Experience.* Melbourne: Palgrave Macmillan.

Jarvis, C. (2012). *Jarvis's Physical Examination and Health Assessment.* Forbes, H., Watt, E., (Australian adapting eds.). Chatswood, NSW: Saunders Elsevier.

McSherry, B. (2008). Mental health and human rights: the role of the law in developing a right to enjoy the highest attainable standard of mental health in Australia. *Journal of Law and Medicine*, 15, 773–81.

Nursing Council of New Zealand (NCNZ) (2011). *Guidelines for Cultural Safety: the Treaty of Waitangi and Māori health in nursing education and practice.* Wellington: NCNZ. Viewed 31 August 2012, <www.nursingcouncil.org.nz/download/97/cultural-safety11.pdf>.

Peplau, H.E. (1952). *Interpersonal Relations in Nursing.* New York: G.P. Putman's Sons.

Ramsden, I. (2002). Cultural safety and nursing education in Aotearoa and Te Waipounamu. Unpublished PhD thesis, Victoria University of Wellington. Viewed 20 August 2012, <http://culturalsafety.massey.ac.nz.

Rapport, N. & Overing, J. (2007). *Social and Cultural Anthropology: the key concepts.* London: Routledge.

Seaton, L. (2010). Cultural care in nursing: a critical analysis. Unpublished PhD thesis, University of Technology Sydney. Viewed 7 August 2012, <http://epress.lib.uts.edu.au/dspace/bitstream/handle/2100/1130/02Whole.pdf?sequence>.

Taylor, K. & Guerin, P. (2010). *Health Care and Indigenous Australians: cultural safety in practice.* Melbourne: Palgrave Macmillan.

Willis, K. & Elmer, S. (2011). *Society, Culture and Health: An introduction to sociology for nurses* (3rd ed.). Melbourne: Oxford University Press.

15

A safe environment

Main points
- A safe environment for mental health care includes legislated occupational health and safety practices, physical, emotional and spiritual safety.
- Protection from harm and responding to issues of sexual and cultural safety require constant vigilance, and are topics for continual practice development.
- The mental health nurse has an important and unique role in managing and creating a therapeutic environment for service user and staff.
- A safe work environment includes ongoing monitoring and management of potential hazards, stress and coping.
- Clinical supervision, mentorship and preceptorship can assist us to reflect on nursing practice and develop professional attributes.

Definitions
Zero tolerance: A non-discretionary or mandatory enforcement policy for violence in the mental health setting.

Harm minimisation: A belief based on the notion that because some people will continue with activities that may cause them harm, reducing harm should take precedence over a prohibition.

Sexual disinhibition: An inability to control or manage sexual urges or impulses.

INTRODUCTION

One of the first things that might come to mind when you think about safety is protection from harm, and it is usually a physical harm that is first envisioned. However, safety in the mental health-care setting is much broader. In addition, safety should imply a protected environment for all persons, not just specific groups. In this chapter, issues of safety such as physical and emotional safety, cultural and sexual safety and therapeutic environments will be discussed. Along the way, tips on how you can create and contribute to a safe environment will be highlighted. This chapter will conclude with an overview and a few ideas for professional development, such as clinical supervision, mentorship and preceptorship.

Throughout this chapter, a case study scenario will be used to describe a multitude of issues relating to a safe environment.

CASE STUDY

Despite almost six months working in the mental health unit, Karli still felt like a 'fish out of water' in some situations. There are now a number of service users on the acute care ward who Karli has come to know quite well; however, some service users continue to avoid her and seek out a more experienced nurse. Yesterday, the afternoon nursing supervisor had asked Karli if she would do an overtime shift. Karli had learnt that doing extra shifts was very tiring, and she now felt more tired than she could remember after completing a sixteen-hour day.

Karli noticed that from 5.00 p.m. all ancillary staff had gone home and the showers in the bathrooms were leaking, making the floors very slippery. The water had even leaked into the hallway, and Karli had sprained her wrist when she fell on the slippery floor. Karli noticed an empty beer bottle in the bathroom as she mopped up the excess water. Someone kept turning up the volume of the cassette recorder in the courtyard, and loud music periodically deafened some of the visitors who were sitting quietly with their family members, which was causing them some concern.

As if things could not get any more disorganised, Karli's second shift developed into a nightmare situation when a young man allegedly attacked an acutely ill young woman of Asian origin in her bedroom. Unfortunately, the young woman spoke very little English and was visibly upset, shaking and crying. It was impossible to determine whether the attack was of a sexual nature or what injuries the young woman might have suffered. Karli wondered how she might get hold of an appropriate interpreter after business hours. The young man was now threatening to set himself alight with a cigarette lighter that he had stolen the day before from a visitor. The fire alarm was triggered and rang out loudly as he waved the open flame over the ceiling sensor.

Karli found that only one other nurse on this particular evening shift had more experience than she did, and she seemed to be busy on the phone with the emergency department, who wanted to send a new person diagnosed with drug-induced psychosis to the ward as soon as possible. On top of the ensuing mayhem, the loud thumping music that continued to play periodically in the courtyard had given Karli a headache that was growing worse by the hour.

SAFETY IN THE MENTAL HEALTH-CARE SETTING
Occupational health and safety

At the centre of all working environments are the health and well-being of people. Therefore, safety in the workplace is about people and their working environment. Quite a lot of mental health nursing care will occur in a health-care facility, so in talking about a work environment, safety will relate to all people within that environment—including health professionals, service user and visitors. Occupational health and safety is defined here as the promotion of health, safety, protection and the prevention of injury and disease in an environment in which people work. The aim of occupational health and safety is to create and maintain a safe environment, and in doing so promote healthy working lifestyles.

Occupational health and safety is developed and regulated through state and federal legislation, and consequently through health-care facility policies, procedures and, ultimately, our activities. While safety is important to the continued well-being of people in all workplaces, it is critical within the mental health-care setting, where physically, emotionally and spiritually vulnerable people may seek refuge and care.

The Commonwealth of Australia determines the federal legislation for occupational health and safety through Comcare, a Commonwealth statutory authority (see <www.comcare.gov.au>). However, each state and territory defines the legislation in relation to its population, environment and current government. For example, the New South Wales *Occupational Health and Safety Act 2011* aims to:

- protect workers and other persons against harm to their health, safety and welfare through the elimination or minimisation of risks arising from work
- provide fair and effective workplace representation, consultation, cooperation and issue resolution in relation to work health and safety
- encourage organisations to take a constructive role in promoting improvements in work health and safety practices
- promote advice, information, education and training
- secure compliance with the legislation through effective and appropriate compliance and enforcement measures

- provide a framework for continuous improvement and progressively higher standards of work health and safety
- facilitate a consistent national approach to work health and safety (see <www.work cover.nsw.gov.au>).

There are a number of occupational health and safety issues that may be of concern to everyone within the mental health-care setting, including noise, manual handling, licensing, workplace substances, hazardous substances, smoke and workplace stress.

The mental health-care setting has specific requirements within occupational health and safety. Overall, there is a need to feel safe at work as well as a need to feel safe in being cared for in or when visiting the mental health-care facility. The issues most likely to lead to feeling safe in the mental health-care setting include:

- confidence in the ability to work with aggression and violence
- protecting others—physically, psychologically and spiritually
- knowledge, skills and experience
- use of teamwork and staffing numbers
- organisational supports and resources, including appropriate policies and protocols.

PHYSICAL AND EMOTIONAL SAFETY
Sexual safety

In Chapter 10 we discussed the value of good sexual relations. An emerging issue in the mental health-care setting, and one that specifically relates to our discussion on the broad aspects of safety, is that of sexual safety. This is defined as the recognition, maintenance and mutual respect of the boundaries between people. Boundaries may be physical, psychological, emotional and spiritual. The position of state Health Departments around Australia is that 'sexual activity is unacceptable' in acute mental health facilities (NSW Health 2005, p. 2).

The broad aims of public mental health services in relation to sexual safety are to:

- provide mental health service providers in all settings with precise guidance and advice on their responsibilities for sexual safety
- provide ongoing policy directions and practical advice
- promote awareness and importance of sexual safety
- provide service user, families and carers with information regarding rights and obligations in relation to the sexual safety of service user
- improve collaboration and strengthen relationships between mental health services and sexual assault services (adapted from NSW Health 2011c; Department of Health, Victoria 2009).

In order to discuss sexual safety, it is useful to first define and discuss what sexual assault is. We can define this type of assault as one where the actions of a person (of any gender) coerce, threaten or force another person (of any gender) into sexual acts against their will. A broader definition of sexual assault from the Australian Centre for the Study of Sexual Assault states that 'sexual assault includes any unwanted sexual behaviour that makes a person feel fearful, uncomfortable or threatened. It includes any sexual activity that a person has not freely agreed to' (<www.aifs.gov.au/acssa>).

Looking back at the chapter case study, Karli was concerned that a young Asian woman may have been sexually assaulted, but initially was unable to determine what had occurred. Sexual assaults that occur in mental health services may be committed by other service users, mental health professionals, visitors or even members of the public (Frisch & Frisch 2010). It is important to remember that sexual assault is an illegal act in any context, and police reporting, attendance and criminal charges may be necessary in some circumstances.

Sexual disinhibition

Unfortunately, sexual assault is not uncommon in the community. In mental health care facilities, sexual disinhibition may occur as a part of mental illness and treatment, instead of being a deliberate act. Therefore, it is important to make the distinction between predatory and calculated criminal behaviour and the actions of someone who is temporarily unable to control their impulses and behaviour. However, this does not necessarily diminish the impact such behaviour may have on the person and/or others.

Sometimes sexually disinhibited behaviour may be a side-effect of medication in a similar manner to the disinhibited behaviour of a person who has drunk too much alcohol. Although such behaviour, talk and impulse may be out of character for a person when well, the person may be unable to restrain themself, and could get involved in sexual activities to which they are not able to give or receive consent. These are often delicate situations, in that while one person is vulnerable, another person may take deliberate advantage of the situation by targeting the vulnerable person because of their uncontrolled sexual disinhibition.

The victim of sexual assault can be anyone, regardless of gender, age or occupation (Savino & Turvey 2011). The mental health-care environment can contain vulnerable people—staff included. Not understanding what constitutes sexual assault, or being unable to access help, causes the cycle of vulnerability to continue. For these and other reasons, it is not unusual for some people not to report sexual assault events, or to report them well after the event has passed.

There are many reasons for the non-reporting of sexual assault, but one factor that stands out for mental health service users is a fear of not being believed. The issue of being believed is linked with reporting of sexual assault generally, but you can imagine that for people who may be hospitalised because of a perceived loss of touch with reality, the assumption of not being believed may well contribute to people not reporting. For this reason, it is critical to listen to and consider what is said.

It is also important to reflect on the potential power imbalance within health-care settings, and to actively address this through good policy and procedures. Persons in positions of power, such as mental health professionals, may knowingly or even unwittingly make disclosure of sexual assault difficult for the service user and/or may even be the cause of the assault. For example, in the chapter scenario, Karli worried that she could not easily determine the nature of the attack on the female service user. However, Karli was already planning on how to assist the service user by accessing interpreter services. Disclosure is also more difficult for those people who are historically disempowered and marginalised, such as women, persons from diverse cultural backgrounds and Indigenous people, because of potential barriers such as language, lifestyle, stereotypes and stigma.

Effective response to sexual assault

- Mental health services have a duty to protect the rights and needs of an individual disclosing sexual assault. This includes believing and listening to what is said, and providing information on an individual's rights.
- Sexual assault is a criminal offence; therefore, for the protection of all concerned, all reports should be investigated and followed up.
- On suspicion that a sexual assault has occurred, senior management must be notified immediately. Senior management is then responsible for coordinating the immediate and ongoing response to the situation; mental health services must contact and consult the local sexual assault service.
- Re-establishing safety is of paramount importance for the victim, other service users and staff. The alleged perpetrator should be separated from the victim.
- Keep notes only of what is actually said, heard and observed. Terms, language (such as jargon and sexually explicit comments) and conjecture, which may be open to different interpretations, are to be avoided.
- Inter-agency meetings between mental health services, the local sexual assault services and the police (where applicable) should be held in the event of a report of sexual assault.
- Incidents of sexual assault should be subject to a critical incidents/sentinel events review. A collaborative management plan for follow up with victims of sexual assault must be in effect.
- Information and resources should be readily available, including pamphlets outlining procedures for complaint and redress, and information on where to find appropriate counselling and legal assistance. These resources should be visible to staff and service users, and available in different community languages (adapted from NSW Health 2005, p. 3; <www.health.vic.gov.au/mentalhealth/cpg>).

Table 15.1 Interventions for sexual assault

Risk assessment	While initial and ongoing risk assessment for aggression, violence, self-harm and suicide should be part of all mental health nursing practice, this must also include an assessment of the potential for sexual assault, as well as vulnerability to sexual assault. The prevention of sexual assaults will depend on how well the risk assessment is managed, and how often it is updated. Aim to be constantly aware of factors that may increase sexual vulnerability and changes that may increase sexual disinhibition.
Environmental management in mental health	Vulnerable people should not be placed in environments that are conducive to the predatory or disinhibited actions of others. The privacy and safety of single bedrooms and proximity to nursing care facility staff must be considered, as well as careful observation and working accessible alarm systems. For those who pose a risk of committing sexual assault intentionally or unintentionally, security such as increased presence of people in communal areas, sensor detectors and cameras, close observation and engagement in activities to discourage predatory thoughts and action may be utilised. Use of lighting and monitoring of the therapeutic environment can assist all clientele.
Promoting safety	Prevention of sexual assault in any form is the goal, and this can be achieved by promoting sexual safety through good and, if necessary, assertive communication; promoting respect for people's boundaries and supporting rights to sexual safety; creation and ongoing development of workable facility policies and procedures; swift, caring, supportive and appropriate interventions for any breaches in sexual safety and ongoing staff education.
Ongoing education and assessment of service	Facility-wide information on prevention and reporting must be made available to anyone who enters the mental health-care facility. All mental health staff should avail themselves of ongoing education and training to prevent, manage and resolve incidents and be up to date with the chain of reporting and outcomes of sexual assault. Detection, assessment and awareness education should be a regular part of all professional development programs.

Other resources on sexual safety you may wish to access include:

- the Victorian Women and Mental Health Network
- the Australian Government's Office for Women
- the Queensland Government's Queensland Health Adult Sexual Health
- the Western Australian Government's Department of Health—Sexual Health.

CULTURAL SAFETY

Vulnerability can occur on many fronts in mental health care, and the subject of cultural safety was discussed in Chapter 14. The following discussion summarises these points from the perspective of a safe environment as well as considering the topic of occupational health and safety.

As stated, a person's culture is an important area where the individual or group can feel unsafe. McEldowney and Connor (2011) claim cultural safety occurs when a nurse is aware and respectful of a person's unique cultural entity, and consciously sets about nurturing the service user's needs, expectations and rights within that understanding of their cultural awareness. In the chapter scenario, Karli's first thought when confronted with a crying and shaking young Asian woman was worry about the language barrier. Considerations of what an attack by a young male meant to this young Asian woman will involve understanding and awareness of her cultural entity, and therefore is much more than a language barrier.

Recognition of and reflection upon our own cultural identity can assist in understanding and managing the effect of personal culture on nursing practice (Holland & Hogg 2010). Nursing actions that are demeaning or disempowering, or that diminish the cultural identity—and therefore the well-being— of an individual must be avoided. However, it is important to realise here that the area of mental health care in itself is a culture with a long history of stereotyping and poor community relations.

Being sensitive about a person's culture is just one part of cultural safety. You can develop a culturally safe approach in your nursing care by:

- reflecting, exploring and examining your cultural realities and attitudes
- using a flexible and open-minded approach in your attitudes towards people from cultures other than your own
- being aware of any health problems that are within the cultural context of historical and social processes for the individual.

ZERO TOLERANCE AND HARM MINIMISATION

In recent years, a number of policies have been developed that indirectly relate to occupational safety and safety in the health-care setting. These include zero tolerance and harm minimisation.

'Zero tolerance' is a term that has been recently associated with mental health-care policy directions, and is relevant to safety and any discussion of violence and aggression and substance abuse. It is defined here as a mandatory or enforceable policy by persons in positions of authority against specific offences or rule-breaking (Bruce & Nowlin 2011). Zero tolerance allows for the enforcement of predetermined punishment, irrespective of individual mitigating circumstances.

There are several situations where you might consider the idea of zero tolerance to be appropriate to prevent even more predatory dangerous behaviours. These might include driving under the influence of alcohol, violence against health-care staff and service users, sexual harassment, sexual assault (child and adult), child pornography, bullying, terrorism and threats (including stalking). Sometimes, however, zero-tolerance policies can have unintended and potentially ambiguous effects that may not provide equity to all, and this is worth careful consideration. For example, in the chapter scenario Karli found an empty beer bottle in the bathroom. The ward in which Karli is working may have a policy of zero tolerance for alcohol and illicit drug use. Karli may spend considerable time in attempting to track down the source of the bottle, only to find that the cleaner had found it outside the ward and had forgotten to dispose of it appropriately before leaving for the day.

The Health Departments of all states and territories in Australia support the goals of zero tolerance to violence in the health-care workplace. For example, in 2003 a mandatory policy for zero tolerance response to violence in the workplace was developed, which was last updated in 2011 (NSW Health 2011b). This policy applies to all persons working or being cared for in the New South Wales health-care system, and is aimed at preventing and managing violence in the workplace. The purpose of this and other state-based policy directives is to 'ensure that in all violent incidents, appropriate action is consistently taken to protect health service staff, patients and visitors and health service property from the effects of violent behaviour' (NSW Health 2011b). For another example of policy produced and provided by state health see NSW Health (2011a).

CRITICAL THINKING

- What are the policies or protocols in your state or territory health service regarding issues such as the beer bottle that Karli found in the bathroom?
- How would you handle this situation?

A quick zero tolerance checklist

- Is there a written policy on zero tolerance in your workplace?
- Do you have access to it and have you read it?
- Is it appropriately supported by other violence-control strategies?
- Is the zero tolerance message clearly displayed in relevant areas such as admissions areas and emergency departments?
- Is there documentation that clearly outlines patient and visitor behavioural requirements, and is this documentation provided to all people, including those receiving care in the community?

- Do all staff, including community health staff, have ready access to a simple violence incident report form?
- Are all staff trained in the reporting procedure and encouraged to report all violent incidents?
- Are all assaults reported to police?
- Are all staff who have been identified as being at risk of violence provided with violence-minimisation and management training?
- Do all staff, including community health staff, have access to urgent assistance in the event of a violence-related emergency?
- Are there guidelines in place for the prevention and management of workplace bullying, and are staff aware of these guidelines?
- Is there a patient alert system in place?
- Are there procedures in place to ensure that file flags are regularly reviewed for relevance, and do all flagged files include an up-to-date management plan? (Adapted from NSW Health 2011b, p. 52)

The current focus of workplace violence prevention centres on the individual 'pathology' of the service user—or, in the case of workplace bullying, the abusive staff member. Thus, in mental health services, we talk of 'aggression management'. However, mounting evidence from health services across Australia and the United Kingdom suggests that the focus should instead be on organisational culture and management style, as these are the key factors that trigger workplace violence (Cleary, Hunt & Horsfall 2010). For example, to speak of 'conflict management' rather than 'aggression management' acknowledges the fact that conflict occurs between people for a host of reasons, and can be attributed to a range of environmental and attitudinal factors. To reconceptualise in this way is to invite a whole-of-organisation response rather than tending to locate problems within individuals.

There is a link between what appears to be increases in individual and group workplace violence and organisational factors, and the potential for these to trigger 'pathological' or criminal behaviour. The future aims in workplace violence are for the development of non-violent organisational structures and management styles. Each health-care facility adopts and continues to develop policy guidelines to enact these policy directives, and it is important for you to take some time in any new work environment to familiarise yourself with these.

Harm minimisation is a strategy adopted by the federal government for its National Drug Strategy policy and direction statements (see <www.health.gov.au>). It is worth briefly defining and discussing this strategy here, as it relates to zero tolerance and safety in the health-care workplace. In the early 1980s, the Australian government adopted the harm-minimisation strategy. The purpose of this strategy was to assist in limiting alcohol and drug abuse. The aim is to reduce supply and demand of illicit drugs and to minimise the harms that are associated with the use of alcohol and drugs in our communities. Harm minimisation is composed of three major strategies: supply reduction, demand reduction and harm reduction.

This strategy has an appeal for behaviours and actions that, while not criminal in type, can lead to self-destruction if not controlled. This includes actions that are unlikely to cease even during periods of prohibition or government control. Examples of harm-minimisation programs may include:

- reduced alcohol drinks such as light beer and light coolers, alcohol-free venues and alcohol-restricted events
- safe sex education and access to counsellors in schools, community information services and at tertiary institutions
- condom use for the prevention of HIV, hepatitis C and STDs made available through vending machines, and easy access to condoms through assorted shopping venues such as supermarkets and local stores instead of just through pharmacies
- methadone maintenance programs to assist opiate-dependent (for example, heroin) people, made available through local health services
- clean needle and syringe exchange programs made available in local communities and through area health clinics.

The underlying message of harm minimisation is that the use of illicit drugs and the misuse of legal drugs can be controlled by learning to use them responsibly and safely. Some people may argue that the drug itself, through tolerance and dependence, will make the user lose control, and so responsible and safe use and behaviour cannot occur. Others may claim that it is poor clinical judgement to think that people (particularly young people) will be deterred from using both illicit and misused legal drugs if they are told they can use them safely or responsibly.

CREATING A THERAPEUTIC ENVIRONMENT FOR SERVICE USER AND STAFF

As nurses, we can manipulate or shape an environment so that it is geared specifically towards mental well-being and safety. Therapeutic environments in mental health care are an important safety intervention. The idea of a safe, caring and health-promoting environment is not new. Terms often associated with therapeutic environments include 'therapeutic milieu', 'milieu therapy' and 'therapeutic community'. All terms except 'therapeutic community' describe or refer to an environment 'designed to meet the emotional and interpersonal needs of clients, help them control problematic behaviour, and assist them in the development of coping skills' (Shives 2012, p. 154). One obvious difference between a therapeutic environment or therapeutic milieu and the therapeutic community is that the former is likely to be hierarchical, based as it is on the medical model, while the latter describes a more collaborative and integrated approach.

A therapeutic community is a particular form of society where the emphasis is on the psycho-social interplays—that is, social and interpersonal relationships. Media portrayals of seedy, unclean facilities run by uncaring, cruel custodial staff from the 1950s to 1970s helped to trigger the broader community's interest in providing better environments and just care for people with a mental illness. The principles of the therapeutic community are balancing the social, psychological and physical needs of people (Mistral, Hall & McKee 2002).

The concept of the consumer actively participating and reciprocating in individual treatment within the mental health-care setting helps to define the term 'milieu therapy'. This term has slowly faded from use in Australia, but the principle continues. You will find that mental health-care textbooks alternate between the terms 'milieu therapy' and 'therapeutic milieu' in a rather confusing manner. What is important, and at the heart of the shifting terminology, is the continuing concept of social solidarity (Carter 1981), as opposed to authoritarianism (such as can be found in medical model hierarchies), in an environment that offers safety, security and consideration of cultural entity.

Safe therapeutic environments and therapeutic milieu should address all of the following:

- They should be purposeful and planned to provide safety from physical danger and emotional trauma. There should be furniture to facilitate a homelike atmosphere, privacy, provisions for physical needs and opportunities for interaction and communication among patients and personnel.
- They should provide a testing ground for new patterns of behaviour, while the consumer takes responsibility for their actions. Behavioural expectations should be explained, including the existing rules, regulations and policies.
- It is important to be consistent when setting limits. This criterion reflects aspects of a democratic society. All people are treated as equally as possible, with respect to restrictions, rules and policies.
- It is vital to encourage participation in group activities and free-flowing communication in which a person has the freedom to express themself in a socially acceptable manner.
- It is important to respect the person and treat them with dignity. Adult-to-adult interactions should prevail, promoting equal status of interactions and exchange of interpersonal information and avoiding any power plays. The person should be encouraged to use personal resources to resolve problems or conflicts.
- An attitude of overall acceptance and optimism should be conveyed. Conflict between staff members must be handled and resolved in some manner, in order to maintain a therapeutic environment.
- It is important to continually assess and evaluate the service user's progress, modifying treatment and nursing interventions as needed. (Adapted from Shives 2012, Chapter 11)

Once, when large, sprawling mental institutions were situated around Australian major cities and 1000-bed facilities were not unusual, the control of the environment was very much the domain of the mental health nurse (Carter 1981). The landscape of mental health-care provision has changed greatly since this time, however, and small acute units attached to large general hospitals now dominate mental health care. The rise of individual mental health units within the confines of the general health system (often large public hospitals) means that nurses now have less control over the environment than previously. Under the structure of the general hospital, the mental health unit has become similar to that of its parent facility and often follows the Medical Model of the mainstream hospital. Mental health-care facilities designed more recently are purpose-built to state and federal Health Department specifications. An example of state policy directions to promote safety issues is as follows:

> All planned new mental health units must have single bedroom accommodation available, with access to en suites. Rooms should be arranged into clusters, which are capable of being separated to provide secure and separate space for males and females. Where possible, existing units should provide areas of single sex accommodation and gender specific toilets and bathrooms. (NSW Health 2005, p. 12)

One of the outcomes of this shift in organisational control was the loss of nursing influence on the mental health-care environment. Possibly due to the Medical Model's over-arching influence, nurses may no longer find themselves in as strong a position to encourage a therapeutic environment. Rather, they may be in a position of responding to more custodial care. Nurses may consequently leave therapeutic interventions to associated groups such as occupational therapists, diversional therapists, psychologists and social workers, depending on the resources available.

CRITICAL THINKING

Looking back at the case study and your considerations of what makes for a therapeutic environment, what could Karli do to improve the environment during her double shift?

- How would you manage the loud music and the flow of people in and around the bedroom areas?
- What ideas do you have that might improve visitor contact with the service users in this unit?
- In your understanding, who is now responsible for the therapeutic environment in which Karli is working?

An example of the adjustment in role perception is evident in the following extract. The Treatment Protocol Project (2004) acknowledged difficulty in defining the construct of therapeutic environment in that there is a lack of agreement and boundaries regarding this term.

It has been suggested that, rather than continue to invest in a concept (therapeutic environment) with obvious difficulties, health professionals should focus explicitly on explaining the clinical functions of in-patient treatment and their role in providing these functions. For in-patient psychiatric care, clinical functions include:

- assuring the patients' safety
- providing the structure needed to facilitate patients' self-care
- planning for discharge and future support needs
- instituting measures aimed at symptom management (Treatment Protocol Project 2004).

NURSE AS ENVIRONMENTAL MANAGER

Environmental factors can contribute to aggression and, in turn, fearful staff and service users will often distance themselves from therapeutic relationships (Dean et al. 2010). Nurses who feel unsafe in their workplace may lack confidence, which can also decrease therapeutic interactions and ultimately lower the quality of nursing care. Environmental issues of safety may include the care setting, such as:

- ward layout
- bed spacing
- overcrowding
- poor sleeping environment
- lack of quiet areas, including family and visitor space
- lack of personal space, privacy and space for personal belongings
- lack of diurnal light changes (via windows, etc.)
- lack of sunlight and fresh air
- lack of security
- excessive air-conditioning
- smoke-filled air
- excessively noisy areas
- pest infestations and damp, dusty, dirty areas
- lack of access, such as stairs, walkways, ramps, handrails, wheelchair access.

Alternatively, environmental factors can contribute to mental health. For example, a calming and low-stimulus environment can assist the person diagnosed with a mood disorder—mania—to relax, slow down and even get some much-needed sleep. Other issues that can promote safety and mental health care include the following:

- clean, comfortable and cared-for surroundings that promote a home-like environment
- use of soothing colour schemes, pictures and decorations
- freedom of movement throughout the facility where possible
- emphasis on family interactions, education and access
- emphasis on respect, collegiality and courtesy in all interactions.

Close observation can present an ideal opportunity to further develop a therapeutic relationship and alliance. However, while perhaps necessary for the ongoing safety of individuals and others, close observation needs to be sensitively and carefully managed by the nurse as a significant safety issue. We may take for granted personal privacy, freedom and personal space. The sudden loss of this can be disconcerting to the consumer at best, and a trigger for aggression at worst. It is important to keep the client informed and reassured of the purpose, timeframe and level of observation while being sensitive to cultural and gender issues at all times.

STRESS AND COPING

Those famous words from the Bible, 'Physician, heal thyself' (Luke 4:23), are critical in the assessment, intervention and management of stress. Without first having dealt with our own stress, it may be impossible to assist someone else. Equally, a safe environment is also one in which stress is recognised and managed.

Workplace stress can occur when physical, emotional, social, spiritual and economic forces are no longer able to be managed by the individual. These might cause conflict and/or a loss of control from a single or multiple events, and may be from single or multiple origins. Stress may manifest as increases in physiological events such as raised blood pressure, pulse and respiration, as well as psychological events such as distress, irritability, panic, inability to concentrate, anger, frustration and labile (rapidly changing) moods.

Through assessing numerous incidents of workplace stress (Happell et al. 2013; Mark & Smith 2012; Ward 2011), researchers have determined that this type of safety issue can progress from early warnings such as increased anxiety and emotional fatigue to sleep disturbances, immune system degradation, depression and withdrawal from colleagues and service users.

In its most severe form, workplace stress can be life threatening, through self-destructive actions, including suicide and homicide. Urgent interventions are required here; however, consider that it may take more than five years for workplace stress to progress to this state. In the United States, the phrase 'going postal' has come to represent the self-destructive potential outcome of chronic and unrelieved workplace stress. The term has come to be used for events where a worker or ex-worker has become extremely angry and loses control to the point of homicidal and suicidal violence after having worked for the US Postal Service. At best, a career is ended, but at worst ongoing uncontrollable rage, grief and homicidal/suicidal events can occur.

Dealing with workplace stress involves implementing strategies aimed at reduction and prevention. These might include task variety, task ownership, collegial and professional support systems and environmental controls. Individually, stress-proofing might include using humour and relaxing (physically, emotionally and mentally), limiting working hours by decreasing overtime and making sure there are more than eight hours between shifts, and talking to your nurse manager or supervisor. In the case study scenario, Karli may have been advised not to take on any overtime until such time as she had looked through her current work and life commitments and had established a work–life balance.

Table 15.2 Ten general tips for reducing stress and improving coping

1	Build self-confidence	Identify and recognise your abilities and weaknesses together, accept them, build on the strengths and where possible overcome the weaknesses, and then do your best with what you have.
2	Eat right, keep fit and rest well	A balanced diet, exercise and appropriate rest will help you to reduce stress and enjoy a healthy life.
3	Ensure time for family and friends	Your relationships need time and effort to be nurtured. If family and friends are taken for granted, they may not be there to share good times and be supportive in difficult times.
4	Give and receive support	Family and friends give and take as relationships develop, and you can unite in times of need.
5	Create a workable budget	Financial problems cause stress and increase anxiety. Over-spending on wants rather than needs may be a source of unnecessary stress. Utilise financial advice where it is warranted.
6	Volunteer	Join an organisation—by being involved in your community, you can gain a sense of belonging, purpose and satisfaction.
7	Manage your stress	Everyone has stressors in life, but learning how to deal with them now when they threaten to overwhelm us helps to maintain our mental health.
8	Find strength in numbers	By sharing a problem with others— particularly those who have had similar experiences—you may find a solution and will feel less isolated.
9	Recognise and deal with moods	Search and use safe and constructive ways to express feelings of anger, sadness, joy and fear.
10	Practise being at peace	Get to know who you are and what makes you really happy, and learn to balance what you can and cannot change about yourself.

Source: Adapted from Canadian Mental Health Association—National Office, <www.cmha.ca>.

Workplace stress is an increasingly common phenomenon that can have enormous implications in the mental health-care setting, where mental health is the priority. Looking out for each other is a great beginning when it comes to managing this potential issue.

PROFESSIONAL DEVELOPMENT
Reflection on practice
The broad aim of reflecting on our nursing practice (reflective practice, or RP) is to explore and improve what we do, thereby making continual changes to our nursing practice (Nelson 2012). As you will have determined throughout your nursing education—both clinically and theoretically—RP is currently very popular. Most nursing education aims to 'encourage both student and registered nurses to analyse and contemplate their practice by embracing the notion of critical reflection' (Nairn et al. 2012, p. 190). The general principles for reflection on nursing practice include:

- observing our thoughts and feelings
- critically thinking about our nursing practice
- creating new practice from thinking about our previous practice.

Reflective practice can assist you to increase your professional development, connect theory with your nursing practice, increase your critical thinking and refine your self-awareness and understanding (Lethbridge et al. 2011). All of these can lead to empowerment and improved mental health-care outcomes.

There are potential pitfalls to avoid in the use of RP, such as confusion, marginalising and distancing ourselves from those outside the group (these being service users and carers in the case of mental health care). So it is important in our reflections to take 'an inclusive view of diverse perspectives' to maximise the benefits of RP (Cotton 2001, p. 518).

The greatest benefits of RP are in the areas of ethical and holistic nursing care (Gustafsson, Asp & Fagerberg 2007) and, as you have seen from previous chapters, these areas are of critical importance to good mental health nursing practice. Reflective practice can help you to focus on specific details, such as 'How can I empower, support, collaborate, share and develop my relationships with the service user?' By focusing RP in this way, and by aiming to improve our ethical and holistic practices, we can continually improve our nursing care.

CLINICAL SUPERVISION
Clinical supervision in mental health care has become an extremely popular topic in recent years. What does it entail and how does a nurse know whether the clinical supervision being received is appropriate, useful and warranted? In this section, we will

> **CRITICAL THINKING**
>
> - How can Karli utilise the principles of reflective practice to improve her current practices?
> - In what ways could anxiety and poor recollection of events (hindsight bias) affect Karli's reflection on her practice and detract from her professional development?

explore models of clinical supervision that may be most useful in the current mental health-care workplace. Hancox & Lynch (2002, p. 6) define clinical supervision as 'a formal process of consultation between two or more professionals. The focus is to provide support for the supervisee(s) in order to promote self awareness, development and growth within the context of their professional development.'

Clinical supervision can provide a system for identifying answers to difficulties in nursing care provision, raise understanding of nursing and improve our nursing practice and nursing environment (Koivu, Hyrkäs & Saarinen 2011). Psychoanalytical processes (see Chapter 13) provide the underlying theoretical frameworks for the development of all clinical supervision models and practices. In summary, the aims of psychoanalysis are to uncover and explore issues by reflecting and analysing. A reasonably broad definition for use here comes from Hancox and Lynch (2002, p. 6, cited in Lynch et al. 2008, p. 19), and is likely to apply to most nursing clinical supervision. Hancox and Lynch state that:

> Clinical supervision is a formal process of consultation between two or more professionals. The focus is to provide support for the supervisee(s) in order to promote self awareness, professional development and growth within the context of their professional environment.

Clinical supervision became popular in the mental health field in the 1960s, and was incorporated into the training schedule for psychiatrists (MacDonald & Ellis 2012). The supervision was predominantly written and taught by doctors for doctors, and contained a large psychoanalytic component (MacDonald & Ellis 2012). At the time, supervision was not well received outside of psychiatry; however, it is difficult to determine whether this was because of the amount of clinical supervision that doctors undertook or due to the experience of clinical supervision.

Clinical supervision is not therapy for nurses, although there are considerable gains to be made by utilising clinical supervision in mental health nursing. Increases in job satisfaction and decreases in the effects of burnout are two frequently cited professional effects (Taylor & Harrison 2010). In terms of providing high-quality nursing care to service user and carers, the effects of clinical supervision are clear. Clinical supervision can offer the nurse:

- a protected learning environment
- peer support
- confidence-building
- reflective practice
- professional nursing development
- a framework for change to nursing practice
- shared information
- raised awareness, insight and autonomy
- refined interpersonal skills
- reduction in nursing stress
- identification of possible solutions.

The advantages for using clinical supervision specifically for mental health nurses are that it:

- emphasises the clinical aspects of mental health nursing
- helps mental health nurses to assess training and research needs
- encourages the recognition and appreciation of the individual consumer and their social situation
- examines the multidisciplinary contribution to comprehensive care
- identifies and develops innovative practice
- creates an ethos that fosters staff retention and morale
- promotes links between research and clinical practice.

On the negative side, there are a number of reasons put forward by authors, researchers and nurse participants for non-involvement in clinical supervision (Koivu, Hyrkäs & Saarinen 2011). These include the following:

- a similar scheme already functioning in the workplace
- good peer support already being available.
- a lack of time
- a lack of knowledge about clinical supervision
- confidentiality and anonymity concerns
- a lack of continuity of supervision
- misinterpretation as a therapy.

Clinical supervision can be assessed for both structural and quality aspects. These include the amount of supervision, punctuality and reliability, availability, constructive critical feedback, encouragement, educational value, and clinical guidance and support. Other assessment points are explained by Lynch et al. (2008) as a safe supportive environment, enhancing critical evaluation of practice, raised professional understandings, identification of solutions to problems and overall improvement in practice. Outcomes of clinical supervision may be assessed as personal or organisational. Outcomes of a personal nature may include raised self-esteem and self-confidence, increased enthusiasm and an increased sense of coping. Organisational outcomes could include collegiality, increased staff morale and improved interpersonal relationships.

MODELS OF SUPERVISION

Clinical supervision is in fact an 'umbrella term' meaning that a wide variety of models and structures are used to provide clinical supervision (McKenna et al. 2010). A model needs to describe the function of the role of clinical supervision, identify the components in the supervisory relationship and outline the process of the relationship. Clinical supervision models and structures fall into three broad categories: the supervisory relationship type, the descriptive function of clinical supervision role and the process of supervisory relationship (Lynch et al. 2008). The areas within models most attractive to nursing thus far are those containing normative aims, formative aims and restorative aims, such as the seven tasks model shown in Figure 15.1.

Individual or group supervision

Just as there are many different models of supervision, there are a number of ways to approach clinical supervision for nurses. These can include individual or group supervision, supervision via video teleconferencing and online supervision. Before beginning clinical supervision, there are a number of possible advantages and disadvantages for the individual or group to consider regarding the use of clinical supervision. These issues have been outlined by Van Ooijen (2000, p. 12), and are listed in Table 15.3.

CRITICAL THINKING

Imagine that you are Karli, and that two days after the shift described in the chapter scenario you are to meet with your clinical supervisor.

- What might you especially want to discuss in the session?
- How will clinical supervision assist you to make sense of the shift and reflect on ways that you may have supported and guided service users in your care?
- What effect might clinical supervision have on your reaction and management of the young female service user who was very distressed, or on the occupational health and safety issues encountered throughout the scenario?

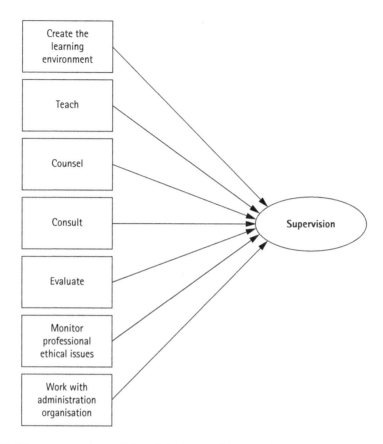

Figure 15.1 The seven tasks model: a clinical supervision model

Source: Holloway & Carroll (1999, p. 76).

Mentorship and preceptorship

The early stages of the transition year for the new graduate nurse may be fraught with situations in which the nurse may suffer from a lack of confidence, a feeling of being lost and tired, and stress over the new position. In the chapter scenario, Karli was no longer a newcomer to the mental health workplace; however, she was still developing her skills at establishing therapeutic relationships with the service users. The use of a nurse mentor can greatly assist the new nurse in developing confidence and in melding the theory and practice of nursing in mental health-care settings.

A mentor is defined as a person who can provide support, guidance, coaching and role modelling to the new nurse (Smith, McAllister & Crawford 2002). Mentorship is more often associated with formal, long-term relationships, and can be an effective means of increasing the retention of 'highly skilled nurses' within an organisation

Table 15.3 Advantages and disadvantages of individual and group clinical supervision

Individual clinical supervision

Advantages	Disadvantages
There is less likelihood of breaching confidentiality.	There may be prohibitive expenses in time and resources.
People tend to feel more comfortable in one-to-one situations.	Room for advancement and change may be overlooked because of the development of unwitting collusion between the supervisor and supervisee.
Issues may be discussed in greater depth and focus.	Problematic issues might be overlooked.
There is a greater opportunity to develop a strong rapport that involves ongoing development, honesty and trust in a one-to-one situation	The focus may dwell on fringe or unhelpful issues relating to the supervisor rather than the supervisee.
	Mutual appreciation may stifle ongoing development.
	Issues of a difficult nature may overwhelm the supervisor without a collegial outlet.

Group clinical supervision

Advantages	Disadvantages
There is more economical use of time, personnel and resources.	There may not be sufficient time to address each individual's needs.
Where commonality in themes occur, isolated thoughts and feelings tend to disappear.	Some group members may be overwhelmed and/or intimidated by more vocal members.
A learning environment is inclusive for all group members (good for inexperienced supervisors).	The dynamics of the group may not be conducive to clinical supervision (obstructional, non-reflective, lacking vision for change, destructive, scapegoating, competitive, overly challenging, obsessive with own dynamics).
A greater range of gender, socio-economic, life, career and professional experiences may stimulate greater discussion and discovery.	The group may consciously or unconsciously intimidate individual members.
A group situation can lend itself to role-play and other techniques for explaining circumstances and exploring strategies for interventions.	The sharing of personal attributes and/or deficiencies may raise excessive anxieties in some people being supervised.
	Honesty, trust, privacy and confidentiality may be problematic.

(Tourigny 2005, p. 68). The mentor relationship is often a longer-term relationship (three to six years) and the nurse being mentored may be given a choice of mentors who are suitable to their professional goals and aspirations. Preceptorship, however, is most often short-term and is a skills-based relationship where the assignation of the preceptor to the preceptee is often predetermined by expressed interest from the experienced preceptor nurse and by roster availability, rather than any attempt to match personality or other individual traits (Smedley, Morey & Race 2010; Firtko et al. 2005).

The benefits of having a mentor are considerable in terms of putting knowledge into practice, making friends and gaining an understanding of the workplace, as well as for thinking about career directions (Barker 2006). Nurse mentors are clinically competent and confident experienced nurses who are able to forge a valuable relationship with the new nurse, and thereby ease the passage from novice to a more proficient and professionally socialised nurse.

Unfortunately, Karli found herself on a shift where only one other nurse was more experienced in mental health care than she was. Low staffing levels and the growing use of agency and casual nursing staff may make this a reality on occasions. Although the mentor is an important asset, the process can be emotionally and physically draining, and can require a significant investment in the role (Veeramah 2012). Current workloads and skill base of our experienced nursing workforce may not be supportive of the mentor role; consequently, relatively new nurses such as Karli may reassess their role in mental health care.

The terms 'mentor' and 'preceptor' are often used interchangeably by nurses, but these roles are quite different. A preceptor is defined here as a teacher–student, task-oriented role that is time-limited and formal in structure and supervision (Lynch et al. 2008, p. 15). The provision of a preceptor is linked with successfully traversing the transition into a new workplace by nursing researchers (Kantar 2012) and 'new staff members expressed anger and frustration when an effective preceptor relationship was not developed' (Fox, Henderson & Malko-Nyhan 2005, p. 197).

Preceptorship increasingly is found to be a useful strategy for clinical education and applying theory to nursing practice (Burns et al. 2006). Not only can the nurse preceptor assist the new nurse with how to start using what they have learnt, but they can also act as an incentive to stay in the workplace. Effective preceptorship requires dedicated time, assistance in workload management, designation of space, monetary remuneration for preceptorship, preparation for the preceptor role, issues within the structure of a one-to-one relationship and a learning environment. Looking back at the scenario, would Karli have benefited from a mentor and/or a preceptor, or simply a more appropriate skill mix in the rostering system?

Clinical supervision should not be confused with mentorship or preceptorship. They are different, and are utilised for different purposes (often for new graduates or registered nurses and for those returning to the workplace after a substantial break). Table 15.4 highlights some important differences between mentor/preceptorship and clinical supervision.

Table 15.4 Linking mentorship, preceptorship and clinical supervision

Stages of professional development →	Undergraduate nursing students	Period of preceptorship following qualification	Primary practice	Advanced practice
Needs from mentors and supervisors	Mentorship and clinical teaching	Preceptorship and clinical supervision	Clinical supervision	
Providers of mentorship, preceptorship and clinical supervision	Clinical staff, mentors, educators	Experienced nurses, managers	Registered nurse, clinical nurse specialist, clinical nurse consultants, nurse practitioners	
Methods of provision	1 peer group support 2 group supervision 3 network supervision			

Source: Adapted from Butterworth, Faugier & Burnard (1998, p. 218).

CONCLUSION

A safe environment for mental health care is an important prerequisite to developing interpersonal and therapeutic relationships, leading to good nursing care outcomes. This chapter has explored a number of historical and contemporary categories, such as physical and emotional safety, zero tolerance and harm minimisation. How we create a therapeutic environment where people can feel safe and supported is outlined in our discussions of therapeutic settings. Discussions on managing the mental health-care environment were followed by sections on managing stress, coping and professional development such as clinical supervision, mentoring and preceptoring. This chapter concludes with the hope that, now you have read these explorations, your graduate nurse experiences in mental health care (if you choose to practise in this field) will avoid some of the difficulties experienced by Karli in the case study scenario.

REFERENCES

Barker, E.R. (2006). Mentoring: a complex relationship. *Journal of the American Academy of Nurse Practitioners*, 18, 56–61.

Bruce, M.D. &. Nowlin, W.A. (2011). Workplace violence: awareness, prevention, and response. *Public Personnel Management*, 40(4), 293–308.

Burns, C., Beauchesne, M., Ryan-Krause, P. & Sawin, K. (2006). Mastering the preceptor role: challenges of clinical teaching. *Journal of Pediatric Health Care*, 20(3), 172–83.

Butterworth, T., Faugier, J. & Burnard, P. (eds) (1998). *Clinical Supervision and Mentorship in Nursing* (2nd edn). Cheltenham: Stanley Thornes.

Canadian Mental Health Association—National Office. Website. Viewed 20 February 2013, <www.cmha.ca>.

Carter, F.M. (1981). *Psychosocial Nursing: theory and practice in hospital and community mental health* (3rd edn). New York: Macmillan.

Cleary, M., Hunt, G.E. & Horsfall, J. (2010). Identifying and addressing bullying in nursing. *Issues in Mental Health Nursing*, 31: 331–5.

Cotton, A.H. (2001). Private thoughts in public spheres: issues in reflection and reflective practices in nursing. *Journal of Advanced Nursing*, 36(4), 512–19.

Dean, A.J, Gibbon, P., McDermott, B.M., Davidson, T. & Scott, J. (2010). Exposure to aggression and the impact on staff in a child and adolescent inpatient unit. *Archives of Psychiatric Nursing*, 24(1), 15–26.

Department of Health, Victoria (2009). Promoting sexual safety, responding to sexual activity, and managing allegations of sexual assault in adult acute inpatient units: Chief Psychiatrist's guideline. Viewed 20 February 2013, <www.health.vic.gov.au/mentalhealth/cpg>.

Firtko, A., Stewart, R. & Knox, N. (2005). Understanding mentoring and preceptorship: Clarifying the quagmire. *Contemporary Nurse*, 19, 32–40.

Fox, R., Henderson, A. & Malko-Nyhan, K. (2005). 'They survive despite the organizational culture, not because of it': a longitudinal study of new staff perceptions of what constitutes support during the transition to an acute tertiary facility. *International Journal of Nursing Practice*, 11, 193–9.

Frisch, N.C. & Frisch, L.E. (2010). *Psychiatric Mental Health Nursing* (4th edn). New York: Delmar Thomson Learning.

Gustafsson, C., Asp, M. & Fagerberg, I. (2007). Reflective practice in nursing care: embedded assumptions in qualitative studies. *International Journal of Nursing Practice*, 13, 151–60.

Hancox, K. & Lynch, L. (2002). *Clinical Supervision for Mental Health Professionals*. Melbourne: Centre for Psychiatric Nursing Research and Practice.

Happell, B., Reid-Searl, K., Dwyer, T., Caperchione, C.M., Gaskin, C.J. & Burke, K.J. (2013). How nurses cope with occupational stress outside their workplaces. *Collegian*, in press. Viewed 20 February 2013, <http://acquire.cqu.edu.au:8080/vital/access/manager/Repository/cqu:8919>.

Holland, K. & Hogg, C. (2010). *Cultural Awareness in Nursing and Health Care: an introductory text* (2nd ed.). London: Hodder Arnold.

Holloway, E. & Carroll, M. (ed.) (1999). *Training Counselling Supervisors: strategies, methods, and techniques.* Thousand Oaks, CA: Sage.

Kantar, L.D. (2012). Clinical practice of new nurse graduates in Lebanon: challenges and perspectives through the eyes of preceptors of clinical supervision by hospital nurses. *Journal of Continuing Education in Nursing*, 43(11), 518–28.

Koivu, A., Hyrkäs, K. & Saarinen P.I. (2011). Who attends clinical supervision? The uptake of clinical supervision by hospital nurses. *Journal of Nursing Management*, 19, 69–79.

Lethbridge, K., Andrusyszyn, M.A., Iwasiw, C., Laschinger, H.K.S. & Fernando, R. (2011). Structural and psychological empowerment and reflective thinking: is there a link? *Journal of Nursing Education*, 50(11), 636–45.

Lynch, L., Hancox, K., Happell, B. & Parker, J. (2008). *Clinical Supervision for Nurses*. Oxford: Wiley-Blackwell.

MacDonald, J. & Ellis, P.E. (2012). Supervision in psychiatry: terra incognita? *Current Opinion in Psychiatry*, 25, 322–6.

Mark, G. & Smith, A.P. (2012). Occupational stress, job characteristics, coping, and the mental health of nurses. *British Journal of Health Psychology*, 17(3), 505–21.

McEldowney, R. & Connor, M.J. (2011). Cultural safety as an ethic of care: a praxiological process. *Journal of Transcultural Nursing*, 22(4), 342–9.

McKenna, B., Thom, K., Howard, F., & Williams, V. (2010). In search of a national approach to professional supervision for mental health and addiction nurses: The New Zealand experience. *Contemporary Nurse*, 34(2): 267–76.

Mistral, W., Hall, A. & McKee, P. (2002). Using therapeutic community principles to improve the functioning of a high care psychiatric ward in the UK. *International Journal of Mental Health Nursing*, 11, 10–17.

Nairn, S., Chambers, D., Thompson, S., McGarry, J. & Chambers, K. (2012). Reflexivity and habitus: opportunities and constraints on transformative learning. *Nursing Philosophy*, 13(3), 189–201.

Nelson, S. (2012). The lost path to emancipatory practice: towards a history of reflective practice in nursing. *Nursing Philosophy*, 13(3), 202–13.

New South Wales Health (2005). *Guidelines for the Promotion of Sexual Safety in NSW Mental Health Services* (2nd edn). Sydney: NSW Department of Health.

—— (2011a). Your Health—Rights and Responsibilities: a guide to patients, carers and families. Sydney: NSW Health. Viewed 20 February 2013, <www0.health.nsw.gov.au/policies/pd/2011/PD2011_022. html>.

—— (2011b). *Zero Tolerance Response to Violence in the NSW Health Workplace*. Sydney: NSW Health. Viewed 20 February 2013, <www.health.nsw.gov.au/policies/PD/2005/PD2005_315.html>.

—— (2011c). *Sexual Safety in NSW Mental Health Services Project*. Viewed 3 July 2013, <http://www0. health.nsw.gov.au/mhdao/sexual_safety.asp>.

New South Wales Occupational Health and Safety Act 2011. Viewed 20 September 2012, <www.legislation.nsw. gov.au/maintop/view/inforce/subordleg+674+2011+cd+0+N>.

Savino, J.O. & Turvey, B.E. (2011). *Rape Investigation Handbook* (2nd edn). San Diego, CA: Elsevier.

Shives, L.R. (2012). *Basic Concepts of Psychiatric–Mental Health Nursing* (8th edn). Philadelphia, PA: Wolters Kluwer/Lippincott Williams & Wilkins.

Smedley, A., Morey, P. & Race, P. (2010). Enhancing the knowledge, attitudes and skills of preceptors: an Australian perspective. *Journal of Continuing Education in Nursing*, 41(10), 451–61.

Smith, L.S., McAllister, L.E. & Crawford, C.S. (2002). Mentoring benefits and issues for public health nurses. *Public Health Nursing*, 18(2), 101–7.

Taylor, M. & Harrison, C.A. (2010). Introducing clinical supervision across Western Australian public mental health services. *International Journal of Mental Health Nursing*, 19, 287–93.

Tourigny, L. (2005). A critical examination of formal and informal mentoring among nurses. *Health Care Manager*, 24(1), 68–76.

Treatment Protocol Project (2004). *Acute Inpatient Psychiatric Care: a source book*. (4th edn). World Health Organization and the Centre for Mental Health and Substance Abuse. Sydney: Brown Prior & Anderson.

Van Ooijen, E. (2000). *Clinical Supervision: a practical approach*. Edinburgh: Churchill Livingston.

Veeramah, V. (2012). What are the barriers to good mentoring? *Nursing Times*, 108(39), 12–15.

Ward, L. (2011). Mental health nursing and stress: maintaining balance. *International Journal of Mental Health Nursing*, 20(2): 77–85.

16

Mental health issues across the health-care sector

Main points

- Mental health challenges are common within the general community, and even more common within the general health-care system.
- Nurses will find themselves working with people experiencing mental illness and mental health challenges, regardless of the setting in which they choose to practise.
- Nursing embraces the notion of holistic care, so psychological and social aspects must be as important to their role as the more physical aspects.
- Nurses have a responsibility to provide the best available care for people experiencing mental health challenges.
- Nurses frequently describe difficulty in, or negative attitudes towards, caring for people with mental health challenges.
- Psychiatric consultation–liaison nursing is a sub-specialty of mental health nursing that provides expert consultation to assist with the management of mental health challenges within general hospitals.

Definitions

Comorbidity: This term refers to the existence of two or more diagnosed illnesses in the one person at the one time. A person may experience a physical illness and a mental illness, or more than one mental or physical illness, at the same time.

Mainstreaming: The co-location of mental health services within the general health-care system, to reduce discrimination by minimising the perceived differences between mental illness and physical illness (see Chapter 4).

Prevalence: The frequency of the existence of a specific diagnosis within a specific population at a specific point in time.

INTRODUCTION

As discussed in Chapter 4, mainstreaming has altered the structure of mental health service delivery in Australia and many other countries. Many large institutions have been closed, and care and treatment of people with mental illness now generally occur in the community or in-patient psychiatric units in general hospitals. This means that nurses working in all health settings now have more contact with people experiencing mental health challenges (Sharrock & Happell 2007).

There is a close relationship between mental health and physical health, and the recognition of and early intervention in mental health challenges will enhance more positive physical outcomes. This chapter will address the prevalence of mental health challenges with the general health system.

Many nurses don't think they are well prepared to provide high-quality care for people experiencing mental health challenges (Sharrock & Happell 2007). It is argued that undergraduate nursing programs do not devote enough time or status to teaching the theory and practice of mental health nursing, and therefore nurses don't have the opportunity to develop the skills and knowledge they need (Happell & Cutcliffe 2011).

Mental illness is common, and it is even more common in hospitals and other health-care settings than in the general population (Happell & Platania-Phung 2005). So, as stated in Chapter 1, wherever you choose to work as a nurse in the future, you will find yourself caring for people with mental illness and mental health challenges. It is very important that you are sufficiently skilled and confident to do so.

The aim of this chapter is to inform you about mental health challenges within the general health-care system, and to highlight the important role of nurses in providing care to meet the health-care needs (including mental health) for people experiencing mental illness. Relax: you will not be expected to be an expert mental health nurse, but hopefully you will have the skills and confidence to provide care and treatment within the scope of your expertise. More specifically, this chapter will provide an overview of:

- the prevalence of mental health challenges within the general community
- the prevalence of mental health challenges within the general health-care system
- comorbidity
- the relationship between physical and mental health and illness
- the impact of physical ill-health on psychological well-being
- common mental health challenges in health-care settings.

MENTAL ILLNESS IN THE GENERAL COMMUNITY

There is an increasing understanding that mental health challenges are common in the general community. The most recent National Survey of Mental Health and Well-being of Adults (Slade et al. 2009) found that one in five Australians had experienced a mental illness at some time during the twelve months prior to the survey. The most common were anxiety disorders, substance misuse and depression.

Nearly two-thirds of people with such mental health challenges do not seek any type of health services to assist with them. However, from time to time they may access health services for physical challenges. General health-care settings therefore provide an excellent opportunity to recognise and address mental illness within people who might otherwise not receive treatment at all.

MENTAL ILLNESS AND AGE

Mental illness does not affect people of all ages in the same way. Surveys estimate the prevalence of mental health challenges in children and adolescents to be at 13–20 per cent. Attention deficit hyperactive disorder (ADHD), depression and conduct disorder are the most commonly diagnosed (Department of Health and Aged Care 2000).

Depression is the most common mental health challenge in older people, affecting 10–15 per cent of the population aged 65 and above. In the nursing home population, this figure more than doubles to approximately 30 per cent. As well, one in fifteen adults aged over 65, one in nine between 80 and 84 and one in four people aged above 85 have moderate to severe dementia (Zhang et al. 2010).

While dementia in older people is generally acknowledged, depression is much less so, and often goes undiagnosed. This may be because we expect older people to be less positive about their lives—after all, they are no longer able to enjoy many of the activities that were part of their lives in their 'younger days'. These assumptions can be dangerous. Depression is about more than not being as happy or lively as you used to be. It is a serious disorder that should not simply be regarded as a normal part of ageing.

Depression can also have significant physical consequences. For example, older people with depression are nearly three times more likely to sustain a fall than those without (Delbaere et al. 2010). Untreated depression can also lead to suicide (McQueen 2012). You may be surprised to learn that the suicide rate for persons over the age of 65 is generally as high or higher than the rate for all ages. Although evidence suggests depression is the major cause of suicide in the older people, aged persons are often not assessed for their suicide risk (McQueen 2012).

COMORBID MENTAL DISORDERS

The term 'comorbidity' refers to having more than one diagnosed mental health illness. It can refer to a person experiencing a physical and mental health illness at the same time, such as schizophrenia and diabetes, or to the occurrence of two or more mental health illnesses at the same time, such as depression and substance abuse. Comorbidity is common, and applies at all age levels. About one in four people with an anxiety, affective or substance misuse issue has at least one other mental health challenge. Substance misuse commonly co-occurs with mental health challenges. (Slade et al. 2009).

Trends of comorbidity are different for males and females. The coexistence of anxiety and affective disorders is most common in females, while anxiety or affective disorder combined with substance abuse disorder is more common in males. More than half the people diagnosed with a depressive disorder have suffered at least one additional mental health challenge, with the rate slightly higher for men than women (Slade et al. 2009).

Mental health challenges and physical health challenges also often occur together, particularly when the person experiences a terminal illness such as cancer or an illness such as AIDS. Understandably, these conditions significantly impact on quality of life, and in the case of AIDS there is the added burden of stigma and discrimination (World Health Organization 2005).

PREVALENCE OF MENTAL ILLNESS IN THE GENERAL HEALTH CARE POPULATION

Because physical and mental illnesses commonly co-occur, people receiving care from general hospitals are more likely to have a mental illness. Physical and mental illnesses may:

- occur simultaneously, either taking place by chance or sharing a common cause— for example, a motor vehicle accident may result in significant physical injuries and severe psychological distress, leading to depression
- be a complication of a physical illness—for example, the diagnosis of a terminal illness may result in the person becoming severely depressed
- be the cause of a physical illness.

Hospitalisation is not usually a pleasant experience. Along with concerns about the physical health challenge itself, there are usually a number of other things people worry about, including:

- the impact of time away from employment or study
- the care of children, significant others, family, pets
- financial considerations, such as rent or bills that need to be paid
- impact on friendships, relationships and social events
- boredom.

CRITICAL THINKING

Have you ever been hospitalised for major surgery or a significant physical illness? If so, we ask you to reflect on that experience. If not, we ask you to talk to someone you know well who has had this experience. Use the following questions for yourself or the other person to consider:

- How did you feel about your predicament at the time?
- Were you concerned that you might die or be permanently disabled by the experience?
- If so, what were some of the main concerns you had about this ordeal (for yourself or others)?
- Would you describe yourself as anxious? Depressed?
- How did your family and significant others respond to your situation?
- How did nurses and other staff respond to you?
- What things made you feel worse?
- What things made you feel better?

CRITICAL THINKING

List the top ten things that you would be likely to worry about or miss if you were suddenly to be hospitalised (particularly for an extended period of time).

- What would you need to do to reduce your concern, both before your admission and during your hospitalisation?
- What could nurses do to assist in alleviating your concerns during this time:
  - before going into hospital
  - during hospitalisation
  - to prepare for discharge from hospital?

There is also the impact of the illness or injury itself. For example, imagine that you sustained an injury requiring the amputation of a limb, or were diagnosed with a long-term or life-threatening illness such as diabetes or cancer. These situations are very distressing, and can cause people to act and behave differently. Support and compassion under these circumstances are vitally important, and nurses are well placed to provide this type of care. Understandably, there is a tendency for nurses to concentrate on physical needs, but people have psychological and emotional needs too, and these must not be ignored.

The importance of psychological care was clearly illustrated in a personal account of recovery from serious injury. Moore (1991) recalls the emotional issues that affected him during his period of recovery. Moore, a medical practitioner, gained significant insight into the importance of emotional and psychological factors during the healing process. In his own words:

> Physical recovery and its associated therapeutic supports are not the main problem: you heal what you can and you adapt to or accept the rest. But it's not that simple in the emotional, spiritual and psychological areas. From the deeper parts of a damaged person's being, the heart and soul can be dumped in the casualty department of life and languish there neglected while all around the busy world of physical resuscitation efficiently goes on. (Moore 1991, p. 142)

From his own experience, while the physical care he received could not be faulted, the neglect of the emotional aspects of his situation hindered his recovery, both as a 'damaged man' and as a person.

CRITICAL THINKING

Consider the impact of the above example if the person also had the symptoms of a mental illness. In addition to the injuries sustained, the person is hearing voices telling him that the staff are trying to harm him, that the food is poisoned and that the accident itself was part of a plan to silence him. Think about how fearful the experience would be, and consider:

- how you would react to the knowledge that this person had these symptoms
- how important the way you communicated and related to this person would be
- what strategies you might use to alleviate fear and improve trust with this person.

In the case of mental health challenges, the issues are generally even more pronounced. Although health professionals may not always be receptive to the emotional needs of a person with a physical illness, they are at least able to understand the concept of physical illness. Mental illness, on the other hand, continues to remain misunderstood, and is often feared by the general population.

PREVALENCE OF MENTAL HEALTH CHALLENGES IN THE GENERAL HEALTH–CARE SYSTEM

It is difficult to accurately determine how common mental health challenges are in health-care settings. Comparisons between research findings cannot easily be made for the following reasons:

- Different definitions of mental illness are used.
- Different scales and tools are used to diagnose mental illness.
- Some prevalence rates are based on mental illness symptoms (self-reported or observed), rather than formal diagnoses.
- Symptoms of depression may be confused with symptoms of physical illness.
- Symptoms of mental illness may not be detected in some people.
- People who decline to take part in research may be more likely not to have a psychological condition, and people offered treatment as part of participation in a study may be more likely to take part, thereby increasing the likelihood that the sample will not be representative of the hospital or physical illness population.

However, it appears from the available research that the rates of mental illness are significantly higher in the general health-care system. Despite depression and anxiety being common, there is limited evidence of psychological treatment being made available.

Nursing homes have particularly high rates of mental illness, partly due to the closure of long-stay psychiatric hospital wards and the relocation of people diagnosed with dementia to nursing homes (Kramer et al. 2009). Older adults who have a disability or who are not self-sufficient have a heightened risk of developing a mental illness (Aris et al. 2009).

This frequently creates significant challenges for nurses working in these settings. However, nurses need to be more responsive to service users' symptoms and needs. Improved mental health services in nursing homes would improve quality of life for a great proportion of residents and nursing home staff. As the Australian population continues to age, the mental health care of older people will become a pressing concern.

ACCESSING TREATMENT FOR MENTAL HEALTH CHALLENGES

The National Survey of Mental Health and Well-being found that of all persons who had one or more of the common mental disorders, nearly two-thirds had not used any form of health service in the previous twelve months. Those who sought treatment tended to do so from a general practitioner (29.4 per cent) rather than a specialist mental health professional (6 per cent), such as a psychiatrist, psychologist or mental health worker (Slade et al. 2009).

In simple terms, this means that only 6 per cent of people with a diagnosable mental illness receive mental health services, leaving a large pool of unmet needs. It is also likely that many more people would have accessed the general health-care system, and not had their mental health needs recognised and treated—a golden opportunity that unfortunately is not often fulfilled. The importance of all health professionals having an understanding of common mental illnesses and their potential consequences is therefore crucial to achieving effective and high-quality health care.

IMPACT OF MENTAL ILLNESS ON PHYSICAL HEALTH

The relationship between physical illness and injury is clear. We know that severe cardiac conditions, if untreated, are likely to cause death. We also know that people involved in serious motor vehicle accidents can die if they are left without intervention. The relationship between mental illness and death is not so clear. However, although less obvious, it does exist. The evidence demonstrates the link between mental illness and poor physical health. For example, cardiovascular and respiratory diseases are more likely to lead to death among the people diagnosed with a mental illness than among those without (Happell et al. 2011).

People diagnosed with mental illness die approximately 25 years earlier than the general population, and this figure seems to be increasing (Brown et al. 2010). Many factors contribute to this, including the side-effects of anti-psychotic medications, poorer diet, lower levels of physical activity, increased rates of smoking and substance misuse, economic and social disadvantage and reduced access to services (Happell et al. 2011) .

The side-effects of psychotropic medication are strongly related to physical health concerns, particularly cardiovascular disease and diabetes. There is a strong risk of developing metabolic syndrome, including diabetes or pre-diabetes, obesity, high blood pressure and high cholesterol. The resulting risks of serious cardiovascular disease are very high (Brunero & Lamont 2009).

Mental health challenges have also been identified as a major risk factor for self-harm. Between 60 and 90 per cent of young people who attempt suicide are believed to have the symptoms of clinical depression, meaning that detection and early intervention with depression could profoundly affect the rates of suicide and attempted suicide. In the same way, people in general hospitals who have depression are more likely to experience suicide intent and are more likely to act on their thoughts if they also have a substance misuse disorder (Arria et al. 2009). This clearly demonstrates not only the serious impact of mental illness on physical health, but the important role of detection and early intervention in preventing disturbing and avoidable outcomes.

While it might not be so obvious, it is believed that mental illness is often an indirect cause of death, because it exacerbates long-term disability and is associated with habits that lead to ill-health, including poor diet, alcohol misuse, smoking and sedentary lifestyle (Happell et al. 2011); therefore, it contributes to disease onset and severity.

Depression has become a leading cause of disease and disability in the world, and its impact is considered likely to increase substantially in the future (World Health

Organization 2005). In Australia, we already know that major depression has an adverse impact on health (Slade et al. 2009). Depression has been associated with a diminished level of physical functioning, including physical illness and difficulties with independent living.

MENTAL HEALTH CHALLENGES AND HEALTH CARE

Undoubtedly, mental health challenges influence physical health. There is some evidence of a link between psycho-social factors (i.e. low perceived emotional support, denial, difficulty in coping) and the development and severity of chronic and long-term diseases (i.e. coronary heart disease, HIV/AIDS and cancer). This means that nursing interventions that lead towards creating a supportive environment can influence health outcomes. It might seem a small thing to you, but a caring attitude, being a good listener and attending to the psychological needs of the people with whom you work can significantly influence their recovery from illness or injury.

People experiencing mental health challenges do not receive the same standard of care as people experiencing physical disorders. Kelly's story in the case study below provides a telling example of this. The concepts of stigma and discrimination provide some explanation for this. Kelly's actions that led to the death of her daughter do not conform to society's view of motherhood. Mothers should care for and protect their children, not subject them to risk or danger. Many nurses may find it very difficult to care for Kelly, much less to openly communicate with her with the aim of commencing a therapeutic relationship. It is very easy for this to lead to avoidance or short-cuts in providing health care.

CASE STUDY

Kelly is a 28-year-old woman who has been admitted to the orthopaedic unit following a motor vehicle accident in which she sustained compound fractures to both femurs and the tibia and fibula of her right leg. Kelly was speeding on the wrong side of a four-lane highway. Her one-month-old daughter was in the car without restraints; on impact, she was thrown from the car and ultimately died as a result of extensive head injuries. Kelly is believed to have told the ambulance officers that the baby was evil and needed to die.

In the unit, Kelly is very withdrawn with her family and with hospital staff. The nursing staff are horrified by the situation and blame Kelly for her daughter's death. A number of nurses have stated that they do not want to look after Kelly because 'she doesn't deserve it'. When they have to attend to her, most nurses avoid eye contact with Kelly, conversation is short and to the point, and they appear to be in a hurry to leave. Some staff refuse to enter her room or to care for her. Soon Kelly refuses to see her family, and does not talk to staff at all.

Critical thinking

- Why do you think that Kelly does not communicate well with staff?
- What impact do you think staff behaviour might have on Kelly's attitudes to them?
- What psychological impacts do you think the death of Kelly's daughter and the circumstances in which it occurred might have on Kelly?
- How do you think Kelly's family and friends will react to the baby's death?
- How do you feel about caring for Kelly?
- What nursing approach and interventions do you feel might benefit Kelly's well-being and recovery?

Service users with mental health challenges often do not behave according to the traditional 'sick role' (Zolnierek 2009). For example, they do not always cooperate with the requests of health professionals, and can be considered difficult. The reactions of staff to their behaviour may often make the challenge worse. These people run the risk of being neglected or abused because nurses and other health professionals do not feel confident in meeting their needs, and frequently avoid them, giving them less attention than they would if the challenges were purely physical.

CRITICAL THINKING

Consider Kelly's situation.

- Do you think the approach of staff would be different if Kelly's daughter had been appropriately restrained and her daughter's death had been a 'true accident'?
- Do you think Kelly is experiencing discrimination? If so, why do you think this might be happening?

As nurses, we continue to be humans. We all have our views about which actions and behaviours are acceptable and which are not. However, we need to be aware of the human rights of all people in our care, and acknowledge that they deserve high-quality and effective health care. It is likely that Kelly will be clearly aware that some staff do not want to be in the room with her. Given this, she is unlikely to openly communicate with these staff. Communication may be an important part of Kelly's recovery, both physically and emotionally.

The symptoms of mental illness can appear as 'normal' or expected reactions to hospitalisation or illness. Hospitalisation and illness are often distressing, and may cause the person to act and behave in ways that are not usual. It is therefore not uncommon for service users and health professionals to see symptoms of mental illness as the result of hospitalisation or the physical condition itself. For example, changes in behaviour in older people may be seen as an inevitable part of getting old. Depression is often not treated in older people because it is considered part of ageing (as discussed earlier in this chapter), or as being less important than the person's physical state.

In summary, it is reasonable to assume that people with mental illness or significant mental health challenges do not generally receive the same standard of care and treatment for either their physical or mental conditions. However, improved identification will not solve the challenge. Improving care and treatment must be the important next step.

MEETING THE PSYCHOLOGICAL AND MENTAL HEALTH NEEDS OF SERVICE USERS

Nurses must play an important role if current practices are to be improved. Nursing is the largest professional health-care group, and is likely to have the most contact with people experiencing mental illness. Nurses can help to detect mental health challenges and provide effective care to minimise their impact (Sharrock & Happell 2007). Nursing embraces the notion of holistic care, which means nurses are not solely focused on the physical and medical approach, and can introduce psychological and social aspects to their care. This provides the basis for a more rounded approach, which acknowledges and respects people as total beings rather than component parts. Because of this, nurses are well placed to assess for signs and symptoms of mental distress. This can enable symptoms of depression and anxiety, for example, to be recognised and the appropriate treatment to be sought. Nurses may also contribute to the assessment and treatment of social health and emotional functioning.

As noted above, detection alone is not enough. Nurses have the opportunity to positively influence the hospitalisation experience, engage in early intervention and undertake some basic strategies for people with mental health challenges. Because they have the most contact with service users of any health professional, nurses are also the main source of encouragement for self-care and physical activity. Emphasis on physical activity is of particular importance, given evidence that physical activity appears to enhance mental health and well-being (Happell et al. 2011).

NURSES' ATTITUDES TOWARDS SERVICE USERS WITH MENTAL HEALTH CHALLENGES

While it has been argued that nurses have a significant role to play in providing care for people experiencing mental health challenges, it is also evident that we have a long way to go before this potential can be realised. Nurses who have not specialised in the psychiatric/mental health area tend to express a lack of enjoyment in caring for service users with eating disorders, schizophrenia and those who have committed deliberate self-harm as the result of a mental health challenge (Sharrock & Happell 2007). Similarly, emergency nurses are not clear whether their role should include care for service users with mental health challenges.

Nurses sometimes avoid service users experiencing mental health challenges because of feelings of fear and powerlessness, and often because caring for these people tends to take more time. This is not meant to suggest that nurses without specialist mental health nursing qualifications do not provide effective holistic care. They often do, and their efforts are frequently not recognised or acknowledged. However, Australian research (Sharrock & Happell 2007; Sharrock et al. 2006) has suggested that, because of their fear and sense of powerlessness, many nurses do not enjoy caring for people with mental health challenges, and this makes them more likely to avoid the person or minimise the care they provide, as demonstrated in the example of Kelly in the case study above.

This situation poses considerable concern to the nursing profession, which prides itself on the provision of holistic care to all persons requiring the assistance of the health-care system. The reasons why this situation has occurred are varied and complex. First, there is no doubt that nurses share many of the stereotypical views of the wider society towards people experiencing mental health challenges. The fear of, and discomfort with, people experiencing mental health challenges cannot help but influence their attitudes towards providing care for these people (Happell & Cutcliffe 2011).

As discussed in Chapter 1, the current system of nursing education has been widely criticised for not providing enough scope to address the theory and practice of mental health nursing (Wynaden 2010). Because of this, nurses generally may feel less confident in providing mental health care than they do with physical health care. Undergraduate students generally consider themselves less prepared to work in a mental health setting than in other clinical settings, even after they have completed the mental health nursing component (Happell 2008).

CRITICAL THINKING

During your clinical placement on a surgical unit, you were asked to act as primary nurse for a service user named Connie. Connie has just returned from surgery to repair deep lacerations to her wrists. During the handover, a nurse states that Connie is a PD (this means she is diagnosed with borderline personality disorder), she's a revolving door case and maybe one day she will do the job properly and we won't have to go through this crap any more.

- How do you feel about this statement?
- What sort of attitude towards people experiencing a mental illness (or, more specifically, a personality disorder) does this statement reflect?

- How do you feel such an attitude might influence how Connie is cared for in this unit?
- How do you feel about providing care for Connie?
- How is Connie likely to feel about accessing health services in the future?

CASE STUDY: CONNIE'S STORY

Consider the experience from Connie's point of view—her story:

> I had a lot of bad stuff happen to me when I was growing up and I learned to cope by going numb. The only way I could come back to reality sometimes was to cut myself so I could feel again—bring myself back to life. One time I was in hospital because I had cut my arm and I overheard one of the nurses saying: 'Oh for God's sake, no sooner do we fix her up than she's back in here. Why doesn't she just do the job properly and save us all the bother.' I felt so horrible, so guilty, like there were people who needed help and I didn't deserve any help. I already felt like I didn't deserve anything.

PSYCHIATRIC/MENTAL HEALTH CONSULTATION–LIAISON NURSING

Consultation–liaison (CL) psychiatry is a branch of psychiatry that developed in the United States after World War I. The nursing role in CL psychiatry was first introduced in the United States during the 1960s as a result of a movement towards holistic and service user-centred nursing care and the trend towards greater numbers of people with mental illness being cared for in the general hospital system.

The development of the role in Australia has been slower and more recent. However, there is evidence of an increase in the number of CL roles for nursing. CL nurses have now become a special interest group of the Australian College of Mental Health Nurses, and have been holding annual national conferences since 2003.

Consultation–liaison psychiatry developed from recognition that people with mental health challenges did not receive the care and treatment they required within general hospitals. It is a service provided to service users who are admitted for a physical issue but are also experiencing mental health challenges. CL psychiatry was implemented as a way to provide the mental health expertise of mental health professionals to colleagues without skills in this field. The CL service is provided either through direct consultation with the service user or indirectly, through support, education and advice to other health professionals responsible for the care and treatment of the service user.

An example of direct consultation may involve a psychiatrist or psychiatric registrar from the CL team meeting with the person, conducting a mental health state assessment, making a diagnosis and recommending treatment. A CL nurse providing direct consultation may conduct a mental status and nursing assessment, and recommend specific nursing interventions that would enhance the person's overall care. The following example (adapted from Sharrock & Happell 2002) is developed from a 'real-life' direct consultation by a CL nurse.

An example of indirect consultation might involve the conduct of an educational session. For example, the staff on a medical unit have noticed that they are admitting more service users with a comorbid diagnosis of schizophrenia. They contact the CL nurse, seeking information. Given the large number of staff on the unit, the CL nurse conducts an education session to provide more information about the condition, treatment and care associated with the diagnosis of schizophrenia.

THE ROLE OF THE PSYCHIATRIC CONSULTATION–LIAISON NURSE

Despite the increase in roles, there is no agreed framework for CL practice in mental health. Therefore, these roles have not necessarily developed in a uniform or consistent manner. The following have been identified as examples of situations where the assistance of a CL nurse would be appropriate and potentially beneficial:

- service users whose psychiatric care needs were intense or challenging to the expertise of a generalist nurse or had a significant systemic impact (for example, service users with delirium and dementia, drug and alcohol issues, adjustment issues related to personality factors, somatoform disorders and psychosis)
- service users whose symptoms were difficult to manage in a general ward (for example, risk of self-harm, absconding, refusing treatment or aggression)
- service users with long-term health challenges requiring supportive counselling and monitoring
- service users requiring one-to-one mental health nursing care ('specials'); specials are generally indicated where persons are otherwise considered likely to cause harm to themselves or others
- service users transferred from mental health in-patient settings (including forensic mental health services)
- service users detained as involuntary patients under the relevant mental health legislation (including those on community treatment orders)
- service users requiring electro-convulsive therapy.

Reading all this may make you think: 'What do I need mental health skills for? I'll just call the CL nurse!' Please reconsider. CL nursing is an important way to support general nurses in caring for people experiencing a mental illness and mental health challenges (Sharrock et al. 2006); however, this does not mean that all we need is a CL nurse and

CASE STUDY

Tina is a 26-year-old married woman who was referred to the psychiatric consultation–liaison nurse (PCLN) three days after surgery for the removal of an ovarian tumour. Tina began experiencing episodes of anxiety on her first post-operative day. The results of the pathology had not been obtained due to external difficulties. There was a slim chance the tumour was malignant.

The CL nurse was requested by Tina's primary nurse to assist Tina with her anxiety episodes. The referring nurse also wanted to know how she could help.

Tina was interviewed in the presence of her husband Keith (with Tina's permission). Tina was upset by the unexpected delay of her results. She experienced her first 'anxiety attack' one day post-operatively. She described 'funny feelings all over', dizziness, weakness in the legs, feelings of fear and loss of control. She tried relaxation strategies, but couldn't overcome thoughts of dying. She was also worried about her small business, which she had left to be managed by her partner at a very busy time.

The staff reported that Tina was recovering quite well, but became very uptight once the results were delayed. Her anxiety was worse at night, and she was having difficulty sleeping, but she did not want to take any sleeping pills.

Tina was assessed on the basis of information from herself, her family, the staff and the clinical file. She was provided with supportive counselling and education. Education included alternative relaxation techniques, supported by written material for future reference. Tina was given an opportunity to practise relaxation techniques in the presence of the CL nurse.

Tina was provided with the telephone number of the PCLN so she could make contact after discharge to discuss how things were going. She was also provided with information on community resources that she could choose to access.

The CL reported back to the team regarding Tina's assessment and suggested management plan. The medical officer agreed to prescribe night sedation if required. Written and verbal information was given to staff to help them support Tina when she became anxious—for example, by talking her through her relaxation techniques as required.

Tina was discharged as planned after receiving the pathology results that revealed a benign tumour. She contacted the CL nurse the next week, reporting a settling of her anxiety. She indicated she did not want to follow up as an out-patient. Tina was encouraged to be mindful of her vulnerability to anxiety and to seek help early if the anxiety attacks returned. She resolved to look further at her anxiety, and had purchased a self-help book and relaxation tape recommended by the PCLN.

Critical thinking

- Identify the approaches the CL nurse used in working with Tina.
- How do you think these approaches might have assisted Tina with her recovery?
- Consider Tina's situation without the involvement of the CL nurse. How do you think the outcomes might have been different?

the challenge is solved. Not all hospitals have mental health CL nurses, and for those that do it is simply not possible for this role to meet all needs. There is often only one CL nurse for a large, busy hospital. Nurses need some skills and knowledge to identify a challenge in the first place. Also, the CL nurse is only able to consult; they do not take over the role of providing care, which remains with the treating team. While you are not expected to become an expert mental health nurse during your undergraduate course, the skills and knowledge you are now developing will make a difference to the type and standard of care you are able to provide. It is important that you take this component of your course as seriously as you do all other aspects, even if you don't think that mental health nursing is 'your thing'.

IMPLICATIONS FOR NURSING

Mental health is just as important as physical health, and high-quality nursing care means that all health-care needs should be addressed. Mental health challenges or issues are demonstrated in different ways for different people. For example, some people experiencing anxiety might be quiet and withdrawn, while others might be argumentative and refuse to cooperate with staff.

To ensure you adequately address the mental health needs of service users in the general hospital system, it is important that you:

- conduct a thorough assessment on admission, which includes assessment of mental health status and other relevant information (for example, drug and alcohol usage)
- communicate openly and therefore help to create a trusting relationship
- demonstrate a caring and non-judgemental attitude so that service users are more likely to communicate all relevant health (including mental health) issues to you
- familiarise yourself with the resources and supports offered by the organisation. For example, is there a psychiatric consultation–liaison service available? If there is, it is important that you are knowledgeable about the process for accessing this service. Investigate whether the service uses screening tools routinely or where mental health issues (such as depression) are suspected.
- inform the nurse in charge of the ward or unit if you have any specific concerns about the mental health of service users
- ensure the way you relate to and care for people is not compromised by the knowledge or suspicion that they have a significant mental health challenge. Remember that they are people first and foremost, and that physical needs do not disappear or become less important because of mental health challenges.
- do not avoid people who appear to be experiencing mental illness.

One of the reasons nurses often give for avoiding people with mental illness is that they don't know what to do or how to communicate, or they are concerned that what they may say might worsen the challenge. For example, there is a common concern that asking a person if they are suicidal might put the idea in someone's head. The following are some tips to assist in communication:

- Unless you are intentionally insensitive or rude, you are very unlikely to worsen a situation with words.
- You are far more likely to worsen the situation by not communicating.
- Do not argue or disagree with a person who is hallucinating and/or experiencing high levels of anxiety.
- Be direct; don't beat around the bush. If it is important to ask a person whether they are hearing voices, for example, then ask them directly—just as you would ask them whether they were experiencing pain.

CRITICAL THINKING

Consider times when you have experienced emotional or psychological distress.

- How did people react to your distress?
- What impact did the response you received from others have on you?
- What type of communication style helped?
- What kind of communication style did not help?

Completing this exercise should assist you to develop a communication style that will be welcomed not only by people experiencing a mental illness, but all people for whom you provide care during your nursing career. It is likely that you, like most people, value availability and open communication during periods of distress. While some people feel the need to try to solve the personal challenges of their friends or families by providing advice, often we want someone to listen while we talk through our challenges and move towards the discovery of our own solutions. This is no less true for people experiencing a mental illness. It is not necessary for you to solve the challenge, but rather important to be available and to listen to people as they communicate their distress to you.

CONCLUSION

Mental illness and mental health challenges are common throughout the general community, and particularly common within the health-care system. Mental health can influence health outcomes. It is therefore very important that nurses are aware of, and pay attention to, the mental health needs of service users across all health-care settings. An open and non-judgemental approach to service users will provide a basis for effective communication. Nurses need to be aware of their own values and opinions, and how these might influence the people for whom they care.

REFERENCES

Aris, M.A.B., Draman, S.B., Rahman, J.B.A. & Shamsuddin, N.B. (2009). Functional disabilities and associated factors among elderly patients in primary care clinics. *International Medical Journal*, 16(4), 251–6.

Arria, A.M., O'Grady, K.E., Caldeira, K.M., Vincent, K.B., Wilcox, H.C. & Wish, E.D. (2009). Suicide ideation among college students: a multivariate analysis. *Archives of Suicide Research*, 13(3), 230–46.

Brown, S., Kim, M., Mitchell, C. & Inskip, H. (2010). Twenty-five year mortality of a community cohort with schizophrenia. *British Journal of Psychiatry*, 196(2), 116–21.

Brunero, S. & Lamont, S. (2009). Systematic screening for metabolic syndrome in consumers with severe mental illness. *International Journal of Mental Health Nursing*, 18(2), 144–50.

Delbaere, K., Close, J.C.T., Heim, J., Sachdev, P.S., Brodaty, H., Slavin, M.J., Kochan, N.A. & Lord, S.R. (2010). A multifactorial approach to understanding fall risk in older people. *Journal of the American Geriatrics Society*, 58(9), 1679–85.

Department of Health and Aged Care (2000). *National Action Plan for Promotion, Prevention and Early Intervention for Mental Health*. Canberra: Mental Health and Special Programs Branch, Commonwealth Department of Health and Aged Care.

Happell, B. (2008). The importance of clinical experience for mental health nursing—part 1: undergraduate nursing students' attitudes, preparedness and satisfaction. *International Journal of Mental Health Nursing*, 17(5), 326–32.

Happell, B. & Cutcliffe, J. (2011). A broken promise? Exploring the lack of evidence for the benefits of comprehensive nursing education. *International Journal of Mental Health Nursing*, 20(5), 328–36.

Happell, B. & Platania-Phung, C. (2005). Mental health issues within the general health-care system: implications for the nursing profession. *Australian Journal of Advanced Nursing*, 22(3), 41–7.

Happell, B., Platania-Phung, C., Gray, R., Hardy, S., Lambert, T., McAllister, M. & Davies, C. (2011). A role for mental health nursing in the physical health care of consumers with severe mental illness. *Journal of Psychiatric and Mental Health Nursing*, 18(8), 706–11.

Kramer, D., Allgaier, A., Fejtkova, S., Mergl, R. & Hegerl, U. (2009). Depression in nursing homes: prevalence, recognition, and treatment. *International Journal of Psychiatry in Medicine*, 39(4), 345–58.

McQueen, M. (2012). Depression, suicide and the elderly. *Canadian Nursing Home*, 23(1), 24–7.

Moore, A. (1991). *Cry of the Damaged Man: a personal journey of recovery*. Sydney: Picador.

Robson, D. & Gray, R. (2007). Serious mental illness and physical health problems: a discussion paper. *International Journal of Nursing Studies*, 44(3), 457–66.

Sharrock, J. & Happell, B. (2002). The role of a psychiatric consultation liaison nurse in a general hospital: a case study approach. *Australian Journal of Advanced Nursing*, 20(1), 39–44.

—— (2007). Competence in providing mental health care: a grounded theory analysis of nurses' experiences. *Australian Journal of Advanced Nursing*, 24(2), 9–15.

Sharrock, J., Grigg, M., Happell, B., Keeble-Devlin, B. & Jennings, S. (2006). The mental health nurse: a valuable addition to the consultation–liaison team. *International Journal of Mental Health Nursing*, 15(1), 35–43.

Slade, T., Johnston, A., Browne, M.A.O., Andrews, G. & Whiteford, H. (2009). 2007 National Survey of Mental Health and Wellbeing: methods and key findings. *Australian and New Zealand Journal of Psychiatry*, 43(7), 594–605.

World Health Organization (2005). *Mental Health: policy issues in mental health care—selected reports from the WHO Health Evidence Network*. Copenhagen: WHO Regional Office for Europe.

Wynaden, D. (2010). There is no health without mental health: are we educating Australian nurses to care for the health consumer of the 21st century? *International Journal of Mental Health Nursing*, 19(3), 203–9.

Zhang, Y., Chow, V., Vitry, A.I., Ryan, P., Roughead, E.E., Caughey, G.E., Ramsay, E.N., Gilbert, A.L., Esterman, A. & Luszcz, M.A. (2010). Antidepressant use and depressive symptomatology among older people from the Australian Longitudinal Study of Ageing. *International Psychogeriatrics*, 22(3), 437.

Zolnierek, C.D. (2009). Non-psychiatric hospitalization of people with mental illness: systematic review. *Journal of Advanced Nursing*, 65(8), 1570–83.

Index

Printed and bound by CPI Group (UK) Ltd, Croydon, CR0 4YY

23/10/2024

01777685-0004